Handbook of
Sexual Dysfunction

Medical Psychiatry

Handbook of Sexual Dysfunction

edited by

Richard Balon
Wayne State University
Detroit, Michigan, U.S.A.

R. Taylor Segraves
Case Western Reserve University
Cleveland, Ohio, U.S.A.

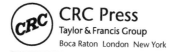

CRC Press
Taylor & Francis Group
Boca Raton London New York

CRC Press is an imprint of the
Taylor & Francis Group, an **informa** business

CRC Press
Taylor & Francis Group
6000 Broken Sound Parkway NW, Suite 300
Boca Raton, FL 33487-2742

First issued in paperback 2019

© 2005 by Taylor & Francis Group, LLC
CRC Press is an imprint of Taylor & Francis Group, an Informa business

No claim to original U.S. Government works

ISBN-13: 978-0-8247-5826-4 (hbk)
ISBN-13: 978-0-367-39298-7 (pbk)

This book contains information obtained from authentic and highly regarded sources. While all reasonable efforts have been made to publish reliable data and information, neither the author[s] nor the publisher can accept any legal responsibility or liability for any errors or omissions that may be made. The publishers wish to make clear that any views or opinions expressed in this book by individual editors, authors or contributors are personal to them and do not necessarily reflect the views/opinions of the publishers. The information or guidance contained in this book is intended for use by medical, scientific or health-care professionals and is provided strictly as a supplement to the medical or other professional's own judgement, their knowledge of the patient's medical history, relevant manufacturer's instructions and the appropriate best practice guidelines. Because of the rapid advances in medical science, any information or advice on dosages, procedures or diagnoses should be independently verified. The reader is strongly urged to consult the relevant national drug formulary and the drug companies' and device or material manufacturers' printed instructions, and their websites, before administering or utilizing any of the drugs, devices or materials mentioned in this book. This book does not indicate whether a particular treatment is appropriate or suitable for a particular individual. Ultimately it is the sole responsibility of the medical professional to make his or her own professional judgements, so as to advise and treat patients appropriately. The authors and publishers have also attempted to trace the copyright holders of all material reproduced in this publication and apologize to copyright holders if permission to publish in this form has not been obtained. If any copyright material has not been acknowledged please write and let us know so we may rectify in any future reprint.

Library of Congress Cataloging-in-Publication Data available on application

Visit the Taylor & Francis Web site at
http://www.taylorandfrancis.com

and the CRC Press Web site at
http://www.crcpress.com

Foreword

When it comes to human nature, there is something about complexity that most people find troubling. Magazines and newspaper articles are fond of announcing, with a flourish, that a "brain center" has been discovered that explains violence, sexual desire, overeating, or why we don't keep New Year's resolutions. Similar articles inform us that the cause of infidelity is purely a product of evolutionary principles, or that a single neurotransmitter is the cause of gambling.

As the co-editors of this splendid new volume point out in their preface, psychiatry has not escaped this popular trend toward biological reductionism. The discovery of the genome and the remarkable advances in the neurosciences have fueled the desire to find discrete causes of complicated human behaviors. Simple biological causes call for simple pharmacologic treatments, and a "magic pill" is the panacea with which psychiatry is enamored at this historical moment. To a remarkable extent, this reductionist trend within psychiatry as a whole is even more striking when we examine the recent trends in the understanding and treatment of sexual disorders. The irony, of course, is that no area of human behavior is more mysterious than sexuality. Moreover, if one wanted to confirm the value of the principle of multiple causation in psychiatric disturbance, one could do no better than to start with sexual disorders as the prime exemplar of this principle. As several of the authors in this collection of outstanding contributions point out, approaching the complexities of sexual desire by studying problems with genital congestion are likely to produce a limited yield.

Balon and Segraves have assembled an international group of experts who share a broad biopsychosocial perspective in their understanding of human sexual dysfunction. To their credit, they in no way give short shrift to biological causes and pharmacologic treatments. Indeed, readers of this book will gain a sophisticated understanding of how physiological factors contribute to sexual problems and how to integrate sound medication strategies in their treatments. What is particularly admirable is that the authors who contribute to this volume are deeply committed to the concept of breadth in the understanding and treatment of sexual dysfunctions, and they convincingly persuade the reader why a broad-based approach is necessary.

Handbook of Sexual Dysfunction comes at an auspicious moment within psychiatry. Going against the grain, it restores a biopsychosocial perspective to the understanding and treatment of sexual dysfunction. It also provides the clinician reader with a practical, commonsense guide to treatment planning that treats the patient as an individual rather than a disease entity. I know of no other text in the field that can match this state-of-the-art treatment of the subject. Both students and experienced clinicians will find it of enormous value.

Glen O. Gabbard, M.D.
Brown Foundation Chair of Psychoanalysis
and Professor of Psychiatry
Director, Baylor Psychiatry Clinic
Baylor College of Medicine
Houston, Texas

Preface

The area of treatment of sexual disorders has undergone an enormous expansion during the last few decades. The introduction of pharmacological treatment of these disorders (e.g., sildenafil for erectile dysfunction or antidepressants for paraphilias) rekindled the interest of physicians from different disciplines (psychiatrists, urologists, gynecologists) in sexual dysfunctions. Physicians are finding these disorders amenable to pharmacotherapy. However, the new developments in the area of "sexual pharmacology" have unfortunately also led to a biological reductionism in the field. In the past, most physicians viewed the etiology of sexual dysfunctions/disorders as mainly psychological, rooted in internal conflicts, deep-seated anxiety, and so on. In the present time, physicians in many disciplines view sexual dysfunctions as mostly, if not purely, of biological origin and discard any notion of psychological factors in the etiology of sexual problems. The initial hype about the success rates of sildenafil certainly contributed to this notion. However, clinicians who treat sexual dysfunctions/disorders on a daily basis know that in sexual functioning, psychology and biology are intertwined in a very complicated way.

In light of that, we feel a text that balances these two not contradictory but complementary etiological views would be highly desirable. A synthesis of biology and psychology in the area of etiology, pathophysiology, and treatment of sexual dysfunction is sorely needed in the field. This book intends to fill this void.

We also hope that this text will spark greater interest in the often necessary dual approach to treatment of these disorders/dysfunctions among psychiatrists and other specialists. Finally, as psychiatrists who are interested in all aspects of well being of our patients, we hope that this book will help to improve the quality of life and sexual functioning of our patients.

Richard Balon
R. Taylor Segraves

v

Contents

Contributors

Richard Balon, M.D. *Department of Psychiatry and Behavioral Neuroscience, Wayne State University, Detroit, Michigan, USA.*

Rosemary Basson, M.B., B.S., M.R.C.P. *UBC Departments of Psychiatry and Obstetrics & Gynaecology, B.C. Centre for Sexual Medicine, Vancouver General Hospital, Vancouver, BC, Canada.*

Yitzchak M. Binik, Ph.D. *Departments of Psychology, McGill University and McGill University Health Center (Royal Victoria Hospital), Montreal, Quebec, Canada.*

Stephanie Both, Ph.D. *Leiden University Medical Centre, Leiden, The Netherlands and University of Amsterdam, Amsterdam, The Netherlands.*

Walter Everaerd, Ph.D. *University of Amsterdam, Amsterdam, The Netherlands.*

Jeffrey W. Janata, Ph.D. *Case Western Reserve University School of Medicine, University Hospitals of Cleveland, Cleveland, Ohio, USA.*

Alina Kao, B.A. *Department of Psychology, McGill University, Montreal, Quebec, Canada.*

Samir Khalifé, M.D. *Faculty of Medicine, McGill University and Department of Obstetrics and Gynecology, Sir Mortimer B. Davis Jewish General Hospital, Montreal, Quebec, Canada.*

Sheryl A. Kingsberg, Ph.D. *Case Western Reserve University School of Medicine, University Hospitals of Cleveland, Cleveland, Ohio, USA.*

Ellen Laan, Ph.D. *University of Amsterdam, Amsterdam, The Netherlands.*

Roy J. Levin, Ph.D. *University of Sheffield, Sheffield, UK.*

Ian MacInnes, B.Sc.   *University of Sheffield, Sheffield, UK.*

William L. Maurice, M.D., F.R.C.P.C.   *Department of Psychiatry, University of British Columbia, Vancouver, British Columbia, Canada.*

Cindy M. Meston, Ph.D.   *University of Texas at Austin, Austin, Texas, USA.*

Cynthia S. Osborne, M.S.W.   *Johns Hopkins University School of Medicine, Baltimore, Maryland, USA.*

Kimberley A. Payne, B.A.   *Department of Psychology, McGill University, Montreal, Quebec, Canada.*

Michael A. Perelman, Ph.D.   *The New York Presbyterian Hospital, Weill Medical College of Cornell University, New York, New York, USA.*

Caroline F. Pukall, Ph.D.   *Departments of Psychology, Queen's University, Kingston, Ontario, Canada and McGill University, Montreal, Quebec, Canada.*

R. Taylor Segraves, M.D., Ph.D.   *Metrohealth Medical Center and Case Western Reserve University School of Medicine, Cleveland, Ohio, USA.*

H. B. M. Van de Wiel   *Groningen University Medical Centre, Groningen, The Netherlands.*

Marcel D. Waldinger, M.D., Ph.D.   *Leyenburg Hospital, The Hague, The Netherlands; and Utrecht Institute for Pharmaceutical Sciences and Rudolf Magnus Institute for Neurosciences, Utrecht University, Utrecht, The Netherlands.*

W. C. M. Weijmar Schultz   *Groningen University Medical Centre, Groningen, The Netherlands.*

Thomas N. Wise, M.D.   *Johns Hopkins University School of Medicine, Baltimore, Maryland, USA.*

Kevan Wylie, M.D.   *Royal Hallamshire Hospital, Sheffield, UK; Porterbrook Clinic, Sheffield, UK; and University of Sheffield, Sheffield, UK.*

1

Introduction: Treatment of Sexual Disorders in the 21st Century

R. Taylor Segraves

Metrohealth Medical Center and Case Western Reserve University School of Medicine, Cleveland, Ohio, USA

Richard Balon

Department of Psychiatry and Behavioral Neuroscience, Wayne State University, Detroit, Michigan, USA

In the last decades of the 20th century, major changes have occurred in our under-standing, conceptualization, and treatment of sexual problems. Much of this change was heralded in by the development of oral therapies for the treatment of erectile disorders, the off-label usage of serotonergic antidepressants to treat rapid ejaculation, the increasingly common use of unapproved use of androgens to increase libido in women with hypoactive sexual desire disorder, and the combined use of anti-androgens and serotonergic antidepressants to treat paraphilias. The wide spread usage of effective biological therapies for sexual disorders has contributed to the increasing emphasis on biological models concerning etiology, often to the neglect of psychological factors. In the 1960s, it was commonly assumed that most sexual problems were psychogenic in etiology (1). However, the advent of effective biological therapies has shifted the focus to organic causes of erectile dysfunction (2). These changes in assumed etiology have had profound effects on treatment and conceptualization of the origins of sexual disorders. Many patients who used to be treated by behavioral therapy are now being treated pharmacologically. The rapid development of biological models of therapy has brought valuable help to many individuals who previously had minimal treatment choices. However, a number of factors including the large number of men who dont refill sildenafil prescriptions indicate that pharmacotherapy alone may not always be sufficient (3). To date, there is insufficient data to indicate when pharmacotherapy alone, psychotherapy alone, or combined therapy is indicated for most of the sexual disorders.

A comparable situation in general psychiatry exists in the treatment of depression and obsessive-compulsive disorders. In each of these conditions, both pharmacological and psychological treatment approaches have been shown to be effective, and the most efficient clinicians select and combine therapies for the individual patient (4–7). Our experience in treating depression and obsessive-compulsive disorders may provide useful models for the treatment of sexual disorders. An example of an useful model is the study comparing nefazodone to cognitive-behavioral analysis system of psychotherapy to the combination of these two modalities (8). Although the monotherapies were efficacious, they were not significantly different from each other. However, the combination of the two modalities was significantly better than either monotherapy. Actually, the combination resulted in a highest ever treatment response rate in clinical trials of chronic major depression. As Heiman (9) pointed out, the implications for treatment of sexual dysfunction are compelling, though we need to clarify which medications and psychological therapies might be compared and combined.

The rest of this chapter will briefly summarize the history of the development of treatment for sexual problems and the recent knowledge about the epidemiology of sexual dysfunction, and discuss problems with current nomenclature.

EVOLUTION OF CURRENT TREATMENT APPROACHES

In the 1960s, psychiatric treatment of sexual problems was predominantly psychoanalytic psychotherapy. In the mid- to late-1960s, behavioral therapists began publishing clinical series documenting the successful treatment of sexual problems by the use of classical conditioning techniques. Indeed, the start–stop technique for the treatment of rapid ejaculation was first described by Semans in 1956 (10). However, the major use of behavioral techniques to treat sexual problems began after the publication of "Human Sexual Inadequacy" by Masters and Johnson in 1970 (11). In the 1980s, case reports began appearing in the psychiatric literature about using monoamine oxidase inhibitors and low dose antipsychotic drugs to treat rapid ejaculation (12). However, the use of psychiatric drugs to treat rapid ejaculation became much more common after the introduction of the selective serotonin reuptake inhibitors.

Urologists have made important contributions to the treatment of erectile dysfunction. Both the Small-Carrion and inflatable penile prostheses were introduced in the 1970s. Although patents for vacuum erection devices were obtained as early as 1917, the introduction of the vacuum erection pump by Osborn in 1974 resulted in this being a common solution for many men before the introduction of other treatment options. Alprostadil intracorporal injections were introduced in the 1980s. However, the popularity of treatment approaches decreased dramatically with the introduction of sildenafil in 1998 and the subsequent introduction of tadalafil and vardenafil. Now a man could take an effective oral agent that allowed sexual behavior to occur in a more natural way. Understandably, as the primary etiology of erectile dysfunction for majority of aging men is vascular (13,14), the main focus of therapeutic oriented research of erectile dysfunction has been the vascular dysfunction/insufficiency area. The previously touted use of androgens in erectile dysfunction has been abandoned as it became clear that androgen administration does not improve erectile dysfunction in eugonadal men (15). Interestingly, testosterone replacement in men with age-related mild hypogonadism is not effective in reversing symptoms of hypogonadism (in contrast to the same situation in older men) (15).

The successful introduction of sildenafil contributed to the search for pharmacological treatments for female sexual disorders. Initially, many companies did clinical trials in women with substances that had proven successful in treating erection problems. In general, these trials were unsuccessful. The one exception is a clitoral vacuum erection device, which has FDA approval (16,17). Another approach is the study of androgens to stimulate desire in women. Off-label use of androgen preparations increased significantly after the work by Gelfand and Sherwin (18,19) demonstrated that supraphysiological levels of testosterone increased libido in postmenopausal women (20). The use of androgen preparations to treat desire problems in women is currently undergoing clinical trials. As Rosen (21) pointed out, many large pharmaceutical trials of female sexual dysfunction are unfortunately hindered by various methodological problems, such as the lack of use of physiological outcome measures and the lack of consensus classification system for female sexual dysfunction in determining inclusion and exclusion criteria. There is also no precise and stable definition of normal sexuality available. Definition is also of dubious clinical usefulness.

The lack of success in search for efficacious pharmaceuticals for treatment of sexual dysfunction in women led to the examination and use of various botanical or herbal, and other substances in these indications (22,23); for review see Ref. (24). As Rowland and Tai (24) caution us, the effects of herbals tend to be limited, relatively nonspecific, poorly studied, and associated with unpredictable or unknown side effects.

The recent focus on pharmacological and other biological treatments of sexual dysfunction unfortunately takes away attention and emphasis from psychological treatments. However, as Heiman (9) points out, psychological treatments are efficacious (though their demonstrated efficacy is frequently limited) and needed (for various reasons, such as optimization of psychological treatments, patient choice, low frequency of side effects, etc.). Heiman (9) also cautions that the prescription of a physiologic treatment that ignores the fact that human sexuality is infused with individual meaning may invite further interference with sexual functioning.

EPIDEMIOLOGY OF SEXUAL DYSFUNCTION

Numerous population surveys in this and other countries indicate a high prevalence of sexual problems in the general population. These surveys indicate that ~40% of women have evidence of psychosexual dysfunction. The corresponding number for men is ~30% (25). We have more evidence concerning the prevalence of sexual problems in men than women although the data base in both groups is rapidly growing. Correlates of erectile dysfunction in men include diabetes, vascular disease, age, and cigarette smoking. Serum dehydroepiandrosterone and high-density lipoprotein cholesterol were found to be negatively correlated with erectile problems (26). Depression was correlated with erectile function in cross sectional studies, whereas passive personality traits tended to predict who would develop impotence in a prospective study (27). Studies in other countries have, in general, found somewhat similar rates of erectile dysfunction in the same age population and also that erectile dysfunction tends to correlate with the presence of diabetes, higher age, cardiovascular disease, and depression (15,28–32).

It is important to note that depression is not the only mental disorder associated with sexual dysfunction(s). Sexual dysfunction occurs in course of schizophrenia (33,34) or anxiety disorders (35).

Some recent studies went beyond collecting pure epidemiological data and studied the impact of sexual dysfunction on men suffering from various sexual dysfunctions. For instance, Moore et al. (36) described that younger men suffering from erectile dysfunction reported comparatively less relationship satisfaction, greater depressive symptomatology, more negative reactions from partners, and less job satisfaction than older men. They concluded that older men experience less difficulty than younger men adjusting to life with erectile dysfunction. Symonds et al. (37) interviewed men with self-diagnosed premature ejaculation. In their relatively small sample, they found that men with premature ejaculation had a sense that premature ejaculation was causing (not exclusively) lower self-esteem and had impact on forming a relationship. Findings of these two studies underscore the complexity of sexual dysfunctions/disorders and their connection to an overall functioning and well-being.

A population study of US females aged 18–65 (25) found that ~33% of US females reported low libido, trouble with orgasm, or difficulty with lubrication for at least 1 month in the previous year. Other surveys have reported similar findings. Hawton (38) studied sexual activity in a community sample in Oxford, United Kingdom and found that 17% reported never experiencing an orgasm and only 29% reported experiencing orgasm at least 50% of the time. Marital satisfaction was the major predictor of sexual activity and satisfaction. Dunn (39,40) also reported several population studies in the United Kingdom. Approximately 40% of the women reported a sexual problem, the most common being difficulty reaching orgasm. A recent population survey in Sweden (41) of sexual behavior in women aged 18–74 found that the most common problems were low desire followed by orgasm and arousal difficulties. They also reported considerable co-morbidity between sexual disorders. Some (42) questioned the methodology of epidemiological studies of sexual dysfunction as too simplistic and medicalized.

Laumann et al. (43) have recently completed a survey of 27,500 men and women aged 40–80 in 29 countries. In Northern European countries, lack of sexual interest was reported in 25.3% of women. Problems with orgasm and pain were reported in 16.9% and 17.7%, respectively. In men, low libido was reported in 12%, erectile dysfunction in 12%, and rapid ejaculation in 20.6%. Similar values were reported for other world regions, with minor differences in prevalence among different regions.

NOMENCLATURE

There are a number of cogent criticisms of the current nomenclature system. The system developed to diagnose psychosexual disorders has been adopted to classify disorders presumed to be organic in etiology (44). Duration and severity criteria for diagnosis are unclear. Many of the diagnoses overlap, and the criteria for diagnosing female sexual disorders have been criticized. To put all of this in perspective, a brief description of the history of the diagnostic system will follow. The Diagnostic and Statistical Manual of Mental Disorders (DSM) was developed in the United States although it is employed by professional in other countries as well. The DSM is supposed to correspond to the International Classification of Diseases (ICD). The DSM-I was developed in 1952. The DSM-II was developed to correspond with the ICD-8. Psychosexual disorders in the DSM-II were grouped under one diagnostic entity, genitourinary disorders. The DSM-III was developed to reflect changes in diagnosis and still remains compatible with the ICD-9. The nomenclature developed by William Masters, Helen Singer Kaplan, and Harold Lief had tremendous impact on the development of classifications of psychosexual disorders in DSM-III. This manual listed inhibited sexual desire, inhibited sexual excitement, inhibited female orgasm, inhibited male orgasm, premature ejaculation, functional dyspareunia, functional vaginismus, and ego-dystonic homosexuality. In DSM-IIIR, ego-dystonic homosexuality was deleted and sexual aversion disorder was added. The names of certain diagnoses were changed. For example, inhibited sexual desire became hypoactive sexual desire disorder. Sexual arousal disorder and male erectile disorder were substituted, respectively, for inhibited male and female sexual arousal disorders. Throughout, changes in criteria sets have been minimal. In DSM-IV, most of the names and criteria sets resemble DSM-IIIR. The requirement that a disorder be diagnosed only if it causes significant personal distress was added to put a high threshold for diagnosis (45). The DSM based classification remains unclear. For instance, it intermingles terms of sexual dysfunction(s) and sexual disorder(s) in an unclear manner.

Current nomenclature includes hypoactive sexual desire disorder, sexual aversion disorder, sexual arousal disorder, dyspareunia, vaginismus, premature ejaculation, erectile disorder, and male and female orgasmic disorders. In addition, each diagnosis is sub-typed into acquired or lifelong and global or situational. Several groups have suggested modification to the criteria sets for female sexual disorders (46).

EVOLVING MODELS

Most of the clinicians involved in the treatment and/or research of sexual dysfunctions/disorders are probably not very satisfied with the current nomenclature, which is mostly unidimensional and not including all nuances and aspects of sexual problems. The nomenclature does not deal with psychological, relational, and situational factors of human sexuality. Some of these issues, especially the ones related to female sexuality, are discussed in more detail in several chapters of this book (see for instance the Chapters 3 and 6).

A 26-year-old male who complains being distressed because ejaculating within 30–60 sec after penetration during sex with his wife, but reports no rapid ejaculation while masturbating technically meets the diagnostic criteria for premature ejaculation. Nevertheless, the diagnosis of premature ejaculation does not fully describe the scope and psychology of his sexual dysfunction. The same could be implied in the case of 67-year-old married male who started to compulsively masturbate about 2 years ago. He thinks about other men being around at times while masturbating, or at times he masturbates just "without any thoughts," in various places, for example, while driving. Is his diagnosis sexual disorder not otherwise specified? Or obsessive-compulsive disorder? Do these diagnoses-labels help the clinician in any way?

The recent diagnostic system, paraphrasing Winston Churchill, is probably the worst diagnostic system except for all those that have been tried. It certainly could be improved. Recently, Fagan (47) proposed a systematic way in which clinician organize the mass of information about sex. We discuss it in more details for two reasons—it clearly demonstrates that human sexuality, as other areas, requires a more complex and sophisticated descriptive/diagnostic system, and it illustrates one of probably many possible approaches.

Fagan suggests using the system of four perspectives, or four different ways to view a clinical case, which was originally developed by McHugh and Slavney (48) for all psychiatric disorders. He believes that these four perspectives are a more complex way of viewing clinical information and then communicating that information to clinicians, colleagues, and the individual with the clinical problem or disorder.

These four perspectives are:

1. The disease perspective
2. The dimension perspective
3. The behavior perspective
4. The life story perspective.

The disease perspective is categorical, the patient either has or does not have the disease. As Fagan (47) points out, this is the foundation of the medical model, but not the entire story. This perspective turns to physiology, anatomy, and medicine to learn about patient's sexual problem.

The dimension perspective focuses on measurement (dimensional gradation and quantification). Examples of the objects of measurements are intelligence quotient, behavioral patterns, mood, or personality traits.

The behavior perspective focuses on the behavior of an individual who is goal directed, or teleological. Fagan explains that the behavior perspective is to cognitive-behavioral clinician what the disease perspective is to physician.

Finally, the life story perspective is what "most people associate with psychotherapy." It relies on the narrative told by the patient to give some meaning and direction to their life.

Fagan emphasizes that "no single perspective is, in itself, more valuable than any other," and each perspective can contribute to the formulation. His proposal helps, in part, to deal with several issues. First, human sexuality is much more complicated than just achieving reliable erection and, as noted, the medical diagnosis does not include psychological, relational, and other factors. Second, not all sexually disordered behavior has a psychiatric diagnosis. Third, sexual diagnosis is an alternate and developing construct. Fourth, sexual diagnosis does not imply causality.

Fagan suggests that one should select the primary perspective that "best fits the patient and then integrate the other perspectives into the formulation and treatment to make use of the additional contributions they may provide." He also emphasizes that perspectives are conjunctive and not disjunctive.

Fagan feels that using the four perspectives is more helpful in delineating sexual problems/dysfunctions/disorders and conceptualizing their treatment. Many will probably find this proposal too complex or not complex enough, overly inclusive or not inclusive enough, not practical enough or too practical. However, we feel that it is an interesting and thoughtful proposal, which may further stimulate and help the debate about the diagnostic issues in the area of sexual dysfunctions/disorders.

MEDICALIZATION OF SEXUALITY

The recent developments in "sexual pharmacology" only reinforced some to warn us about the medicalization of sexual dysfunction and human sexuality in general. We believe that the treatment of sexual dysfunctions/disorders belongs to the realm of medicine. However, we also believe that the "sexual pharmacology" and total medicalization of sexuality does not provide the best understanding of the complexities of human sexuality and is not always in the best interest of our patients.

Bancroft (42) among others cautions just about a few important issues connected to medicalization of human sexuality. He points out that male sexuality has been medicalized for most of the 20th century, and that medical profession has paid more attention to female sexuality lately (interestingly, this increased interest seems to parallel with the increased interest of the pharmaceutical industry in female sexuality).

Bancroft points out that the interface between psychological processes and physiological response, especially in women, is not well understood. He discusses the numerous male–female differences in sexuality. He also asks, "when is a sexual problem a sexual dysfunction," as many times impaired sexual interest or response in women is psychologically understandable and thus rather an adaptive response to a problem in the sexual relationship rather than sexual dysfunction.

Medicalization of sexual dysfunction and human sexuality has been beneficial to some extent in expanding part of our understanding of human sexuality and its impairment(s), and in expanding our treatment armamentarium. However, it also poses dangers in a form of trivialization of human sexuality and secondary suppression of exploring other avenues of our understanding of human sexuality.

CONCLUSION

From the discussion of the history of the field, the evolution of nomenclature, and emerging data on epidemiology, it is clear that this is a field in rapid evolution. Most of the impetus for this change came from the discovery of effective oral therapies for male sexual disorder and the subsequent search for similar therapies for women. This has contributed to better studies of the epidemiology of these disorders and to debates about the proper nomenclature. In addition, clinicians have begun trying to find which psychological, pharmacological, or combined approach is most suited to treat these disorders (49,50).

The purpose of this book was to assemble experts in treatment of each disorder into one text so that this text could serve as a treatment guide for students and practicing clinicians. Ultimately, we hope that those who will benefit the most are our patients. Patient sexual satisfaction may be associated with many health factors, including a reduced risk for subsequent new severe disabilities (51).

REFERENCES

1. Segraves RT, Schoenberg HW, Zarins CK, Camic P, Knopf J. Characteristics of erectile dysfunction as a function of medical care system entry point. Psychosom Med 1981; 43:227–234.
2. Bodie JA, Beeman WW, Monga M. Psychogenic erectile dysfunction. Int J Psychiatry Med 2003; 33:273–293.
3. Leiblum S. After sildenafil: bridging the gap between pharmacologic treatment and satisfying relationships. J Clin Psychiatry 2002; 63(suppl 5):17–22.
4. Craighead WE, Hart AB, Craighead LW, Ilardi SS. Psychosocial treatments for major depressive disorders. In: Nathan PE, Gorman JM, eds. A Guide to Treatments that Work. New York: Oxford University Press, 2002:245–262.
5. Dougherty DD, Rauch SL, Jenike MA. Pharmacological treatments for obsessive compulsive disorder. In: Nathan PE, Gorman JM, eds. A Guide to Treatments that Work. New York: Oxford University Press, 2002:387–410.
6. Franklin ME, Foa EB. Cognitive behavioral treatments for obsessive compulsive disorder. In: Nathan PE, Gorman JM, eds. A Guide to Treatments that Work. New York: Oxford University Press, 2002:367–386.
7. Nemeroff CB, Schatzberg AF. Pharmacological treatments for unipolar depression. In: Nathan PE, Gorman JM, eds. A Guide to Treatments that Work. New York: Oxford University Press, 2002:229–244.
8. Keller MB, McCullough JP, Klein DN, Arnow B, Dunner DL, Gelenberg AJ, Markowitz JC, Nemeroff CB, Russell JM, Thase ME, Trivedi MH, Zajecka J. A comparison of nefazodone, the cognitive behavioral-analysis system of psychotherapy, and their combination for the treatment of chronic depression. N Engl J Med 2000; 342:1462–1470.
9. Heiman JR. Psychologic treatments for female sexual dysfunction: are they effective and do we need them? Arch Sex Behav 2002; 31:445–450.
10. Semans JH. Premature ejaculation: a new approach. South Med J 1956; 49:353–358.
11. Masters WH, Johnson VE. Human Sexual Inadequacy. Boston: Little Brown, 1970.
12. Segraves RT. Effects of psychotropic drugs on human erection and ejaculation. Arch Gen Psychiatry 1989; 46:275–284.
13. Sullivan ME, Keoghane SR, Miller MA. Vascular risk factors and erectile dysfunction. BJU Int 2001; 87:838–845.
14. Shabsigh R, Fishman IJ, Schum C, Dunn JK. Cigarette smoking and other vascular risk factors in vasculogenic impotence. Urology 1991; 38:227–231.
15. Seidman SN. The aging male: androgens, erectile dysfunction, and depression. J Clin Psychiatry 2003; 64(suppl 10):31–37.
16. Billups KL, Berman L, Berman J, Metz ME, Glennon ME, Goldstein I. A new non-pharmacological vacuum therapy for female sexual dysfunction. J Sex Marital Ther 2001; 27:435–441.
17. Segraves RT. Female sexual disorders: psychiatric aspects. Can J Psychiatry 2002; 47:419–425.

18. Sherwin BB, Gelfand MM, Brender W. Androgen enhances sexual motivation in females: a prospective, crossover study of sex steroid administration in the surgical menopause. Psychosom Med 1985; 47:339–351.

19. Sherwin BB, Gelfand MM. The role of androgen in the maintenance of sexual functioning in oophorectomized women. Psychosom Med 1987; 49:397–409.

20. Gelfand MM. The role of androgens in surgical menopause. Am J Obstet Gynecol 1999; 180:325–327.

21. Rosen RC. Sexual function assessment and the role of vasoactive drugs in female sexual dysfunction. Arch Sex Behav 2002; 31:439–443.

22. Meston CM, Worcel M. The effects of yohimbine plus L-arginine glutamate on sexual arousal in postmenopausal women with sexual arousal disorder. Arch Sex Behav 2002; 31:323–332.

23. Ferguson DM, Steidle CP, Singh GS, Alexander JS, Weihmiller MK, Crosby MG. Randomized placebo-controlled, double-blind, crossover design trial of the efficacy and safety of *Zestra for Women* in women with and without female sexual arousal disorder. J Sex Marital Ther 2003; 29(suppl 1):33–44.

24. Rowland DL, Tai W. A review of plant-derived and herbal approaches to the treatment of sexual dysfunctions. J Sex Marital Ther 2003; 29(3):185–205.

25. Laumann EO, Paik A, Rosen RC. Sexual dysfunction in the United States. J Am Med Assoc 1999; 281:537–544.

26. Feldman HA, Goldstein I, Hatzichristou DG, Krane RJ, MacKinlay JB. Impotence and its medical and psychosocial correlates: results of the Massachusetts Male Aging Study. J Urol 1994; 151:54–61.

27. Araujo AB, Johannnes CB, Feldman HA, Derby CA, MacKinlay JB. Relation between psychosocial risk factors and incident erectile dysfunction: prospective results from the Massachusetts Male Aging Study. Am J Epidemiol 2000; 152:533–541.

28. Akkus E, Kadioglu A, Esen A, Doran S, Ergen A, Anafarta K, Hattat H. Turkish Erectile Dysfunction Prevalence Study group: Prevalence and correlates of erectile dysfunction in Turkey: a population-based study. Eur Urol 2001; 41:298–304.

29. Bonierbale M, Lancon C, Tignol J. The ELIXIR study: evaluation of sexual dysfunction in 4557 depressed patients in France. Curr Med Res Opin 2003; 19(2):114–124.

30. Braun M, Wassmer G, Klotz T, Reifenrath B, Mathers M, Engelmann U. Epidemiology of erectile dysfunction: results of the 'Cologne Male Survey.' Int J Impot Res 2000; 12:305–311.

31. Moreira EB Jr, Bestane WJ, Bartolo EB, Fittipaldi JA. Prevalence and determinants of erectile dysfunction in Santos, southeastern Brazil. Sao Paulo Med J 2002; 120:49–54.

32. Nicolosi A, Moreira ED Jr, Shirai M, Bin Mohd Tambi MI, Glasser DB. Epidemiology of erectile dysfunction in four countries: cross-national study of the prevalence and correlates of erectile dysfunction. Urology 2003; 61:201–206.

33. Aizenberg D, Zemishlany Z, Dorfinan-Etrog P, Weizman A. Sexual dysfunction in male schizophrenic patients. J Clin Psychiatry 1995; 65:137–141.

34. Raja M, Azzoni A. Sexual behavior and sexual problems among patients with severe chronic psychoses. Eur Psychiatry 2003; 18:70–76.

35. Kotler M, Cohen H, Aizenberg D, Matar M, Loewenthal U, Kaplan Z, Miodownik H, Zemishlany Z. Sexual dysfunction in male posttraumatic stress disorder patients. Psychother Psychosom 2000; 69:309–315.

36. Moore TM, Strauss JL, Herman S, Donatucci CF. Erectile dysfunction in early, middle, and late adulthood: symptom patterns and psychological correlates. J Sex Marital Ther 2003; 29:381–399.
37. Symonds T, Roblin D, Hart K, Althof S. How does premature ejaculation impact a man's life? J Sex Marital Ther 2003; 29:361–370.
38. Hawton K, Gath D, Day A. Sexual function in a community sample of middle-aged women with partners: effect of age, socioeconomic, psychiatric and gynecological and menopausal factors. Arch Sex Behav 1994; 23:375–395.
39. Dunn KM, Croft PR, Hackett GI. Association of sexual problems with social, psychological and physical problems in men and women: a cross sectional population survey. J Epidemiol Community Health 1999; 53:144–148.
40. Dunn KM, Croft PR, Hackett GI. Satisfaction in the sex life of a general population sample. J Sex Marital Ther 2000; 26:141–151.
41. Fugl-Meyer KS. Epidemiology of female sexual dysfucntion. Paper presented at Female Sexual Forum. Boston, Massachusetts, 2001.
42. Bancroft J. The medicalization of female sexual dysfunction: the need for caution. Arch Sex Behav 2002; 31:451–455.
43. Laumann E, Nicolosi A, Glasser DB, Paik A, Buvat J, Gingell C, Moreira ED Jr, Hartmann U, Brock G, Wang T. Prevalence of sexual problems among men and women aged 40 to 80 years: results of an international survey. Poster presentation at 2nd International Consultation on Erectile and Sexual Dysfunction. June 28–July 1, 2003, Paris, France.
44. Segraves RT. Emerging therapies for female sexual disorders. Expert Opin Emerg Drugs 2003; 8:515–522.
45. Segraves RT. Historical and international context of nosology of female sexual disorders. J Sex Marit Ther 2001; 27:205–207.
46. Basson R, Berman J, Burnett A, Derogatis L, Ferguson D, Fourcroy J, Goldstein I, Graziottin A, Heiman J, Laan E, Leiblum S, Padma-Nathan H, Rosen R, Segraves K, Segraves RT, Shabsigh R, Sipski M, Wagner G, Whipple B. Report of the international consensus development conference on female sexual dysfunctions: definitions and classifications. J Urol 2000; 163:888–893.
47. Fagan PJ. Sexual disorders. Perspectives on diagnosis and treatment. Baltimore, Maryland: Johns Hopkins University Press, 2004.
48. Mc Hugh PR, Slavney PR. The perspectives in psychiatry. 2nd ed. Baltimore, Maryland: Johns Hopkins University Press, 1998.
49. Bartlik B, Legere R, Anderson L. The combined use of sex therapy and testosterone replacement therapy in women. Psychiatr Ann 1999; 29(1):27–33.
50. Wylie KR, Hallam Jones R, Walter S. The potential benefit of vacuum devices augmenting psychosexual therapy for erectile dysfunction: a randomized controlled trial. J Sex Marital Ther 2003; 29(3):227–236.
51. Onder G, Penninx BWJ, Guralnik JM, Jones H, Fried LP, Pahor M, Williamson JD. Sexual satisfaction and risk of disability in older women. J Clin Psychiatry 2003; 64:1177–1182.

2

Combination Therapy for Sexual Dysfunction: Integrating Sex Therapy and Pharmacotherapy

Michael A. Perelman

The New York Presbyterian Hospital,
Weill Medical College of Cornell University, New York, NY, USA

INTRODUCTION: THE FALSE DICHOTOMY

The 20th century marked huge strides in our knowledge of sexual disorders and their treatments, however, advancements were followed by periods of reductionistic thinking. Etiology was conceptualized dichotomously, first as psychogenic and then organic. Early in the 20th century, Freud highlighted deep-seated anxiety and internal conflict as the root of sexual problems experienced by both men and women. By mid-century, Masters and Johnson (1) and then Kaplan (2) designated "performance anxiety" as the primary culprit, while providing a nod to organic factors. Together, they catalyzed the emergence of sex therapy, which relied on cognitive and behavioral prescriptions to improve patient functioning. For the next two decades, a psychological sensibility dominated discussions of the causes and cures of sexual dysfunctions (SDs). However, during the late 1980s, there was a progressive shift toward surgical and predominantly pharmaceutical treatments for male erectile dysfunction (ED). By the 1990s, urologists had established hegemony, with the successful marketing of various penile prostheses, as well as intracavernasal injections (ICI) and interurethral insertion (IUI) systems [e.g., Caverject (Pharmacia, Teapak, NJ, USA), Muse (Vivus, Mountainview, CA, USA)]. The monumentally successful 1998 sildenafil launch (Pfizer, New York, NY, USA) and its subsequent publicity at the end of the 20th century symbolized the apex of biologic determinism. Most physicians and most of the general public saw SD and its treatment solely in organic terms.

    The new millennium finds us moving forward toward a more enlightened and sophisticated paradigm where the importance of both organic and psychogenic factors is appreciated for their role in predisposing, precipitating, maintaining, and reversing SD. The pharmaceutical industry has developed other phosphodiesterase-5 inhibitor (PDE-5) based treatments for ED as evidenced by the successful 2003 launches of vardenafil (Bayer, New Haven, CT, USA and

GSK, Philadelphia, PA, USA) and tadalafil (Lilly, Indianapolis, IN, USA and ICOS, Seattle, WA, USA). All three FDA-approved PDE-5 inhibitor compounds are selling well worldwide, and new pharmaceutical delivery systems for treating SD are in development. The FDA has approved EROS (UroMetrics, Inc., Anoka, MN, USA), a mechanical device, for the treatment of female SD (FSD). Indeed, multiple products (pharmaceutical, nutriceutical, and mechanical) are being introduced, or are in development, to treat a host of complaints under the market driven heading of "FSD." Despite this juggernaut of pharmaceutical activity, a renewed sensitivity to psychosocial issues is emerging and a more balanced perspective is shaping our discussions of the understanding and treatment of male and female SD. These discussions are the focus of symposia at important international meetings (American Urological Association, World Health Organization, International Society for the Study of Women's Sexual Health, etc.). Yet, they are underwritten (directly or indirectly) by the same pharmaceutical companies that develop and manufacture the drugs, which essentially catapulted a biologic medicalized view of SD onto the world stage, to the exclusion of psychosocial sensitivity. This rebalancing of perspective, reflected a growing consensus of thought, catalyzed by mental health professionals (MHPs). These MHPs have once again successfully advanced the obvious concept: psychosocial factors are also critical to the understanding of sexual function and dysfunction. Sexual pharmaceuticals can very frequently restore sexual capacity. Yet, rewarding sexual function is experienced only when psychosocial factors also support restored sexual activity. Medicine today emphasizes an evidence-based research. There is a seeming inherent tension between this concept and the qualitative "art and science" of psychotherapy (3). This chapter will attempt to bridge that gap by discussing combination treatments (CTs) for SD, where the use of sex therapy strategies and treatment are integrated with sexual pharmaceuticals. There is a synergy to this approach, which is not yet supported by empirical evidence, but is rapidly gaining adherents which over time will document its successful benefits. Although there has been an explosion of research regarding the efficacy of PDE-5s for ED in the last 5 years, there is no doubt in this author's mind that combination therapy (CT) will be the treatment of choice for all SD, as new pharmaceuticals are developed for desire, arousal, and orgasm problems in both men and women. Yet, owing to the paucity of current data available for other sexual disorders, this chapter will primarily emphasize CT for ED.

MODELS FOR TREATING SEXUAL DYSFUNCTION

Sex Therapy

Sex therapy theory and technique were derived from the pioneering works of both Masters and Johnson (1) and Kaplan (2). Initially Masters, a gynecologist, used an innovative 2 week, mixed-gender, co-therapy team, quasiresidential approach.

Sex therapy rapidly morphed into weekly sessions provided within a solo MHP's office based practice. Treatment continued to emphasize "sensate focus exercises" and the reduction of performance anxiety. By the 1980s, sex therapy reflected a cognitive-behavioral theoretical bias, while typically utilizing Masters and Johnson variations, such as Kaplan's, four phase model of human sexual response: desire, excitement, orgasm, and resolution (1,4,5). The models were not necessarily linear and causes could become effects. For instance, an ED might cause diminished desire. However, generally speaking, sex therapy was and is, the diagnosis and treatment of disruptions in any of these four phases and/or the sexual pain and muscular disorders. These dysfunctions occurred independent of each other, yet they frequently clustered.

Sex therapy was based on the development of a treatment plan conceptualized from the rapid assessment of the immediate and remote causes of SD while maintaining rapport with the patient (6,7). The sex therapist assigned structured erotic experiences carried out by the couple/individual in the privacy of their own homes. These exercises were designed to correct dysfunctional sexual behavior patterns, as well as positively altering cognitions regarding sexual attitudes and self-image. This "home play" modified the immediate causes of the sexual problem, allowing the individual to have mostly positive experiences and created a powerful momentum for successful treatment outcome. Interventions aimed at correcting or challenging maladaptive cognitions were incorporated into the treatment process (8). The individually tailored exercises acted as "therapeutic probes" and were progressively adjusted until the individual or couple was gradually guided into fully functional sexual behavior (4,6). However, each dysfunction had its own cluster of immediate causes. Certain exercises were typically used with a particular dysfunction. For example, almost all men with premature ejaculation (PE) were taught the "stop–start" technique, because failure to recognize and respond properly to sensations premonitory to orgasm, characterized that syndrome.

Patients might be single or coupled. The single patients were seen alone, but their new sexual partner might join them in treatment, once an ongoing relationship was formed. Couples were usually seen conjointly, however, during the evaluation phase of treatment, they were typically seen alone for at least one session of history taking. Other individual sessions were reserved for management of resistance where it may be more strategic to discuss the obstacles to success privately. To facilitate the success of this rapid approach, individuals/couples at times needed to explore other aspects of their relationship and/or intrapsychic life. Nevertheless, establishing sexual harmony typically remained the primary focus. Despite the concrete goal orientation, the therapeutic context was humanistic, emphasizing good communication, intimate sharing, and mutual respect.

Sex therapy was an "efficacious" treatment for primary anorgasmia in women, some erectile failure in men, and was "probably efficacious" for secondary anorgasmia, . . . , vaginismus in women and PE in men (9). Clinical experience supported efficacy in treating hypoactive sexual desire, sexual aversions, dyspareunia, and delayed orgasm in men (9). Despite its potency, there were and are drawbacks to this approach, particularly from a cost-benefit standpoint. Although considered as a "brief treatment" within a mental health context, it typically required many appointments with a trained specialist and a high degree of motivation on the part of the patient. Historically, healthcare systems have discarded labor intensive, expensive approaches once "easier" and more rapid alternatives were available. Sex therapy receded as a treatment of choice during the 1990s, as medical and surgical approaches performed by urologists established hegemony over the treatment of ED, in particular. The pinnacle of this transition was reached during 1998, with the launch of sildenafil.

Medical Treatments for Erectile Dysfunction

The 1980s saw a progressive shift away from psychological treatments of SD to an emphasis on surgical and medical solutions for improving sexual health. Simultaneously, there was a progressive shift within the medical community and public at large, towards viewing the etiology of SD as organic, rather than the psychogenic understanding emphasized by sex therapists. Use of improved sophisticated diagnostic procedures, such as duplex sonography and cavernosograms (although not necessarily improving treatment) added credibility and imprimatur to the importance of organic pathogenesis (10). This was particularly true in the area of ED, where urologists established dominance, with the successful marketing and use of various intracavernosal and intraurethral systems. Although highly touted by urologists, the treatment efficacy of these products was offset by their intrusiveness into the patient's bodies and reduction in spontaneity, their patterns of use required.

Initially, there were few oral treatments for ED, being used by urologists, such as yohimbine based products, trazodone, and bupropion. They had only modest proerectile capability (11). Pharmaceutical companies were inspired to pursue oral treatments with the promise of less intrusiveness and even greater profits. The first visible evidence of fulfilling that promise was the sildenafil launch. Subsequent to Pfizer's success, multiple companies simultaneously pursued clinical trials of easy-to-use treatments for male SD. Among others, these included additional PDE-5 type compounds and other oral treatments, such as ixense (TAP Holdings, Deerfield, IL, USA), and topically applied compounds (MacroChem, Lexington, MA, USA). Additionally, PT-141 (Palatin Technology, Cranbury, NJ, USA) is a nasally administered peptide that is under development, which is presumed to work through a central nervous system mechanism.

Currently, there are three highly efficacious PDE-5, FDA-approved treatments for ED: sildenafil, vardenafil, and tadalafil. Reviews of long-term extension studies and published accounts of use in clinical practice show that sildenafil's effectiveness was maintained with long-term treatment. "Significantly improved erectile function was demonstrated for sildenafil compared with placebo for all efficacy parameters analyzed ($P < 0.02$ to 0.0001), regardless of patient age, race, body mass index, ED etiology, ED severity, ED duration, or the presence of various co morbidities. Long-term effectiveness was assessed in three open-label extension studies (12)." Vardenafil (launched in 2003) "is a potent, selective PDE-5 inhibitor, which improved erectile function in a broad population of men with ED and in characteristically challenging-to-treat groups such as diabetic and post prostatectomy patients (13)." Tadalafil also launched in 2003, when taken, "as needed before sexual activity and without restrictions on food or alcohol intake, significantly improved erectile function. It allowed a substantial proportion of patients to achieve a normal IIEF erectile function domain score, exhibited a broad window of therapeutic responsiveness and was well tolerated in a representative population of patients with broad-spectrum erectile dysfunction (14)."

NEW SEXUAL PHARMACEUTICALS: SUCCESS OR FAILURE

Success of the New Treatments

The new PDE-5 inhibitors have resulted in more people being treated than ever, with high success rates. There is much greater awareness of sexual and psycho-sexual issues surrounding dysfunction, simultaneous with a reduction of the stigma previously associated with ED. Treatment is now conducted by an expanding number of helping professionals, primarily PCPs. Treating ED is now a billion-dollar business with millions of men treated and many helped.

Barriers to Treatment Success

Approximately 90% of men who seek assistance for ED are treated with PDE-5s, all of which are reasonably safe (15). All are completely contraindicated with concomitant nitrate use; with some additional warnings and/or contraindications attached to use of alpha-blockers. Generally, PDE-5 inhibitors are highly effective, restoring erections in $\sim$70% of men, yet there is a growing body of evidence suggesting that the frequently quoted 20–50% drop-out rate for medical treatments is true for PDE-5 treatment as well (15). Why? The adverse event profile is excellent for all three PDE-5s, with few patients terminating treatment, because of adverse events. Of course, not all discontinuation of sexual pharmaceuticals are due to failure or complications. There are some who tried the medications out of curiosity and never intended to continue using a PDE-5. There are some reported cases of men with psychogenic ED experiencing a "cure" after temporary use of a PDE-5 (16).

Reciprocally, some people will discontinue PDE-5 because of the severity of their ED. For these individuals, the pharmaceuticals simply do not work. Regardless of the mode of administration, a certain percentage of the population will not experience restored capacity, because the degree of organicity is so profound as to overwhelm the salutary effects of the drug. In particular, some diabetics and radical prostatectomy survivors may need more powerful medical treatments.

Importantly, PDE-5 treatments do have significant psychosocial limitations and consequences which have created "born-again" roles for sex therapists, albeit more complex and sophisticated ones (17). Previously, many presumed that high discontinuation rates were due to the objectionable nature a specific treatment, such as self-injecting the penis. They thought that the introduction of efficacious and safe oral agents would decrease this high drop-out rate (18). However, there is great complexity to the barriers to success story. Although definitely improving, the reported success rate, the ensuing publicity (following PDE-5 launches) still resulted in just a small percentage of people worldwide receiving pharmaceutical therapy. ED treatment, even with its juggernaut of publicity and advertising has penetrated <15% of the estimated market place. In fact, industry information suggested that a geometrically small number of individuals were actually successfully treated and satisfied repeat "customers" (19). Apparently, a limited number of men were treated and a large percentage of those who tried it, apparently discontinued rather abruptly (19). There was also a high relapse rate when medication was stopped. The model for all three PDE-5s, as well as ICI and IUI treatments for ED, was chronic pharmaceutical use in order to relieve symptoms. To date, very little was written about "weaning" patients from pharmaceuticals or effectively maintaining them on lower doses. Concepts of "weaning" and relapse prevention offer opportunities for MHPs (20).

Identifying Psychosocial Barriers to Success

Importantly, pharmaceutical advertising and educational initiatives have altered the delivery of sexual medicine services, especially in the United States. Specifically, these changes in practice patterns resulted in PCPs becoming the principal healthcare providers for men who present with a primary complaint of ED, with urologists typically seeing the more recalcitrant cases. MHPs rarely are the initial treating clinicians anymore. This both helps and contributes to the problem of success and failure. The large number of PCPs treating ED has dramatically increased the number of patients seen, and the accessibility of medical treatment. Unfortunately, the history obtained by PCPs and urologists is frequently limited to an end-organ focus, and fails to reveal significant psychosocial barriers to successful restoration of sexual health. These obstacles or "resistance" represent a significant cause of noncompliance and nonresponse to treatment (2). These barriers manifest themselves in varying levels of complexity, which individually and/or collectively must be understood and managed for pharmaceutical treatment to be optimized (15,20).

Only recently, have physicians begun incorporating sex therapy concepts, and recognized that resistance to lovemaking is often emotional. Clearly, medical treatments alone are often insufficient, in helping couples resume a satisfying sexual life. There are a variety of bio-psychosocial obstacles to be recovered that contribute to treatment complexity. All of these variables impact compliance and sex lives substantially, in addition to the role of organic etiology (20). There are multiple sources of patient and partner psychological resistance, which may converge to sabotage treatment: (i) What is the mental status of both the patient and the partner and how will this impact treatment, regardless of the approach utilized? What is the nature and degree of patient and partner psychopathology (such as depression)? What are the attitudinal distortions causing unrealistic expectations, as well as endpoint performance anxiety? (ii) What is the nature of patient and partner readiness for treatment? When and how should treatment begin, and be introduced into the couple's sex life? What is his approach to treatment seeking? What should be the pacing of intimacy resumption? The average man with ED waits 2–3 years, before seeking assistance (21). By that time, a new sexual equilibrium has been established within the relationship, which may be resistant to the changes a sexual pharmaceutical introduces. Furthermore, although partner pressure is a primary driver for treatment seeking, some men who sought treatment at their partner's initiation do not necessarily confide in them about the treatment (21). (iii) What is their emotional and attitudinal readiness for change? The sexual history will provide information regarding premorbid and current sexual desire. What is her motivation or desire for sex? What are her concerns regarding his safety? What are her belief systems regarding the treatment process which now enables coitus? Her compliance may be affected be her perception of the treatment being artificial or mechanical: "Is it the sildenafil, or me?" (iv) What is her health status (vaginal atrophy, etc.) and physical readiness for sex; her capacity for lubrication and need for stimulation, etc.? We know from the Massachusetts Male Aging Study that frequency of ED increases with age (22). We know that older men tend to have older, post-menopausal partners. Female partner's additional and sometimes complex medical needs are frequently not addressed in the brief evaluation interview, often conducted by the average physician. (v) What are the relevant contextual stressors in the patient and/or partner's current life, such as work, finances, parents, and children, etc.? (vi) What is the couple's overall quality and harmony of relationship? Interpersonal issues impact outcome through a variety of manifestations? Intimacy blocks and power struggles may cause failure. (vii) What are the patient and partner's sexual script? Overtime, incompatible sexual scripts, interest, and arousal patterns may predetermine SD. For instance, PDE-5s require stimulation, for the man to respond sexually; stimulation is frequently more than merely adequate friction. There are many divergent sexual scripts and a variety of unconventional patterns of sexual arousal (homosexuality, sadomasochism, etc.), which may sabotage arousal. Additionally, over time, there are reality-based alterations in a partner's sexual desirability, which may also affect both arousal and orgasmic response.

Although most of these barriers to success can be managed as part of the treatment, too few physicians are trained to do so (20,23). What is a model for this situation? These various sources of psychological resistance manifest themselves in a diverse manner, which Althof conceptualized as three "scenarios" of psychosocial complexity (15). Each level would lead to an alternative treatment plan. Importantly, this concept can be expanded to conceptualize treatment for all SD, and regardless of who provides care—they all would be CT.

COMBINATION THERAPY: THE ROAD TO SUCCESS

Combining sexual pharmaceuticals and sex therapy is the "oral therapy" of choice to optimize treatment for all SDs. This is true for men with ED, PE, or retarded ejaculation (RE) and will also be true for FSD. Less medication is required when you modify immediate causes while appreciating other psychological obstacles (20). However, CT is by no means a new idea, and sexual medicine is not the first specialty utilizing a broad-spectrum approach to increase efficacy and satisfaction.

Combination Therapy: A Brief Relevant History

During the 1970s, psychiatrists and psychoanalysts argued, with analysts insisting that psycho-pharmaceuticals interfered with analysis. Today, mainstream psychiatry is characterized by a CT of psychotherapy and psychopharmacology. In the 1990s, psychiatrists finally integrated SSRIs synergistically with cognitive-behavior therapy to treat depression. Indeed such a model, frequently practiced in modified form by PCPs, probably dominates the treatment of depression today. There is an emerging literature demonstrating the benefit of combining both pharmacological and psychological treatments for a number of psychiatric conditions (24–26).

In urology and many medical specialties, CT usually referred to a, two or more drug regimen, such as the 2003, AUA guidelines for BPH (27). There already is a history of using CT in sexual medicine. In the 1990s, sex therapists worked with urologists combining either ICI or vacuum tumescence therapy. Turner et al. (28a) found that psychological counseling was necessary to augment a pharmaceutically induced erection, for a man with a psychogenic ED. Kaplan managed "resistance to ICI," helping five couples find satisfaction with pharmaceutical restoration of potency (28b). Hartmann and Langer (29) integrated injection therapy and sexual counseling concluding that a combined approach was beneficial. Colson described the results of a study integrating cognitive-behavior therapy and ICI technique. Of their patients, 51% were still able to experience satisfactory sexual intercourse after discontinuing injection therapy (30). Lottman et al. (31), integrated short-term therapy with intracavernosal injections and counseling, improving erectile function and facilitating couples communication. Wylie et al. (32) reported a successful combining of "vacuum treatment" and couple's therapy for primarily psychogenic ED patients using a group approach.

Multiple case reports have summarized the benefits of combining sexual pharmaceuticals with cognitive or behavioral treatments for ED (33–37). There were
also multiple articles recommending the combination of medical and psychological
approaches to the treatment of ED (15,20,32,38,39). Unfortunately, at this point
there are no well-designed randomized control studies focused on integrated
approaches to the treatment of SD. However, many are optimistic that the data supporting this approach will be forthcoming. An excellent summary of this material on
CTs, primarily for ED, with a few FSD studies, can be found in Table 10 of the WHO
2nd Consultation on Erectile and Sexual Dysfunction, Psychological and Interpersonal Dimensions of Sexual Function and Dysfunction Committee report (40).

Combination Therapy for Sexual Dysfunction: Integrating Sex Therapy and Sexual Pharmaceuticals

We know, clinically, that many PDE-5 nonresponders will be restored to sexual
health through a CT integrating sex therapy and sexual pharmaceuticals. Yet how
do we conceptualize such a model so that standard treatment algorithms could be
stretched to incorporate this concept? The answer is twofold. We need a schema
for understanding psychosocial obstacles (PSOs) to successful treatment, integrated into a model that executes that understanding.

Combination therapy is the therapeutic modality of choice for any SDs.
Combination therapy refers to a concurrent or step-wise integration of psychological and medical interventions. We have previously described developing
adherence for this approach to ED, with enthusiasm growing within the FSD
treatment community (36). Combination therapy is already being recommended
for PE, and is likely to be recommended for the full range of ejaculatory disorders
(41). Although desire disorders for men and women have a strong psychosocial
cultural component, there is little doubt that sexual "desire" has biological underpinnings and is likely to be distributed on the same bell-shaped distribution curve
as other human characteristics. This simply means that all SDs have a biopsychosocial basis and that treatment must incorporate medical and psychological dimensions. Without adequate desire, motivation, and realistic expectations,
treatment outcome is likely to be disappointing and with high discontinuation
rates. Medical interventions do not motivate the sexually reluctant patients or
partners to try treatment, nor do they help overcome psychological obstacles to
success. Reciprocally, it would constitute malpractice to only focus on psychological factors to the exclusion of all possible organic etiology for an individual
seeking assistance. Then, how can an ethical and motivated clinician proceed?

Combination Therapy Guidelines: Who, How, and When?

There are two alternative models for CT: both will likely be adopted within the
framework of sexual medicine, by different clinicians. First, working alone,
PCPs, urologists, psychiatrists, and eventually gynecologists will integrate sex
counseling with their sexual pharmaceutical armamentarium to treat SD. "Sex

counseling" in this situation, is utilizing sex therapy strategies and techniques to overcome psychosocial resistance to sexual function and satisfaction (20). In a second model, the above clinicians will collaborate with nonphysician MHPs (sex therapists), resolving SD(s) through a coordinated multidisciplinary team approach to treatment. The clinical combinations will vary according to the presenting symptoms, as well as the varying expertise of these health care providers. The utilization of these two different models will require three steps. (i) The clinician first consulted by the patient will consider their interest, training, and competence. (ii) The bio-psychosocial severity and complexity of the SD as a manifestation of both psychosocial and organic factors will be evaluated. (iii) The clinician in consideration of the two previous criteria, together with patient preference, will determine who initiates treatment, as well as, how and when to refer. The guidelines for managing the relative severity of the dysfunction will essentially be expanded, but continue to match the type of treatment algorithm described in "The Process of Care" and other step-change approaches (42).

Categorizing Psychosocial Obstacles to Treatment

Whether or not a physician works alone, as in the first model, or as part of a multidisciplinary team, as in the second, will be partially determined by the psychosocial complexity of the case. This CT model adapts Althof and Lieblum's "Proposed Integrated Model for Treating Erectile Dysfunction" (15,40). However, it must be emphasized that this author is advocating a CT model for all SD. The treating clinician would diagnose the patient(s) as suffering from mild, moderate, or severe PSOs to successful restoration of sexual function and satisfaction. This characterization would be based on an assessment of all the available information obtained during the evaluation. This would include an assessment of the issues/factors described in this chapter's earlier section on "Psychosocial Barriers to Success." This assessment would essentially include the psychosocial (cognitive, behavioral, cultural, and contextual) factors predisposing, precipitating, and maintaining the SD. This would be a dynamic diagnosis, continuously reevaluated as treatment progressed. The consulted clinician would continue treatment and/or make referrals on the basis of progress obtained. These PSOs are categorized as follows:

1. *Mild PSOs*: No significant or mild obstacles to successful medical treatment.
2. *Moderate PSOs*: Some significant obstacles to successful medical treatment.
3. *Severe PSOs*: Substantial to overwhelming obstacles to successful medical treatment.

Sexual Dysfunction Treatment Guidelines

Although no objective data determines the criteria for diagnosing these three PSO categories, they will become a useful heuristic device to help clinicians know

when to refer. For instance, "Severe" PSOs may require psychotherapeutic and/
or psychopharmacologic intervention prior to the initiation of treatment utilizing
sexual pharmaceuticals in order to restore sexual functioning and satisfaction.
Most nonmedical MHPs will collaborate with physicians to augment their own
treatments, as sexual pharmaceuticals are likely to provide an ever-increasing
role in MHP's treatment strategies and armamentarium for SD (15,17,20,43).
Additionally, this treatment matrix will provide a useful tool for sex therapist
physicians (usually psychiatrists), when deciding whether to treat themselves,
or seek collaborative assistance. The matrix determining who might treat is
presented in Table 2.1.

Table 2.1 SD Management Guidelines Based on PSO Severity

	Mild PSO	Moderate PSO	Severe PSO
Physician sex coach	Frequently	Often	Rarely
Multidisciplinary team	Frequently	Frequently	Frequently

PSOs = Psychosocial obstacles.

The following discussion illustrates how Table 2.1 could be used in clinical
practice. Clearly, a multidisciplinary team including a sex therapist and multiple
medical specialists could attempt to treat almost every case. Although severe
cases would usually require a greater number of office visits with lower
success rates, than moderate or mild cases. However, a team is a very labor-
intensive approach and frequently unrealistic, both economically and geographi-
cally in terms of available expertise and manpower. However, in the first two
cells, which reflect common scenarios in clinical practice, a physician who first
evaluates a patient suffering from SD, could integrate sex counseling with their
sexual pharmaceuticals, often resulting in a successful outcome.

SEX COUNSELING TIPS FOR CLINICIANS

A sex counseling model is frequently being recommended by CME courses for
physicians, under the rubric of "optimizing" care when using PDE-5 treatments.
As discussed earlier, multiple MHPs have attempted to raise awareness of the
importance of psychosocial factors in the etiology and treatment of ED
(15,17,20,32). However, this sex counseling model will apply to clinicians treating both men and women for the entire range of SDs, not merely those treating
ED. Clinician difficulty with either moderate or severe psychosocial complexity
would lead to appropriate referral and presumably the use of the multidisciplinary
team model.

A recent article, "Sex Coaching for Physicians" provided a comprehensive
discussion for nonpsychiatric physicians on incorporating psychotherapy into
their office practice to enhance sexual pharmaceutical efficacy (20). The article

emphasized augmenting pharmacotherapy with sex therapy when treating ED specifically, or SD generally. Although intended for the nonpsychiatric physician, the article served as a good model for any clinicians interested in integrating use of sexual pharmaceuticals with their sex therapy practice, using a multidisciplinary model. That multidisciplinary approach constitutes the second alternative for "combination treatment" and will be addressed more fully, later in this chapter. The following section on counseling, incorporates key issues from the article in addition to other tips, helpful to clinicians counseling SD patients.

Clearly, clinicians treating SD must consider the psychological and behavioral aspects of their patient's diagnosis and management, as well as organic causes and risk factors. Integrating sex therapy and other psychological techniques into their office practice will improve effectiveness in treating SD. Psychological forces of patient and partner resistance, which impact patient compliance and sex lives beyond organic illness and mere performance anxiety must be understood. The following key areas of therapeutic integration will be highlighted: Focusing the sex history; sexual scripts and pharmaceutical choice; "follow-up" and "therapeutic probe" to manage noncompliance; partner issues; relapse prevention; and referral.

The Focused Sex History

A focused sex history is the clinician's most important tool in evaluating SD, as it is most consistent with the "review of systems" common to all aspects of medicine. This limited history gives clinicians critical information in <5 min. Both sex therapists and physicians juxtapose detailed questions about the patient's current and past sexual history unveiling an understanding of the causes of dysfunction and noncompliance. A good, focused sex history assesses all current sexual behavior and capacity. The interview is rich in detail, providing a virtual "video image," clarifying many aspects of the individual's behavior, feelings, and cognitions regarding their sexuality. A flood of useful material emerged when actively and directly evoked. A focused sex history critically assists in understanding and identifying the "immediate cause"—the actual behavior and/or cognition causing or contributing to the sexual disorder. Armed with this information, a diagnosis could be made and a treatment plan formulated. These sexual details provide important diagnostic leads. Significantly, the sexual information evoked in history taking will help anticipate noncompliance with medical and surgical interventions. Kaplan's "Cornell Model" heuristically used immediate, intermediate, and remote causal layering to help determine timing and depth level of intervention (7). Modifying immediate psychological factors results in less medication being needed for men and women, regardless of their specific SD. Sex therapist's interventions are exercises and interpretations. In general, physicians will intervene with pharmacotherapy and brief "sex counseling," which address "immediate causes" (insufficient stimulation) directly, intermediate issues (e.g., partner) indirectly, and rarely focuses on deeper (e.g., sex abuse) issues. Nonpsychiatric physicians typically manage current obstacles to success, which are both organic and psychosocial in nature. In fact, when deeper psychosocial issues are the primary obstacles, it is usually time for referral (4).

Many clinicians learned about the statistically significant increase in the incidence of depression in individuals with SD. Treatment of SD may improve mild-reactive depression, whereas depressive symptoms might alter response to therapy of SD (44). A clinician's history taking must parse out this "chicken or egg problem": Is SD causing depression, or is depression and its treatment (e.g., SSRIs) causing the SD? Here, the value of direct questioning about sex becomes clear in particular. If clinicians did not ask, the patients may not tell. When asked direct questions, SSRI patients reported an increase, from 14% to 58%, in the incidence of SD vs. spontaneous report (45). True incidence was probably underestimated as PDR data was based on patient spontaneous report (46). To manage adverse effects of medication, physicians must adjust dose or, combine with other drugs, to ameliorate the problem. For instance, many might reduce the SSRI and supplement with bupropion or try sildenafil as a possible adjunct (43,47). Although "alternative medicine" (herbs, etc.) or other treatment approaches might be effective, sex therapy enhances all of these strategies. In particular, teaching immersion in the sexual experience through fantasy is helpful to eroticize both the experience and the partner. However, fantasy could be about anything erotic; masturbatory fantasies are usually quite effective. Fantasy of an earlier time with the current partner may be especially helpful for those who feel guilty about fantasizing in their own partner's presence. Referral to a sex therapist can help when extensive and specific discussions of masturbation are useful to develop, recalibrate and/or restore the sexual response (20).

The focused sex history allows the clinician to initiate therapy with the least invasive method available; literally an "oral therapy." For this author, one question helps pin down many of the immediate and remote causes: "tell me about your last sexual experience?" Common immediate causes of SD are quickly evoked by the patient's response. The most important cause of SD is lack of adequate friction and/or erotic fantasy, in other words, insufficient stimulation. Sex is fantasy and friction, mediated by frequency (20). To function sexually, people need sexy thoughts, not only adequate friction. Although fatigue may be the most common cause of SD in our culture, negative thinking/anti-fantasy, whether a reflection of performance anxiety or partner anger, is also a significant contributor. Of course, the clinician initiating the discussion of sex with the patient, in a mutually comfortable manner, transcends the importance of which question is asked. The clinician follows-up, with focused, open-ended questions to obtain a mental "video picture." Inquiries are made about desire, fantasy, frequency of sex, and effects of drugs and alcohol. Did arousal vary during manual, oral, and coital stimulation? What is the masturbation style, technique, and frequency? Idiosyncratic masturbation is a frequent hidden cause of ED, as well as RE (41a,41b). The clinician becomes implicitly aware of the patient's sexual script and expectations, leading to more precise and improved recommendations and management of patient expectations (20). For instance, a clinician would improve outcome by briefly clarifying whether a patient was better-off practicing with masturbation, or reintroducing sex with a partner? A recently divorced man, who was using condoms for the first time in years, was probably better-off masturbating with a condom rather than attempting sex with his partner, the first time he tried a new sex pharmaceutical.

Patient Preference, Sexual Scripts, and Pharmaceutical Choice

Patients suffering from SD, first express preference when they choose to seek help from a MHP vs. a nonpsychiatric physician. Most MHPs (having ruled out organic etiology) will initially proceed with sex therapy in cases where psychogenic etiology is paramount. For many of these patients, sex therapy will be effective in and of itself. For others, the MHP will facilitate incorporating sexual pharmaceuticals into the treatment process, to help "bypass" or overcome PSOs. The use of sexual pharmaceuticals for these patients may be a temporary recommendation, until a more pro-sexual equilibrium is established for the patient and partner. Reciprocally, pharmacotherapy may be either continuously or intermittently integrated with other attitudinal and behavioral changes necessary for a successful sexual and emotional experience. This will vary based on patient and partner pathologies interacting with the progressive organicity, often secondary to aging. Understanding relapse prevention requires consideration of these issues and factors (16,20,48). How these issues are currently managed by MHPs is illuminated within this chapter's Case Studies.

Owing to multiple factors including the organization of health care delivery, attitudinal beliefs, and pharmaceutical advertising; the majority of patients suffering from ED (when they do seek treatment) are likely to consult their PCP or a nonpsychiatric physician specialist (21). Although a few select physicians (primarily multiskilled psychiatrists) will provide sexual counseling as an exclusive modality when appropriate, most nonpsychiatric physicians will initiate treatment with a PDE-5 regardless of etiology. All three PDE-5s are used worldwide and are now FDA approved in the USA. All have good success rates! Simple cases do respond well to oral agents, with proper advice on pill use, expectation management, and a cooperative sex partner. However, physicians should offer patients choices, especially those who are pharmaceutically naïve. Providing an unbiased, fair-balanced description of treatment options, including pharmaceutical benefits on the basis of the pharmacokinetics, efficacy studies, and the physician's own patients' experience will result in the patient attributing greater importance to the physician's opinion. Incorporating patient preference provides important guidance and will enhance healer/patient relations, minimize PSOs, and improve compliance. Preliminary comparator data, abstracted from the 2003 European Society of Sexual Medicine, suggested, patient preferences reflected, key marketing messages of the respective pharmaceutical companies (49). Prescribing physicians might take advantage of that hypothesis to increase efficacy. If safety and long-term side effects are the primary concern, sildenafil has the oldest/longest database (12). If, pressed by questions regarding hardness of erection; *in vitro* selectivity may or may not translate to clinical reality, yet some patients believe vardenafil provides the best quality erection with the least side-effect (13). What is the physician's experience with their own patients?

By taking a sex history and evaluating the premorbid sexual script (what used to work sexually), a skillful clinician may make an educated guess, as to which pharmaceutical to first prescribe. This transcends, "try it, you'll like it." Knowledge of pharmacokinetics (onset, duration of action, etc.) and sexual script analysis helps optimize treatment, by improving probability of initially selecting the right prescription. Many physicians initiated treatment with sildenafil and will continue to do so. However, psychosocial factors and previous sexual scripts, may suggest a different drug on the basis of pharmacokinetic profile. Partner issues help determine correct pharmaceutical selection on the basis of analysis of the couple's premorbid sexual script and relationship dynamics. Understanding the couples "sexual script" can help the physician fine tune pharmaceutical selection, leading to better orgasm and sexual satisfaction, not merely improved erection (50). Sexual script in this situation refers to style and process of the couple's premorbid sex life (51). For those fortunate enough to have had a good premorbid sex-life, dosing instructions should focus on returning to previously successful sexual scripts—as if medication was not a necessary part of the process. This maximizes patient likelihood of getting adequate stimulation in a manner likely to be comfortable and conducive to partner sensitivities. Awareness of within individual differences improves the quality of recommendations made for that person or couple's sexual recovery. Differences between individuals in sexual style (sex script analysis) can determine which medication might be used by a couple effectively, with less change required in their "normal" sexual interactions. For instance, some couples mutually presume that the man is "in charge" and should initiate and seduce like he used to. As he is planning the sexual encounter, sildenafil or vardenafil might be good choices. However, tadalafil may be preferable, if a more spontaneous response to an externally evoked situation is desired.

Fitting the right medication on the basis of pharmacokinetics to the individual/couple will increase efficacy, satisfaction, compliance, and improve continuation rates. Rather than changing the couples' sexual style to fit the treatment, try to fit the right medication to the couple (50). A sensitive clinician may be tempted to facilitate a relationship of greater egalitarian and psychological balance. However, a symbiotic relationship with decades of history must be respected. For the most part, clients are seeking restoration of sexual function not a "make over," defined and reflecting a "politically correct" professional bias. Success requires consumer sensitivity. For instance a "rejection sensitive" woman may function as the couple's sexual "gatekeeper," yet may never initiate sex. She may require him to respond to explicit initiations or her implicit initiations through signs of sexual receptivity (leg touching in bed, a subtle caress). The astute clinician might ask "Couldn't these merely be signs of partner affection and not subtle sexual initiation?" Yes. However, for such a women, his willingness and ability to be sexual, is experienced positively even if she declines sex. She needs to feel both affirmed and in control. They agree that she is the gatekeeper and she may encourage sexuality, or limit the process to affection. Yet, his initiation is an important aspect of their sexual script and relationship equilibrium. By serving as a source of affirmation for her, it reduces the noxious (toxic) manifestations of her insecurity and rejection sensitivity. They both expect that she will decline some initiations. Yet, if he is only willing and able to initiate once dosed, then sildenafil or vardenafil is a poorer choice. For their relationship, multiple initiations are required, and pre-dosing with longer acting tadalafil may be a better choice. Harmony will be restored and satisfaction will increase. Two to three doses of tadalafil weekly, for a month, might be useful for such men who are essentially "on-call" in order to initially facilitate their capacity. As confidence and capacity improves and predictability increases, dosing could be titrated down or the pharmaceutical even weaned away. If the previous sex script was weekend sex, then a Friday night dose may be sufficient. If he has become resistant to her "controlling dom-ination," then a referral for couples counseling would be appropriate. Although the suggestion of referral may be enough to compel him to try the drug, given the reaction many men have to MHPs. The physician simply makes an educated guess regarding pharmaceutical selection. Follow-up may indicate greater PSO complexity. Then, the case would be better managed utilizing a multi-disciplinary integrated approach, with a sex therapist working collaboratively with the prescribing physician. Later in this chapter, this multidisciplinary method is illustrated with the case of Jon and Linda.

Follow-up and Therapeutic Probe

Discussions of follow-up most vividly illustrate the importance of integrating sex therapy and pharmacotherapy. Urologists, Barada and Hatzichristou improved sildenafil nonresponders by emphasizing patient education (e.g., food/alcohol effect), repeat dosing, partner involvement, and follow-up (52,53). Patient edu-cation about the proper use of sildenafil was crucial to treatment effectiveness. Physicians can increase their success by scheduling follow-up, the first day they prescribe. As with any therapy, follow-up is essential to ensure an optimal treatment outcome. Initial failures examined at follow-up reveal critical infor-mation. The pharmaceutical acts as a therapeutic probe, illuminating the causes of failure or nonresponse (2,15,20). Retaking a quick current sexual history provides a convenient model for managing follow-up. Other components of the follow-up visit include monitoring side effects, assessing success, and considering whether an alteration in dose or treatment is needed. Future comparator trials will help determine which drug works best, for which person(s), under which context. Until then, physicians will likely trust their own judgment and experience. However, physicians must provide ongoing education to patients and their partners, as well as involving them in treatment decisions whenever possible. A continuing dialogue with patients is critical to facilitate success and prevent relapse. The numerous psychosocial issues previously discussed may evoke noncompliance. These are important issues in differentiating treatment nonresponders from "biochemical failures," in order to enhance success rates. Early failures can be reframed into learning experiences and eventual success.

Partner Issues

Regaining potency does not automatically translate into the couple resuming sexual intercourse. Psychological issues may render the best treatments futile. PDE-5 discontinuation or failure rates of 20–40% are not due to adverse events. Resistance to lovemaking is often emotional and the most common "mid-level" psychological causes of SD are relationship factors (15,20,23). As discussed previously, partner dynamics can help determine correct pharmaceutical selection on the basis of analysis of the couple's premorbid sexual script and relationship (50). Yet numerous partner related psychosexual issues may also adversely impact outcome.

Cooperation vs. Attendance

Mild immediate causes of SD are often amenable to brief counseling in the physician's office. Still the most common mid-level relationship causes may present considerable difficulty for the nonpsychiatric physician treating SD within the context of a typically brief office visit. How might this challenge be met? The complexity of this conundrum can be reduced or resolved. The physician's challenge is not necessarily requiring an office visit with the partner, as many CME programs have advocated. Instead, the emphasis should be on evaluating the level of partner cooperation and support. Since Masters and Johnson, sex therapists have recognized that SD is a "couples problem," not just the identified patient's problem (2). However, almost equally long ago, this author and others noted that the key partner treatment issue was supportive cooperation, independent of actual attendance during the office visit (5,20). Generally speaking, encourage partner attendance with committed couples, allowing assessment and counseling for both. However, the issue is never forced. Treatment format is a psychotherapeutic issue and rapport is never sabotaged. Although conjoint consultation is a good policy, it is not always the right choice! A man or woman in a new dating relationship is probably better-off seeing the physician alone, than stressing a new relationship by insisting on a conjoint visit (20,54).

Partner Consultation?

Although CME courses recommended that patient–partner–physician dialogue was best enhanced through patient–partner education during conjoint visits, there was anecdotal evidence that physicians were not regularly meeting with partners of SD patients. This author undertook a 2002 Internet survey of the Sexual Medicine Society of North America, member's practice patterns. These urologists are all sub-specialists in sexual medicine in general, and ED in particular. Although methodologically limited, the results were interesting. The data pointed to a striking disparity between urologist attitude and actual practice. An overwhelming 79% of the responding urologists considered partner cooperation with ED treatment "important," regardless of whether the partner actually attended sessions or not? Yet, only 39% of the responding urologists saw only one partner or less in their last five ED patient's office visits. Nor was there any contact by phone, e-mail, or other means between doctor and partners for 90% of the responding urologists, despite the vast majority of patients were married or coupled. However, there were good reasons for not having a conjoint visit, as long as the importance of partner issues in treatment success was understood. Indeed, many urologists reflected thoughtfully on the burden of the treater to not invade the privacy beyond what was freely accepted by the patient. Urologists noted that the men saw ED as their problem, and were not interested in involving their partner. These urologists gently encouraged partner attendance, but appropriately did not require it (20). So why are pharmaceutical ED treatments so effective? Does this data suggest that partner issues do not impact outcome? No, but it does support the thesis that "partner cooperation" is even more important than "partner attendance." Why are many physicians successful even when not seeing partners? Sex pharmaceuticals with sex counseling and education work for many people, if the partner was cooperative in the first place. Fortunately, many partners of both men and women are cooperative, which partially accounts for the high success rates of medical and surgical interventions. Indeed, most of the cooperation goes unexplored. The cooperation is assumed based on *post hoc* knowledge of success. Importantly, many women were cooperating with their partners, or facilitating sexual activity, independent of their knowledge of the use of a sexual aid or pharmaceutical. In other words, serendipitous matching of sexual pharmaceutical and previous sexual script equaled success: "we did, what we used to do, and it worked." (20,54).

The existence of large numbers of cooperative, supportive women who themselves have partners with mild to severe ED account for much of the success of many ED patients who see their physicians alone, for evaluation and subsequent pharmacotherapy. Many of these partners were never seen by the treating physician, nor was their attendance necessary for success. This is likely to be true for other male and female dysfunctions as well, depending on the degree of psychosocial barriers to success. Obviously, the most pleasant, supportive, cooperative partners would rarely be discouraged from attending office visits with any patient. Ironically, these same patients would probably have successful outcomes even if their partners never attended an office visit. However, good becomes better by evaluating, understanding, and incorporating key partner issues into the treatment process (54).

The patient–partner–clinician dialogue is best enhanced through patient–partner education. Partner attendance during the office visit would allow for such education. Yet, many clinicians do not regularly meet with partners of SD patients. Although working with couples was often recommended: sometimes there was no partner; sometimes the current sexual partner was not the spouse, raising legal, social, and moral sequella. The reality and cost/benefit of partner participation is a legitimate issue for both the couple and the clinician, and not always a manifestation of resistance. Finally, the patient's desire for his partner's attendance may be mitigated by a variety of intrapsychic and interpersonal factors, which, at least initially, must be respected and heeded (15,20).

There are other solutions. When evaluation or follow-up reveals significant relationship issues, counseling the individual alone may help, but interacting with the partner will often increase success rates. If the partner refuses to attend, or the patient is unwilling or reluctant to encourage them; seek contact with the partner by telephone. Ask to be called, or for permission to call the partner. Most partners find it difficult to resist speaking "just once," about "potential goals" or "what's wrong with their spouse." The contact provides opportunity for empathy and potential engagement in the treatment process, which may minimize resistance and improve further outcome. This effective approach could be modified depending on the clinician's interest and time constraints. Clinicians should counsel partners when necessary and possible. They need to be a resource in treating with medication, counseling, and educational materials. Education needs to be a greater part of SD practice, whether provided within a physician's practice or externally by other competent healthcare professionals. Success rates can be enhanced through patient–partner–clinician education, which will reduce the frequency of noncompliance and partner resistance, and minimize symptomatic relapse. Organic and psychological factors causing SD, and noncompliance with treatment, are on a multi-layered continuum. Although some partners will require direct professional intervention, many others could benefit from obtaining critical information from the SD patient and/or multiple media formats both private and public (20,54).

Weaning and Relapse Prevention

In general, the concept of relapse prevention has not been incorporated into sexual medicine. Yet SD is recognized as a progressive disease in terms of underlying organic pathology, which may play a role in altering threshold for response and potential re-emergence of dysfunction. Both McCarthy and Perelman have recommended that the clinician schedule "booster" or follow-up sessions in order to help the patient stay the course and provide opportunity for additional treatment when necessary (20,48). These concepts are derivative of an "addiction" treatment model where intermittent, but continuous care is the treatment of choice. Additionally, utilizing sex therapy concepts in combination with sexual pharmaceuticals offers potential for minimizing dose and temporary or permanent weaning from medication depending on the severity of organic and psychosocial factors. SDs are frequently progressive diseases, but this is especially true for ED. Over time the progressive exacerbation of either organic factors (endothelial disease, etc.) or PSOs may adversely impact a previously successful treatment regimen. Furthermore, although there is no current evidence for tachyphylaxis, neither are there extensive studies beyond 10 years indicating long-term efficacy of PDE-5s. No doubt, escalating dose and providing alternative medications would be most physician's initial response of choice. However, both these processes may be modulated and mediated by sexual counseling and education. Sex therapy and other cognitive-behavioral techniques and strategies could be extremely important in facilitating long-term medication maintenance, and helping to ensure continuing medication success. As such, clinicians caring for ED patients, are well advised to incorporate these counseling techniques into the treatment they provide themselves, or through referral. Each case requires individual consideration in part determined by patient preference regarding level of outcome success desired. Levine (16) presented an interesting discussion on multiple dimensions of treatment success.

When to Refer?

The physicians "time crunch" can be managed, when brief counseling of the SD patient is sufficient. If the partner's support for successful resolution of the SD is not present, then active steps must be taken to evoke it. Sometimes, a conjoint referral for adjunctive treatment to a sex therapist for the partner may also be required (20). Of course, the more problematic the relationship, the more profound the marital strife, the less likely that patient–partner sex education will be able to successfully augment treatment in and of itself. Inevitably, a referral to a MHP would be required, albeit not necessarily accepted successfully. Additionally, there are numerous organically determined reasons making referral to a multiplicity of medical specialists (urologists, gynecologists, neurologists, psychopharmacologists, endocrinologists, etc.) necessary and appropriate. However, elaborating all of them is beyond the scope of this chapter.

Integration vs. Collaboration

Does a multidimensional understanding of a SD always require a multidisciplinary team approach? Clearly, the answer is no. When there is a question of collaboration vs. integration within an individual clinician; how does one decide whether to be a multitalented physician or part of a multidisciplinary team?

There are a variety of sexual medicine thought leaders conversant with both organic and psychosocial predisposing, precipitating, and maintaining factors of SD, including some notable PCPs, psychiatrists, and urologists. Additionally, there is a convergence towards a bio-psychosocial consensus initially reflected by the "Process of Care Guidelines," and elaborate upon, in the published Proceedings of the WHO 2nd International Consultation on Erectile and Sexual Dysfunction (40,42). These publications are the result of multidisciplinary cooperation, with collaborative knowledge being appreciated, independent of specialty of origin. These consensus reports, speak to the importance of integrating medical, surgical, and psychosocial treatments for SD. Sometimes, the physician's treatment is only partially successful, and the lack of psychosocial sensitivity causes an exacerbation of the problem. This may be corrected. Reciprocally, psychotherapists may be fairly criticized for failing to refer quickly enough for medical consultation, in order to benefit from incorporating a sexual pharmaceutical to speed-up the recovery process and reduce the time and cost of treatment. Discussed subsequently is Roberto's ED case, treated by the author and two different urologists; when an expert sexual medicine physician, who had adequate time and motivation, may have managed equally well.

Case Study: Roberto

A 32-year-old Italian man was suffering from primary ED. Roberto had "two hypospadias operations" at ages 3 and 6. He reported "at 8 years old, circumcision removed 'excess skin'." He remembered friends teasing, about his urinating from the "underside." He had primary ED and 2 years ago (as a visiting student), he consulted a US urologist who prescribed sildenafil. The urologist reportedly told Roberto that he would never function normally, because of his congenital hypospadius. Roberto left that consultation devastated, fearing he was sexually handicapped for life. No great surprise, the sildenafil did not work when he used it with masturbation. He was afraid to date women. The same urologist observed on follow-up that Roberto seemed depressed and was not using the sildenafil, or dating. He referred Roberto to the author. Accurate information incorporated within a cognitive-behavioral sex therapy, improved Roberto's self-esteem, reduced his fear of rejection, decreased performance anxiety, and encouraged dating. His confidence was increased through his masturbation, augmented with sildenafil and fantasy. It worked! He began dating and had erections with foreplay.

Vacationing in Italy, Roberto began a sexual relationship with a woman. He went to an Italian urologist who complemented his sex therapy progress, and provided him with samples of sildenafil, vardenafil, and tadalafil. All worked wonderfully, but he preferred tadalafil, because of the 36 h duration of action. He reported that his new girlfriend supposedly "had six orgasms in 27 years with all her boyfriends; yet with me, she had five in one day." He suspected, she knew, he used "sex drugs." They reportedly had sex twice daily. Back in the

USA, he used 1/3, of a 100 mg sildenafil and fantasy about sex in Italy, to mas-
turbate successfully. Roberto was gradually weaned from the sildenafil when he
masturbated. When his girlfriend visited 6 months later, he initially used low dose
sildenafil successfully. Then, she seduced him one night when he had no medi-
cation available. She remained with him in the US. Reportedly, they now have
twice weekly coitus, fully weaned from medication, for the past 5 months. The
author will see him again in 2 months for follow-up to minimize relapse potential.
Roberto recognizes, "it is mostly in the brain." He wisely said, "If we break up or
in a period of stress, okay let me take a pill a couple of times. I will use it as a
crutch once in a while. When I feel less secure or very stressed."

WORKING TOGETHER: A MULTIDISCIPLINARY TEAM APPROACH

The concept is a simple one with a long history; sometimes, two heads are better
than one. Treatment may require a multidisciplinary team in cases of severe dysfunction, and may be recalcitrant to success even under this ideal circumstance.
There are many models for working together. Team approaches and composition
will vary according to clinician specialty training, interest, and geographic
resources. Although some expert physicians work alone, other PCPs, urologists,
and gynecologists have set up "in house" multidisciplinary teams where nurses,
physician associates, and master's level MHPs provide the sex counseling. This
approach has obvious advantages and disadvantages. In cases of more severe
PSOs, the patient(s) will be "referred out" for psychopharmacology, cognitive-
behavioral therapy, and marital therapy in various permutations, provided by
doctoral level MHPs (55–57). However, typically a clinician refers within
their own academic institution, or within their own professional referral
network—a kind of "virtual" multidisciplinary team. Endocrine, gynecologic,
or urologic referrals for the patient or partner may be required, and would
usually be readily available. However, MHPs trained in sex therapy will experience the greatest number of new opportunities for interdisciplinary participation
to enhance and optimize patient response to sexual pharmaceuticals. Identifying
psychological factors does not necessarily mean that nonpsychiatric physicians
must treat them. If not inclined to counsel, or, if uncomfortable, these physicians
should consider referring or working conjointly with a sex therapist. All clinicians should be encouraged to practice to their own comfort level. Indeed,
some PCP will not have the expertise to adequately diagnose PSOs, independent
of their ability or willingness to treat these factors. Awareness of their own limitations will appropriately prompt these physicians to refer their patients for
adjunctive consultation. Physicians who prescribe PDE-5s and future sexual
pharmaceuticals may need adjunctive assistance, referring to sex therapists,
because of their own psychological sophistication or due noncompliance on
their patient's part. Whether the referral is physician or patient initiated, sex
therapists are ready to effectively assist in educating the patient about maximizing their response to the sexual situation. They are able to help re-motivate people

who have failed initial medical treatments, as well as helping patients to adjust to "second and third line" interventions. They help make patients receptive to trying again. Sex therapists are also equipped to help resolve the intrapsychic and interpersonal blocks (resistance) to restoring sexual health (20,42). Some clinicians are uncomfortable discussing sex, and many important issues remain unexplored because of clinician anxiety and time constraints. Sex therapists can manage event and process based developmental factors, which predisposed the patient to manifest the SD. They are trained to manage the most difficult cases involving process-based trauma that are replicated in the current relationship. Sex therapists working adjunctively with the PCP, urologist, or gynecologist could provide all the previously discussed sex counseling, as well as managing PSOs with greater therapeutic depth. Sex therapists can enhance hope, facilitate optimism and maximize placebo response. There can be an increased individualization of treatment format, by fine-tuning therapeutic suggestions, as well as improving response to medication by optimizing timing and titration of dose. Sex therapists have a sophisticated appreciation of predisposing (constitutional and prior life experience), precipitating factors triggering dysfunction, and factors maintaining SD. Finally, sex therapists are skilled in using cognitive-behavioral techniques for relapse prevention. All of these issues impact potential and capacity for successful restoration of sexual health. Delineating all permutations, of multidisciplinary team approaches likely to be utilized for the next decade, is beyond the scope of this chapter. However, a useful glimpse of this process is provided in the following case, where this author collaborated with a PCP, a urologist, and a psychopharmacologist, in a "virtual" multidisciplinary team approach to CT.

Case Study: Jon and Linda

Jon and Linda were referred to the author by Jon's current psychopharmacologist. Jon is a 62 years old financier who has been married to Linda (53 years old) for over 20 years. She began HRT 4 years ago, which successfully stopped her hot flashes. This is his second marriage and her first marriage. They had three teenage children together. Their marriage was marked by periods of disharmony secondary to multiple etiologies. Jon and Linda had a symbiotic relationship where she dominated much of their daily life. She tended to be explicitly critical of him, which he resented but managed passive-aggressively. This, of course, merely exacerbated their marital tension. Linda was particularly sensitive to rejection, and was considerably upset when Jon withdrew from her in response to her criticism. This infuriated her and she provoked confrontations. He eventually responded, becoming loud and aggressive, which initially dissipated his tension. He then felt guilty as she expressed hurt and disappointment in his behavior. This push–pull process would begin anew, characterizing the rhythm of their marriage. Despite all these difficulties in the relationship, both Jon and Linda were fortunate enough to be capable of engaging in successful sex to reduce their stress and anxiety; unlike those needing to be stress free in order to function. Jon and Linda enjoyed high frequency successful coital activity with mutually enjoyable coital orgasms, despite their intermittent marital disharmony over a 15-year period.

Three years ago, Jon started SSRI treatment for depression, secondary to work stress. His depression exacerbated his insecurity about his intelligence and abilities. He developed ED and could not erect, but his sexual desire was still strong. Medication helped his moodiness and reduced his depression. They both wanted Jon on the antidepressant medications, yet their marital conflict increased. His psychopharmacologist tried reducing the SSRI and aug- menting with bupropion. This did not help! If anything, it uncharacteristically, worsened his sex life. They tried switching him from paroxetine to bupropion to escitalopram. During this time, he lost his job, and money problems became worse. He needed to move to a different city in order to find work, uprooting Linda and the kids. He also used a low dose, blood pressure (BP) medication, which had not caused ED, although it was a risk factor. Possibly, the BP medi- cation exacerbated the anti-sexual impact of the SSRI, culminating in his severe ED. His typical male withdrawal from sex and affection once the ED emerged, only exacerbated her rejection sensitivity and deep feeling of abandonment. This left her slightly depressed, but predominantly, critical of him and doubting the viability of their marriage.

His Chicago psychopharmacologist referred them to a well-known NYC urologist, when they first moved from Chicago. The urologist prescribed 50 mg of sildenafil, which was increased to 100 mg. There were multiple attempts at 100 mg, which all failed. The urologist then prescribed "trimix." They used "trimix" ICI, 15 times, resulting in three coital erections and orgasms. Neither Jon, nor Linda liked the "lack of spontaneity." The urologist recommended a penile prosthesis, but Jon declined and terminated that treatment.

Some months later, still on 10 mg of escitalopram, a new, NYC psychophar- macologist referred Jon to this author. Jon and Linda were seen six times con- jointly and three times individually. She was helped to reframe his withdrawal, as insecurity, not rejection or abandonment of her. This reduced her anger and resentment. He was encouraged to be affectionate when not angry at her. Her criticalness was reduced, which led to a reduction in his passive-aggressive behavior. Although not resolving the individual and marital dynamics, these insights increased harmony enough, for a sexual pharmaceutical to become effective. The author recommended tadalafil to Jon's PCP, because of Linda's rejection sensitivity. The drug's longer duration of action allowed him to respond to her receptivity cues, which she "dropped like a hankie." For 1 month, he took tadalafil, Friday and Tuesday. Quoting her: "it covered him for the week." They now use it, as needed, and are back to twice weekly coitus. She said, "I could do a commercial. It's doing a fabulous job. It's a really good drug for us. It is causing greater emotional warmth that leads to physical intimacy." This, of course tends to be true for all the PDE-5s when they work, not just tada- lafil. He reported, "it takes away the uncertainty, allowing me to feel able."

Reportedly, both individual and relationship satisfaction were increased and Jon continued to be followed by his PCP and his psychopharmacologist.

SUMMARY AND CONCLUSION

For those individuals where cost is less of a factor in determining decision-making, consultation with a qualified sex therapist offers a potentially more elegant solution, than merely experiencing a trial of sexual pharmaceuticals, when confronted with SD. Yet, it would be unnecessary to subject everyone to a complex evaluation by a sex therapist in advance of a sexual pharmaceutical prescription and brief counseling by a PCP. In part, patients will seek the treatment they want and prefer. Some will seek herbal supplements purchased on the Internet, whereas others will choose a consultation with a MHP specializing in sex therapy. However, if only due to pharmaceutical advertising, most patients will first consult with a physician who will hopefully possess sex counseling expertise, as well as a prescription pad. This physician would adjust treatment according to the individual and couple's history, sexual script, and intra and interpersonal dynamics.

All clinicians want to optimize the patient's response to appropriate medical intervention. However, it is equally important to not collude with the patient's unrealistic expectations of either his or her own idealized capacities, or an idealization of the treating clinician's abilities. These fantasies are based on ignorance and may reflect unresolved psychological concerns. There are situations when it is appropriate to either make a referral within a team approach or to decline to treat a patient. Significant, process based, developmental predisposing factors, usually speak to the need for resolution of psychic wounds prior to the introduction of the sexual pharmaceutical. A man with ED or RE who avoids sex with his intrusive, domineering spouse, is even less likely to successfully utilize a sexual pharmaceutical; if his idiosyncratic and hidden masturbation pattern, emerged in response to a critical intrusive mother (35). The more determinants of SD are driven by developmental processes, the more likely the patient will benefit from sex therapy in addition to pharmacotherapy. There are situations when it is appropriate to postpone treating the patient for the SD, until psychotherapeutic consultation is able to assist the individual in developing a more reality-based view. Although sometimes this can be done simultaneously, other times, treatment for SD must be postponed.

Sexuality is a complex interaction of biology, culture, developmental, and current intra and interpersonal psychology. A bio-psychosocial model of SD provides a compelling argument for CT integrating sex therapy and sexual pharmaceuticals. Restoration of lasting and satisfying sexual function requires a multidimensional understanding of all of the forces that created the problem, whether a solo physician or multidisciplinary team approach is used. Each clinician needs to carefully evaluate their own competence and interests when considering the treatment of a person's SD, so that regardless of the modality used, the patient receives optimized care. For the most part, neither sex therapy nor medical/surgical interventions alone are sufficient to facilitate lasting improvement and satisfaction for a patient or partner suffering from SD. There will be new medical and surgical treatments in the future. Sex therapists and sex therapy will complement all of these approaches. This author is optimistic, for a future, which uses CT, integrating sexual pharmaceuticals and sex therapy, for the resolution of SD and the restoration of sexual function and satisfaction.

REFERENCES

1. Masters WH, Johnson VE. Human Sexual Inadequacy. Boston: Little Brown, 1970.
2. Kaplan HS. The New Sex Therapy. New York: Brunner/Mazel, 1974.
3. Norcross JC, Guest Editor. Psychotherapy: Special Issue: Empirically Supported Therapy Relationships: Summary Report of the Division 29 Task Force. Vol. 38, No. 4, Winter, 2001.
4. Kaplan HS, Perelman MA. The physician and the treatment of sexual dysfunction. In: Usdin G, Lewis J, eds. Psychiatry in General Medical Practice. New York, NY: McGraw-Hill, 1979.
5. Perelman MA. Premature ejaculation. In: Lieblum S, Pervin L, eds. Principles and Practice of Sex Therapy. New York, NY: Guilford Press, 1980.
6. Perelman MA. The urologist and cognitive behavioral sex therapy. Contemp Urol 1994; 6:27–33.
7. Perelman MA. Commentary: Pharmacological agents for ED & the human sexual response cycle. J Sex Marital Ther 1998; 24:309–312.
8. Zilbergeld B. The New Male Sexuality. New York: Bantam Books, 1992.
9. Heiman JR, Meston CM. Empirically validated treatment for sexual dysfunction. In: Rosen R, Davis C, Ruppel H, eds. Annual Review of Sex Research. Mount Vernon, IA: The Society for the Scientific Study of Sexuality, 1998.
10. Perelman MA. Rehabilitative sex therapy for organic impotence. In: Segraves T, Haeberle E, eds. Emerging Dimensions of Sexology. NY: Praeger Publications, 1984.
11. Rosen RC, Ashton A. Prosexual drugs: empirical status of the "New Aphrodisiacs." Arch Sexual Behav 1993; 22:521–543.
12. Carson CC, Burnett AL, Levine LA, Nehra A. The efficacy of sildenafil citrate (sildenafil) in clinical populations: an update. Urology 2002; 60(suppl 2B).
13. Hellstrom W. Vardenafil: a new approach to the treatment of erectile dysfunction, Curr Urol Rep, Curr Sci Inc 2003; 4:479–487
14. Brock GB, McMahon CG, Chen KK, Costigan T, Shen W, Watkins V, Anglin G, Whitaker S. Efficacy and safety of tadalafil for the treatment of erectile dysfunction: results of integrated analyses. J Urol 2002; 168(4).
15. Althof SE. Therapeutic weaving: the integration of treatment techniques. In: Levine SB, ed. Handbook of Clinical Sexuality for Mental Health Professionals. New York: Brunner-Routledge, 2003:359–376.
16. Levine SB. Erectile dysfunction: Why drug therapy isn't always enough. Cleveland Clinic J Med 2003; 70(3).
17. Perelman MA. The impact of the new sexual pharmaceuticals on sex therapy. Curr Psychiatry Rep 2001; 3(3).
18. Goldstein I, Lue T, Padma-Nathan H, Rosen R et al. Oral sildenafil in the management of erectile dysfunction. New Engl J Med 1998; 338:1397–1404.

19. Sand et al. Males, ISSIR 2002.

20. Perelman M. Sex coaching for physicians: combination treatment for patient and partner. Int J Impotence Res: J Sexual Med 2003; 15(suppl 5).

21. Shabsigh R, Perelman M, Laumann E, Lockhart D. Drivers and barriers to seeking treatment for erectile dysfunction: a comparison of six countries. Br J Urol Inter September/October 2004; 1055–1065.

22. Feldman HA, Goldstein I, Hatzichristou DG et al. Impotence and its medical and psychosocial correlates: results of the Massachusetts Male Aging Study. J Urol 1994; 151:51–61.

23. Althof S. When an erection alone is not enough: biopsychosocial obstacles to lovemaking. Int J Impotence Res 2002; 14(suppl 1):S99–S104. Nature Publishing Group 2002.

24. Keller MB et al. A comparison of nefazodone, the cognitive-behavioral analysis system of psychotherapy, and their combination for the treatment of chronic depression. New Engl J Med 2000; 342:1462–1470.

25. Seligman MEP. The effectiveness of psychotherapy: the Consumer Reports study. Am Psychol 1995; 50:965–974.

26. Nathan PE, Gorman JM. A guide to treatments that work. New York: Oxford University Press, 1998.

27. AUA BPH Guidelines Panel. The Management of Benign Prostatic Hyperplasia, American Urological Association Education and Research, Inc. Washington, DC, 2003.

28a. Turner LA, Althof SE, Levine SB, Risen CB, Bodner DR, Cursh ED, Resnick MI. Self-injection of papaverine and phentolamine in the treatment of psychogenic impotence. J Sex Marital Therapy 1989; 15:163–170.

28b. Kaplan HS. The combined use of sex therapy and intra-penile injections in the treatment of impotence. J Sex Marital Therapy 1990; 16:4.

29. Hartmann U, Langer D. Combination of psychosexual therapy and intra-penile injections in the treatment of erectile dysfunctions: rationale and predictors of outcome. J Sex Education Therapy 1993; 19:1–12.

30. Colson MH. Intracavernous injections and overall treatment of erectile disorders: a retrospective study. Sexologies 1996; 5.

31. Lottman PE, Hendriks JC, Vruggink PA, Meuleman EJ. The impact of marital satisfaction and psychological counselling on the outcome of ICI-treatment in men with ED. Int J Impot Res Jun 1998; 10(2):83–87.

32. Wylie KR, Hallam-Jones R, Walters S. The potential benefit of vacuum devices augmenting psychosexual therapy for erectile dysfunction: RCT. J Sex Marital Therapy 2003; 29(3).

33. McCarthy BW. Integrating sildenafil into cognitive-behavioral couple's sex therapy. J Sex Educ Ther 1998; 23:302–308.

34. Segraves RT. Case Report, two additional uses for sildenafil in psychiatric patients. J Sex Marital Therapy 1999; 25:265–266.

35. Perelman MA. Integrating sildenafil and sex therapy: unconsummated marriage secondary to ED and RE. J Sex Education Therapy 2001; 26:13–21.

36. Perelman MA. FSD partner issues: expanding sex therapy with sildenafil. J Sex Mar Ther 2002; 28(s):195–204.

37. Lieblum S, Pervin L, Cambell E. The treatment of vaginismus: success and failure. In: Leiblum SR, Rosen RC, eds. Principles and Practice of Sex Therapy: Update for the 1990s. New York: Guilford Press, 1989:113–140.

38. Hawton K. Integration of treatments for male erectile dysfunction. Lancet 1998; 351:728.
39. Rosen RC. Medical and psychological interventions for erectile dysfunction. Toward a combined treatment approach. In: Leiblum SR, Rosen RC, eds. Principles and Practice of Sex Therapy. 3rd ed. New York: Guildford Press, 2000.
40. Lue TF, Basson R, Rosen R et al (eds) Sexual medicine: sexual dysfunction in men and women. Health Publications, Paris, 2004.
41a. Perelman M, McMahon C, Barada J. Evaluation and treatment of ejaculatory disorders, in atlas of male sexual dysfunction [Ed: Lue, T.], Current Medicine, Inc., Philadelphia, Pennsylvania, 2004.
41b. Perelman MA. Retarded ejaculation. Current Sexual Health Reports, 2004: 95–101.
42. Goldstein I. The process of care model for evaluation and treatment of erectile dysfunction. Int J Impotence Res 1999; 11:59–74.
43. Nurmberg G. Treatment of antidepressant-associated sexual dysfunction with sildenafil. J Am Med Assoc 2003; 289:56–64.
44. Seidman SN, Roose SP, Menza MA, Shabsigh R, Rosen RC. Treatment of erectile dysfunction in men with depressive symptoms: results of a placebo-controlled trial with sildenafil citrate. Am J Psychiatry 2001; 158:1623–1630.
45. Balon et al. J Clin Psychiatry 1993; 54:209.
46. Physicians' Desk Reference 57, Edition 2003, Thomson PDR, Montvale, NJ, 2003.
47. Segraves RT, Croft H, Kavoussi R, Ascher JA. Bupropion sustained release (SR) for the treatment of hypoactive sexual desire disorder (HSDD) in nondepressed women. J Sex Marital Ther 2001; 27(3):303–316.
48. McCarthy B. Relapse prevention strategies and techniques with erectile dysfunction. J Sex Mar Ther 2001; 27(1):1–8.
49. Summer F et al. Which PDE-5 inhibitor do patients prefer? A comparator randomized multicenter study of sildenafil, tadalafil and vardenafil. Presented at 6th Congress of the European Society for Sexual Medicine, Istanbul, Turkey, 2003.
50. Perelman MA. Pharmaceutical choice and sexual script analysis. Br J Urol Inter 2005; In press.
51. Gagnon J, Rosen R, Leiblum S. Cognitive and social science aspects of sexual dysfunction: sexual scripts in therapy. J Sex Marital Therapy 1982; 8(1):44–56.
52. Barada JA. Successful Salvage of "Sildenafil (Sildenafil) Failures": Benefits of Patient Education and Re-Challenge with Sildenafil. Presented at the 4th Congress of the European Society for Sexual and Impotence Research, Sept. 30–Oct. 3, 2001, Rome, Italy.
53. Hatzichristou D. Sildenafil failures may be due to inadequate instructions and follow-up: a study of 100 non-responders. Int J Impotence Res 2001; 13:32.
54. Perelman MA. Pharmaceutical choice and sexual script analysis. Br J Urol Inter 2005; In press.
55. Albaugh J et al. Health care clinicians in sexual health medicine: focus on erectile dysfunction. Urologic Nursing 2002; 22(4).
56. Gittelman M. Personal communication, 2003.
57. Padma-Nathan H. Personal communication, 2003.

3

Female Hypoactive Sexual Desire Disorder

Rosemary Basson

UBC Departments of Psychiatry and Obstetrics & Gynaecology,
B.C. Centre for Sexual Medicine, Vancouver General Hospital,
Vancouver, BC, Canada

INTRODUCTION

The term "female hypoactive sexual desire disorder" clearly focuses on lack of sexual desire, as opposed to lack of interest or motivation (reasons/incentives), to be sexual. It encourages the belief that sexually healthy women agree to sex or initiate it mostly because they are aware of sexual desire—before any sexual stimulation begins. Indeed, this is in accordance with the traditional model of human sexual responding of Masters, Johnson, and Kaplan. In that model, after an unspecified time of awareness of desire, arousal occurs. As we will see, this conceptualization contradicts both clinical and empirical evidence—women in established relationships infrequently engage in sex for reasons of sexual desire (1–6). That sense of desire, or need, or "hunger" is nevertheless felt once subjectively aroused/excited. When that arousal is insufficient or not enjoyed, motivation to be sexual typically fades. In other words, although not usually the prime reason for engaging in sex, enjoyable subjective arousal is necessary to maintain the original motivation. So, lack of subjective arousal is key to women's complaints of disinterest in sex. However, their distress is typically presented in terms of "absent desire," as, again stemming from Masters and Johnson's model, the focus of arousal complaints has been on genital congestion rather than the subjective experience. This is despite the fact that psychophysiological studies of women with chronic arousal complaints show genital congestion in response to erotic videos that is comparable to healthy controls (see Chapter 6). This imprecision presents a major dilemma to both clinicians and the women requesting their help.

Any formulation of a hypoactive sexual desire/interest disorder must take into account the normative range of women's sexual desire across cultures (7), age, and life cycle stage (8). For instance, the postpartum period is normally sexually subdued (9). Desire for sex typically lessens with relationship duration and increases with a new partner (6).

Women's sexual enjoyment and desire for further sexual experiences were acknowledged early last century. Before that time, there had been variable denial or intolerance and endeavors to curb women's sexuality. Unfortunately, subsequent to that acknowledgement, came the assumption that women's sexual function mirrors men's experiences. Two particular aspects are fundamentally different. First, the majority of sexually healthy women do not routinely sense sexual desire before sexual stimulation begins; and second, women's sexual arousal is not simply a matter of genital vasocongestion. These misconceptions have led to:

1. the perception that as many as 30–40% of women in nationally representative community studies have abnormally low sexual desire (10–13);
2. current research to find a "desire" drug for women (14);
3. misunderstanding of women's viewpoint of lack of arousal (incorrectly assuming for the majority that genital congestion is impaired) (15);

Thus, lack of subjective arousal has been subsumed under "lack of desire." Women have great difficulty in distinguishing loss of desire/interest, from loss of arousal/pleasure/intensity of orgasm. The comorbidity of desire, arousal, and orgasm disorders is clear (16–24). The only published randomized controlled trial using physiological (or at least close to physiological) testosterone supplementation did not result in any increased "desire" as in having sexual thoughts, over and beyond placebo, but did show increased pleasure and orgasm intensity and frequency. Subjective arousal was not reported, but, given the improvement in pleasure and orgasmic experiences, its improvement is implied (25).

The objectives of this chapter include:

- To identify reasons women willingly initiate/agree to sex—with a view to understanding why some do not.
- To review a model of sexual response that permits motivations (reasons/incentives), for being sexual, over and beyond sexual desire.
- To clarify that it is the woman's arousability (along with the usefulness of sexual stimuli and context) that determines whether she will access sexual desire. In other words, for women, the concept of "responsive desire" or "desire accessed during the sexual experience" may be as or more important than initial desire as measured by sexual thoughts and sexual fantasies.
- To critique the traditional markers of sexual desire as they apply to women—and the questionable relevance of their lack.
- To outline the assessment of low desire and the associated low arousability, thereby identifying therapeutic options.
- To review what is known of the biological basis of women's sexual desire and arousability, including the role of androgens.
- To review psychotherapy, pharmacotherapy, and the biopsychosexual approach to the management of women's lack of sexual interest/desire.
- To make recommendations for clinical practice.

REASONS WOMEN INITIATE OR ACCEPT SEXUAL ACTIVITY WITH THEIR PARTNERS

Both the literature and clinical experience attest to the large number of reasons that sexually motivate women (1–6). Many of these are to do with enhancing emotional intimacy with the partner (2,5,6). Further reasons include increasing the woman's sense of well being, of attractiveness, womanliness—even to feel more normal (26). Simply wanting to share something of herself that is very precious, to sense her partner as sexually attractive (be it his/her strength and power, or ability to be tender/considerate—or both), are further reasons. Incentives that might superficially appear unhealthy are also common, for example, to placate a needy (and increasingly irritable) partner (26), or "do one's duty." When the experience proves rewarding for the woman such that part way through she herself starts to feel—that she, too, would not wish to stop—it becomes unclear whether the original reasons (to placate/do one's duty) are truly unhealthy. The concept of "rewards" or "spin offs" from being sexual is currently being empirically researched.

MODEL OF SEXUAL RESPONSE SHOWING VARIOUS INCENTIVES AND MOTIVATIONS TO BE SEXUAL AND AROUSAL TRIGGERING AND ACCOMPANYING DESIRE

For one or more of the earlier mentioned reasons, a woman choosing to be receptive to sexual stimuli (or to provide them) can subsequently become sexually aroused. The degree of emotional intimacy with her partner that may have even been the major motivating force, is also a very important influence on her arousability to the sexual stimuli. Various other psychological and biological factors will influence this arousability such that the processing of the sexual information in her mind may or may not lead to subjective arousal (27–31). On those occasions she becomes subjectively aroused, providing the arousal remains enjoyable, and the stimulation continues sufficiently long, and she remains focused, then the arousal can become more intense and an urge or "sexual desire" for more of the sexual sensations and emotions is triggered. This accessed or "triggered" sexual desire and the subjective arousal continue together, each reinforcing the other (32,33). A positive outcome, emotionally and physically, increases the woman's motivation to be sexual again in the future (32). (Fig. 3.1).

Sexual desire that appears to be innate or spontaneous and reflected by sexual thoughts/fantasies, awareness of wanting sexual sensations *per se* before any activity actually begins, may or may not augment or sometimes override the previously described cycle (Fig. 3.2). Typically, women are more aware of this type of initial desire early on in their relationships (6). For some women, it continues for decades even with the same partner. But for the majority, it is infrequent (1,3–5).

Some would argue that there is no such thing as apparent innate or spontaneous desire (26). This presupposes that desire is always part of arousal, triggered by a stimulus with a sexual meaning. It is facilitated or inhibited by situational and partner variables, such that sexual motivation will occur only when appropriate sexual stimuli are present and the woman has a sufficiently

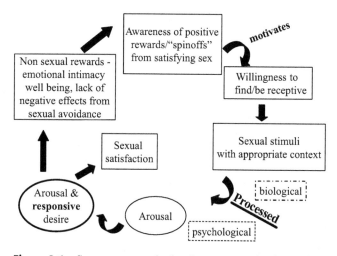

Figure 3.1 Sex response cycle showing many motivations to be sexual, and responsive/ triggered desire. A positive outcome emotionally and physically allows sexual satisfaction (goal set enroute) plus other rewards that motivated initially. Reprinted from Obstet Gynecol 2001; 98:350–353. Basson, with permission from the American College of Obstetricians and Gynecologists.

sensitive sexual response system. The assumption is that the occurrence of sexual motivation, including fantasies, must be the result of sexual information processing of some kind even though in some, or even most cases, the initiating sexual stimulus may not be known. For most people, their sexual response system reacts

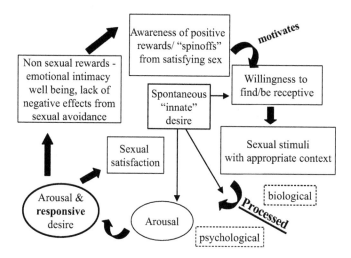

Figure 3.2 Blended sex response cycle: "spontaneous" desire augments or overshadows other motivations and increases arousability. Reprinted from Obstet Gynecol 2001; 98:350–353. Basson, with permission from the American College of Obstetricians and Gynecologists.

with the stimuli in an automatic effortless manner. Thus, sexual desire is sometimes experienced "as if" it were spontaneous (27).

SEXUAL AROUSABLITY

Given the importance of responsive desire as well as any initial desire, when addressing the subject of hypoactive desire disorder, the entity of women's arousability becomes extremely important. Psychological, contextual, and biological factors influence the processing of stimuli in the woman's mind. Psychological factors include those from the past to do with her upbringing particularly any losses, traumas (physical, sexual, emotional), her past interpersonal relationship—both sexual and nonsexual, encompassing cultural and religious attitudes especially restrictions (17,31,34–36). Contextual factors include any current interpersonal difficulties, partner sexual dysfunction, inadequate stimulation, and unsatisfactory sexual and emotional contexts (37–41). Medical conditions, psychiatric conditions, medications, substance abuse may all affect her arousability also (42–45).

TRADITIONAL MARKERS OF SEXUAL DESIRE

Evidence from nationally representative community samples of midlife women confirms that spontaneous sexual thinking is rather infrequent in the majority of sexually healthy women in long-term relationships (38,46,47).

Fantasies, which are a marker of sexual desire in DSM-IV-TR may, in fact, serve as a deliberate means of creating arousal and reinforcing desire. Data confirm the clinical experience that women fantasize to deliberately focus on their sexual feelings and avoid the distractions that are interfering with their sexual response (47).

Awareness of sexual desire is not the most frequent reason women accept or initiate sexual activity (1–6).

ASSESSMENT OF LOW DESIRE/INTEREST AND THE ASSOCIATED LOW AROUSABILITY TO IDENTIFY THERAPEUTIC OPTIONS

The DSM-IV-TR definition of hypoactive sexual desire disorder is problematic because its only focus is on initial desire, does not acknowledge the many reasons that motivate the woman towards sexual activity, and ignores the broad range of frequency of fantasies among sexually healthy women. An international group has recently proposed the following definition for women's sexual interest/desire disorder

> There are absent or diminished feelings of sexual interest or desire, absent sexual thoughts or fantasies and a lack of responsive desire. Motivations (here defined as reasons/incentives), for attempting to

become sexually aroused are scarce or absent. The lack of interest is considered to be beyond a normative lessening with lifecycle and relationship duration (48).

Note that it is the additional lack of responsive desire that indicates dysfunction. The word "interest" was preferred (to "desire") given the aforementioned relative infrequency of desire being the reason/incentive for engaging in sexual activity. However, for practical purposes of literature review, both words were included in the definition.

There is no clear division between assessment and management of desire/interest concerns. The assessment often makes it clear why motivation is lacking, what is amiss with the context, what may be negatively influencing her arousability, and what is unsatisfactory about the outcome. The assessment is biopsychosocial as well as sexual and is aimed at identifying predisposing, precipitating, and maintaining etiological factors. Given the women's sexuality is so contextual and given the known importance of partner factors including emotional intimacy (39,46), and sexual well being of the partner (37,39,49,50), there is need to interview both partners. Ideally, the couple is seen together as well as separately.

The current and past context—biological, psychosocial, as well as sexual—is clarified along with contextual details at the time of onset of the difficulties. The full picture of the woman's sexual response and her partner's response is obtained and importantly the degree of resulting distress is clarified. Predisposing factors are essentially intrapersonal—psychological factors that impair her arousability such as a fear of being vulnerable, guilt or shame regarding sex, past negative sexual experiences, distractions while trying to be sexually responsive, and excessive need for control. Recent careful assessment of consecutive women with low desire found significant disturbance in emotional stability and self-esteem (17). These researchers emphasized how low desire cannot be thought of as a discrete phase disorder. Rather, the evidence is that there is a generalized muting of the sexual response, together with mood instability and fragile self-regulation. Of biological factors reducing arousability, fatigue is perhaps the most common. Although, typically, there may be no definite mood disorder at the onset, women with low desire have a higher lifetime prevalence of depression (17,51,52) and clinical anxiety states (52). Recent studies suggest ~50% of women with depression, experience low desire and arousal, even taking into account the potential lowering of desire from antidepressant medication (45). Debility from chronic disease such as renal failure, medications including most antidepressants, chronic pain, and less commonly, hyperprolactinemia and hypothyroid states are further inhibitors of arousability. The importance of the role of low androgen activity in reducing arousability in some young women with sudden loss of ovarian androgen and in women with pituitary disease where testosterone levels are suddenly reduced, appears secure. However, minimal scientific study exists on the role of low androgen simply in relation to age and natural menopause and will be addressed in detail later.

A hypothesis that women, and men, have a variable proneness to sexual excitement as well as a variable inhibition, is currently being scrutinized (53). This variability may or may not be genetically programmed. Early results suggest that women are more prone to inhibition than men, and this inhibition is more to do with negative consequences of activity, than fear of performance failure. Theoretically, women with higher inhibition proneness are more vulnerable to low desire/interest, whereas high-risk sexual behaviors may be a reflection of low proneness to inhibition.

Lack of appropriate sexual context and sexual stimulation is a frequent precipitating and maintaining cause of low interest/desire. Common examples include too little nongenital caressing and lack of privacy or safety. Interpersonal issues can be both precipitating and maintaining, particularly when there is minimal emotional intimacy with the partner. Expectation of a negative outcome, for example, from dyspareunia or partner dysfunction is a further potent precipitating and/or maintaining factor. Clearly, a number of factors usually contribute. Occasionally, women with an emotionally traumatic past tell of sexual interest only when there is minimal emotional closeness with the partner in question. In other words, there is inability to sustain that interest/desire when emotional intimacy with the partner develops. This is, therefore, a fear of intimacy—not strictly a sexual dysfunction.

A CLOSER LOOK AT THE BIOLOGICAL BASIS OF WOMEN'S SEXUAL DESIRE AND AROUSABILITY INCLUDING THE ROLE OF ANDROGENS

The neuroendocrine basis of sexual desire/interest is poorly understood. The effects on sexuality of medications with known or partially known mechanisms of action suggest that more than 30 neurotransmitters, peptides, and hormones are involved in the sexual response. Currently, the most clinically important include noradrenaline, dopamine, oxytocin, and serotonin via 5HT1A and 5HT2C receptors—all considered to be prosexual. Serotonin acting via most 5HT receptor sites, prolactin, and GABA, are considered sexually negative. The role of dopamine has been investigated particularly in rodents. Dopaminergic input from the ventral tegmental area, particularly to the nucleus accumbens and forebrain is important for cognitive and reward processes. Dopamine administration into the nuclear accumbens has been found to stimulate the anticipatory phase (or appetitive phase) of a sexual activity (54). The paraventricular nucleus and the medial preoptic area of the hypothalamus regulate the anticipatory/motivational phases of rat copulation as well as the physiological changes of genital engorgement. Introducing a male hamster increases the dopamine in the nucleus accumbens in the female hamster along with her increased sexual activity. Even in animals, the effects of experience can be seen—there is more dopamine accumulation and for a longer time period in female hamsters that are sexually experienced than in those who are sexually naïve (55). In oophorized female hamsters, progesterone administration after estrogen priming leads to increased numbers of sex hormone receptors in the medial preoptic area. Interestingly, dopamine administration has the same effect as does environmental change—namely the presence of a male hamster.

Brain imaging of women during sexual arousal shows activation of areas involved in cognitive appraisal of the stimuli, namely the orbital frontal and anterior cingulate areas, and other areas involved in the emotional response to arousal including the rostral anterior cingulate (56). The latter and the posterior hypothalamus also imaged, are involved in the organization and perception of genital reflexes. Of interest, areas in the basal ganglia and temporal lobes that had shown activity in the nonsexually aroused state are no longer imaged during arousal, suggesting that they are involved in tonic inhibition.

Hormones can be measured during the sexual response, but these findings may reflect the consequence of sexual response rather than cause (e.g., oxytocin increases with arousal and prolactin increases after orgasm).

Estrogen is known to affect mood and sleep and so its central action may indirectly influence sexual response. That postmenopausal estrogen therapy causes improvement in well being, sleep, and vasomotor symptoms, is evidence based (5), but there are few scientific data to suggest that sexual benefit is afforded by relief of these particular symptoms. The role of androgen in women's sexual desire and arousability is currently under investigation. Although there is consensus that androgens are needed for sexual response, scientific study of androgen therapy with physiological amounts of androgen is only just beginning. It is also unclear whether the aromatization of testosterone to estradiol within the cell is essential, or whether instead or in addition, activation of the androgen receptor is essential. Areas of high density androgen receptors in women's brains also have high aromatase activity. Thus, the whole question of whether any benefit of testosterone administration to women is actually due to making estrogen more available (by decreasing SHBG) remains unsolved. The major androgens include the proandrogens, dehydroepiandrosterone sulfate (DHEAS), dehydroepiandrosterone (DHEA), androstenedione, plus testosterone (T), and dehydrotestosterone (DHT). Output of adrenal androgen decreases from the early 30s onwards. Ovarian androstenedione is consistently reduced in mid- and later life. Studies are less conclusive regarding ovarian T production after natural menopause, with evidence of both reduced and increased production (58,59). Two recent small studies have shown a gradual decrease of T in women through their 40s with loss of mid-cycle peaks of T and androstenedione (60,61). Studies across the menopause transition show either a minimal decrease or even an increase (62–64). Despite further reduction in adrenal androgen, in some women there may be increased production of ovarian T through the next two decades (59,62). On the other hand, some women show very low levels of ovarian production given the T levels in a large group of older women, after natural or surgical menopause were similar. Both of these groups of women were receiving estrogen therapy (58).

Cross-sectional and cohort studies of sexual response and T values are inconclusive. Either there is no correlation between T levels and sexual variables (65) correlation with estradiol levels but not T (63), or a correlation of free-T with levels of sexual desire (66). There have been several short-term randomized controlled studies of T administration to women complaining of diminished sexual interest and satisfaction. An improved outcome has been found by most but not all of these trials, but the T levels produced were not clearly within the physiological range. The study with levels closest to the physiological (25) was of oophorized women, and showed benefit only in older women receiving 300 μg/day of transdermal T, with corresponding blood levels at or slightly above the normal range for premenopausal women. Of note, the correct range for postmenopausal women is unclear. A very recent study of T administration to premenopausal women did show benefit over placebo, but the free androgen index was above the upper limit for normal premenopausal women (67). Of major importance is the fact that these studies have been only of short duration, and, therefore, safety data are very limited. Moreover, only estrogen replete women have been studied.

Despite documented progressive loss of DHEA and DHEAS in women from late 30s onwards, the results of DHEA supplementation to improve sexual health have been conflicting (68–72).

The term androgen deficiency syndrome has been used recently (73). However, the usual criteria used in endocrinology for establishment of a deficiency state have not been met. These include:

1. Symptoms regularly associated with low levels of the hormone;
2. Relationship of symptoms to the established biological actions of the hormone;
3. Reversal of symptoms on administration of the hormone in doses which are physiological and not pharmacological.

None of these criteria is fully met in the case of "androgen deficiency syndrome" (74). In addition, a specific level of testosterone in women, which can be considered diagnostic of androgen deficiency, has not been established.

Some of this confusion may be in part owing to problems in measuring T, including a lack of assay specificity. Free-T is preferably measured by equilibrium dialysis, but this is rarely available in clinical practice. Free-T correlates more closely with the biological effects of the hormone than does the total because most of the circulating T is bound to SHBG which prevents diffusion into tissues. Unfortunately, the analogue assays for free-T are inaccurate. Free-T can be calculated if the total T, albumin, and SHBG are known. However, at the low levels of T found in women, few assays of total T are reliable. Whichever assay is used, thorough validation is necessary. Another major complicating factor is that much T activity within the cell is derived intracellularly from ovarian adrenal precursors (75). This intracellular T cannot be measured. Estimating T activity from measuring testosterone metabolites is not yet standardized.

There is clearly a clinical dilemma. Clinicians repeatedly see previously responsive women markedly distressed from their lost arousability—none of their formerly useful stimuli are effective. Typically, this is of gradual onset in the late 40s or early 50s. Loss of innate sexual thoughts and fantasies is not the issue. The context of their sexual lives has not changed—they speak of a sexual "deadness". Accurate measurements of T activity and long-term randomized controlled trials of physiological T therapy are very much needed. Clearly, this loss of arousability appertains to just a subgroup of mid-life women— perhaps partially explaining the inconsistencies amongst reports of T levels of women in mid-life and older in the general population.

The free-T can be reduced by $\sim$50% by many oral contraceptive pills and by administration of glucocorticoids (76). There has been little research in these areas that is helpful to clinicians.

The risks of T administration include those that are familiar, for example, greater sebum production, acne, loss of scalp hair, stimulation of facial and other body hair, as well as other potential risks including metabolic dysfunction in some women. This is based on the fact that although in the condition of polycystic ovarian syndrome, it appears that hyperinsulinemia is usually the cause of the hyperandrogenism, there are some reports of situations in which hyperandrogenism causes insulin resistance (77). There is also a risk that other concerns will come to light if women are given testosterone when estrogen deficient, in view of the recent withdrawal of large numbers of women from estrogen therapy owing to the results of the women's health initiative study (78).

MANAGEMENT OF LOW DESIRE/INTEREST: PSYCHOLOGICAL, PHARMACOLOGICAL, AND BIOPSYCHOSOCIAL APPROACH

Psychological Treatments

Psychological therapy is the mainstay of the management of low sexual desire/ interest. Given the mandatory blending of mind and body, making deliberate changes in thoughts, attitudes behavior, leads not only to changed feelings and emotions but altered sexual physiology. Under the term "sex therapy" typically the woman's negative thoughts and attitudes to sex, her distractions during sexual stimulation, the need for more varied, more prolonged, or simply different sexual stimuli, the need for the couple to guide each other; and the usual needs of safety, privacy, and optimal timing of sexual interaction will be addressed. Sensate focus techniques whereby there is a graded transition from touching and caressing that is not specifically sexual to that which is sensual to that which is frankly sexual, may sometimes be included. The approach is one of systematic desensitization common to other behavioral therapies. Cognitive behavioral therapy (CBT) focuses on the restructuring of myths or distorted thinking about sex. Couple therapy may be necessary focusing on interpersonal issues including trust, respect, as well as ways to relate to each other, which foster sexual attraction. Psychodynamic therapy is often recommended to address issues in the woman's past developmental period. Particular attention to family of origin and relationships to parental figures is often needed. A further component is that of systemic therapy/sexual differentiation, that is, the ability to balance desire for contact with the partner vs. desire for uniqueness as an individual. Schnarch (79) suggests that this is extremely important for healthy sexual desire.

In directing the types of interventions, construction of the woman's sex response cycle will clarify the breaks or the sites of weakness (80). When emotional intimacy with the partner is minimal such that motivation and arousability are negatively affected, the couple is advised to receive relationship counseling before or possibly instead of any sex therapy. When problems are due to lack of effective stimuli, contexts, negative thoughts, and attitudes about sex, or nonsexual distractions are present, a combination of CBT and sex therapy is usually given. Similarly, explanation, CBT, and sex therapy can be given when the main issue seems to be expectation of an inevitably negative outcome.

Recent outcome studies include one in 2001 of 74 couples randomized to 12 weeks of CBT or an untreated control group (81). Of the women receiving CBT who met the criteria of hypoactive sexual desire pretreatment, 26% continued to do so at the end of treatment and 36% met the criteria 1 year later. The CBT group experienced significant improvements in sexual satisfaction, perception of sexual arousal, dyadic adjustment, improved self-repertoire, sexual pleasure, and perceived self-esteem, as well as general increase in motivation, mood, and lessening of anxiety. In a noncontrolled study of the same year (82), CBT was assessed in 54 women having a broad spectrum of sexual dysfunction. Fifty-four percent of the women still had the same sexual complaints after treatment, although the overall levels of sexual dysfunction were reduced and there were more positive attitudes towards sex and increased sexual enjoyment and less perception of being a sexual failure. A study of 39 women with low desire in 1993 (83) randomized one group of women to receive standard interventions of sex therapy vs. a group also receiving specific orgasm consistency training. Although both groups improved, benefit was greater in those in the combined group, particularly regarding arousal. A larger study in 1997 of CBT in 365 couples with a range of sexual dysfunction, showed 70% of women improved at 1-year after treatment (84).

Studies have identified factors associated with better prognosis. Those factors include the overall quality of a couple's nonsexual relationship (85), the couple's motivation to enter treatment (86,87), the degree of physical attraction between the partners (85), an absence of major psychiatric disorder (88), attention to systemic issues in the relationship (89), the male partner's motivation to obtain a successful outcome to therapy (90), and the amount of sensate focus experiences the couple complete in their last week of therapy (84).

However, benefit from psychological treatment is to some degree unclear because the outcome measures used reflect male sexual desire but show a broad normative range across sexually healthy women. In addition, subjective arousal and excitement is rarely addressed despite the data confirming its major importance relative to genital congestion, and its close blending with desire.

Nonhormonal Pharmacological Treatment of Low Desire/Interest

The place of pharmacological management for women's complaints of low desire/interest is undecided. This is because of broad normative range of women's appreciation of sexual desire, especially in the long-term relationship; and because of the importance of women's subjective arousal in influencing and triggering their desire and the minimal focus until now on the whole entity of subjective arousal. Thus, the appropriate outcome criteria for a "desire drug" are unclear. Studies with bupropion hydrochloride have suggested benefit over placebo. Of 30 women with active drug, 19 improved during a 12-week double blind placebo-controlled study for nondepressed women having a spectrum of sexual complaints, including low desire/interest (91). A more recent study, again of nondepressed women, this time diagnosed with hypoactive sexual desire, were treated in a single blinded manner and 29% responded to the active drug and none had responded to the initial 4-week placebo phase (14). The entity of sexual interest as well as sexual desire was monitored and shown to improve. Despite these two studies, the clinical experience is of limited benefit from this intervention. Larger placebo-controlled randomized studies of bupropion or other molecules that alter the neurotransmitters known to influence desire and arousability, including dopamine, serotonin, and noradrenaline, are needed.

Hormonal Treatment

Testosterone

Long-term data for safety and benefit of testosterone therapy in women are lacking, but such data are required before long-term use of testosterone can be recommended. Similarly, safety data for the use of testosterone in nonestrogen replaced postmenopausal women are lacking and no recommendation for its use can be made currently. Nor can the supplementation of T to premenopausal women be recommended until such time there exist safety and efficacy data. Unfortunately, any enduring benefit after short-term treatment, although theoretically possible, is unproven. In addition, supplementing T on a temporary basis only, could have adverse effects on the couple if an improvement associated with T therapy is no longer apparent when it is withdrawn.

If despite the above, T supplementation is contemplated, careful assessment must establish absence of ongoing psychological (interpersonal, intrapersonal, contextual, and societal) and/or physical factors negatively affecting sexual interest and arousability. On the basis of available data, no specific testosterone regimen or dose can yet be recommended. The chosen formulation of testosterone must have pharmacokinetic data indicating that it produces blood levels within the normal premenopausal range. Achieving physiological free testosterone levels by transdermal delivery appears to be the best approach.

Contraindications to testosterone therapy include androgenic alopecia, seborrhea, or acne, hirsutism as well as a history of polycystic ovary syndrome, and estrogen depletion. Oral methyl testosterone therapy is contraindicated in women with hyperlipidemia or liver dysfunction. Regular follow up is both clinical—inspection of skin and hair for seborrhea, acne, hirsutism, and alopecia—and biochemical through monitoring of free/bioavailable testosterone and SHBG, keeping these values within the normal range for premenopausal women. Of note, methyl-T is not included in the usual assays for T. Possibly, the target level for older women should be even lower but this remains unclear. Lipid profile and glucose tolerance are also monitored. The current recommendation is to prescribe only for 12 months owing to lack of long-term safety data (92).

Tibolone

Tibolone is a synthetic steroid with tissue selective estrogenic, progestogenic, and androgenic actions. In use in Europe for more than 10 years, tibolone provides some relief from vasomotor symptoms (93), estrogen agonist activity on the vagina (94) and bone (95), but not on the endometrium (96). Tibilone was thought not to have estrogen agonist activity on breast tissue; but a recent, albeit nonrandomized but very large study of postmenopausal hormonal therapy showed a similar increase in breast cancer in women receiving tibolone and those receiving various combinations of estrogen and progestins (97). The typical (presumed beneficial) estrogenic effects on lipids are not seen (98), but it is of note that tibolone does not promote (unwanted) coagulation (96). Prospective randomized trials comparing tibolone to placebo or to various formulations of estrogen and progestin therapy have been done. Although in most (99–101) but not all (102), there was significant improvement in sexual desire/interest in the women receiving tibolone; no study focused on sexually dysfunctional women. Recruitment centered on vasomotor symptoms or bone density. Studies in postmenopausal women with loss of arousability and therefore of sexual interest are needed.

A Biopsychosocial Approach to Therapy

There is a general expectation that modulation of the neurotransmitters involved in sexual arousability and desire from hormonal and nonhormonal therapy, will become available. As there are psychological and interpersonal sequelae of medical disruption of the sexual response, benefit beyond placebo may only be seen if a holistic biopsychosexual treatment approach is used. For instance, loss of arousability and desire in breast cancer survivors is strongly linked to ovarian failure induced by chemotherapy (103). These women report that their former means of sexual stimulation to arousal are no longer effective. Couples describe how local (vaginal) nonsystemic estrogen can allow painless but rather perfunctory intercourse. Most need encouragement to bring back their former sexual contexts and stimuli that were discarded once they no longer worked. Usually, the partner needs to be heard regarding his/her feelings of rejection. Both partners need information on the role of ovarian hormones. Partial replacement of the woman's lost ovarian androgens, rarely helps on its own.

RECOMMENDATIONS FOR CLINICAL PRACTICE

- Assessment needs to be biopsychosocial, as well sexual (Table 3.1).
- Consider predisposing, precipitating, and maintaining factors.
- Endeavor to see the couple together and separately.
- Create a model of the woman's sexual response cycle showing the various breaks or areas of weakness.
- Interpersonal issues need to be addressed first.
- When abuse is elicited in the history, determine whether recovery has taken place. When this is not complete, defer addressing sexual issues and make appropriate referral.
- When negative outcome needs specific treatment (e.g., chronic dyspareunia), address that in parallel with addressing the low desire. Meanwhile, normalize and encourage nonpenetrative sex.
- Psychological therapies are the mainstay of treatment and include sex therapy, sensate focus therapy, CBT, psychodynamic treatment, couple treatment, and promotion of the individual as a separate self.
- There are no firm nonhormonal pharmacological recommendations at this time. However, clinical experience and a recent study (104) suggest increased arousability to sexual cues from administering bupropion to nondepressed women diagnosed with hypoactive sexual desire/ interest, again in keeping with the lowering of desire if arousability is impaired.
- When arousability and accessed desire sharply declines in conjunction with a known cause of reduction of androgens (e.g., younger premenopausal women with loss of all ovarian function), consider investigational testosterone therapy using a formulation that produces physiological as opposed to pharmacological levels. Hopefully, there will be such formulation in the near future.
- Remember safety data regarding T treatment are only short-term and only for the estrogen replete woman. There are no data on T supplementation to premenopausal women whereby the achieved androgen levels have been strictly physiological.

Table 3.1 Components of a Comprehensive Sexual, Medical, and Psychosocial History

	Biological	Psychosocial	Sexual
Symptoms	Current general health	Current mood, mental health	The sexual difficulties in her own words
Present context (precipitating/maintaining)	Medications/substance abuse, fatigue, presence of nonsexual pain	Nature and duration of current relationship. Societal values/beliefs impacting the sexual problems	Context when activity is attempted—type of sexual stimulation, the woman's feelings towards her partner, safety, and privacy
Past context (predisposing/precipitating)	Past medical history	Particularly for lifelong problems, developmental history, including relationships with caregivers, siblings, traumas, and losses	Past sexual experiences alone and partnered, wanted, coercive, abusive
Onset (precipitating)	Medical, psychiatric details at time of onset of sexual problems	Psychosocial circumstances including relationship at time of onset of sexual problems	Sexual details at onset of dysfunctions
Full picture of her current sexual response	Details regarding effects of medical condition on sexual activity, e.g., cardiac compromise	Personality factors including control issues, ability to express nonsexual emotions	Rest of the sexual response cycle including pain
Role of the partner (precipitating/maintaining)	Partner's medical health	Partner's mood and mental health, partner's reaction to sexual problems	Partner's sexual response cycle including pain
Distress	Level of distress regarding medical issues	Level of distress regarding psychosocial issues	Reaction to the sexual difficulties, level of distress

- Analogue assays for free-T are currently unreliable—but total T alone is insufficient owing to SHBG bound T being relatively unavailable to the tissues. Thus, modifying T formulations designed for men is fraught with difficulties due to lack of reliable laboratory monitoring.
- If and when hormonal and pharmacological treatments become available, a biopsychosocial approach to treatment will still be needed. Secondary dysfunctions, changed expectations, adaptations to the low arousability, and disinterest will have occurred. These may negate any potential benefit.

CONCLUSION

There are many reasons why women are sexual. A broad normative range in sexual desire exists between women and across life stages. The extreme importance of sexual arousability—used here to mean the factors influencing the mind's information processing of the sexual stimulation—directs the assessment and management of distress resulting from disinterest in sex. The subject is larger and more complex than a "hypoactive sexual desire disorder." Desire, as in sexual thoughts and fantasies is helpful, but is neither sufficient nor essential for on-going healthy sexual interest.

REFERENCES

1. Lunde I, Larson GK, Fog E, Garde K. Sexual desire, orgasm, and sexual fantasies: a study of 625 Danish women born in 1910, 1936 and 1958. J Sex Educ Ther 1991; 17:111–115.
2. Hill CA, Preston LK. Individual differences in the experience of sexual motivation: theory and measurement of dispositional sexual motives. J Sex Res 1996; 33(1):27–45.
3. Galyer KT, Conaglen HM, Hare A, Conaglen JV. The effect of gynecological surgery on sexual desire. J Sex Marital Ther 1999; 25:81–88.
4. Schultz WCM, van de Wiel HBM, Hahn DEE. Psychosexual functioning after treatment for gynecological cancer and integrated model, review of determinant factors and clinical guidelines. Int J Gynecol Cancer 1992; 2:281–290.
5. Regan P, Berscheid E. Belief about the state, goals and objects of sexual desire. J Sex Marital Ther 1996; 22:110–120.
6. Klusmann D. Sexual motivation and the duration of partnership. Arch Sex Behav 2002; 31(3):275–287.
7. Cain VS, Johannes CB, Avis NE, Mohr B, Schocken M, Skurnick J, Ory M. Sexual functioning and practices in a multi-ethnic study of midlife women: Baseline results from SWAN. J Sex Res 2003; 40(3):266–276.
8. Dennerstein L, Lehert P. Sexual functioning, mid age and menopause: a comparative study of 12 European countries. Menopause 2004; 11(6):778–785.
9. De Judicibus MA, McCabe MP. Psychological factors and the sexuality of pregnant and postpartum women. J Sex Res 2002; 39(2):94–103.

10. Laumann EL, Paik A, Rosen RC. Sexual dysfunction in United States: prevalence and predictors. J Am Med Assoc 1999; 10:537–545.
11. Fisher WA, Boroditsky R, Bridges M. Measures of sexual and reproductive health among Canadian women. Can J Human Sexuality 1999; 8(3):175–182.
12. Kontula O, Haavio-Mannila E. Sexual pleasures. Enhancement of sex life in Finland. Aldershot: Dartmouth, 1995:1971–1992.
13. Fugl-Meyer AR, Sjögren Fugl-Meyer K. Sexual disabilities, problems and satisfaction in 18 to 74-year-old Swedes. Scand J Sexol 1999; 2(2):79–105.
14. Segraves RT, Croft H, Kavoussi R, Ascher JA, Batey SR, Foster VJ, Bolden-Watson C, Metz A. Bupropion sustained release (SR) for the treatment of hypoactive sexual disorder (HSDD) in nondepressed women. J Sex Marital Ther 2001; 27:303–316.
15. Laan E, Everaerd W. Determinants of female sexual arousal: psychophysiological theorian data. Annu Rev Sex Res 1995; 6:32–76.
16. Sjögren Fugl-Meyer K, Fugl-Meyer AR. Sexual disabilities are not singularities. Int J Impot Res 2002; 14:487–493.
17. Hartmann U, Heiser K, Rüffer-Hesse C, Kloth G. Female sexual desire disorders: subtypes, classification, personality factors, a new direction for treatment. World J Urol 2002; 20:79–88.
18. Basson R, McInnes R, Smith MD, Hodgson G, Koppiker N. Efficacy and safety of sildenafil citrate in women with sexual dysfunction associated with female sexual arousal. Gend Based Med 2002; 11(4):367–377.
19. Cyranowski JM, Andersen BL. Schemas, sexuality, romantic attachment. J Personality Soc Psychol 1998; 74(5):1364–1379.
20. Derogatis LR, Schmidt CW, Fagan PJ, Wise TN. Subtypes of anorgasmia via mathematical taxonomy. Psychosomatics 1989; 30(2):166–173.
21. Segraves KB, Segraves RT. Hypoactive sexual desire disorder: prevalence and comorbidity in 906 subjects. J Sex Marital Ther 1991; 17(1):55–58.
22. Rosen RT, Taylor JF, Leiblum SR. Prevalence of sexual dysfunction in women: results of a survey study of 329 women in an outpatient gynecological clinic. J Sex Marital Ther 1993; 19:171–188.
23. Meston CM. Validation of the female sexual function index (FSFI) in women with female orgasmic disorder and in women with hypoactive sexual desire disorder. J Sex Marital Ther 2003; 29:39–46.
24. Trudel G, Ravart M, Matte B. The use of the multi axis diagnostic system for sexual dysfunctions in the assessment of hypoactive sexual desire. J Sex Marital Ther 1993; 19(2):123–130.
25. Shifren JL, Braunstein GD, Simon JA, Casson PR, Buster JE, Redmond GP, Burki RE, Ginsburg ES, Rosen RC, Leiblum SR, Caramelli KE, Mazer NA. Transdermal testosterone treatment in women with impaired sexual function after oophorectomy. N Engl J Med 2000; 7; 343(10):682–688.
26. Kadri N, McHichi Alami KH, Mchakra Tahiri S. Sexual dysfunction in women: population based epidemiological study. Arch Womens Ment Health 2002; 5(2):59–63.
27. Everaerd W, Laan E. Desire for passion: energetics of sexual response. J Sex Marital Ther 1995; 21:255–263.
28. Cyranowski JM, Andersen BL. Schemas, sexuality, romantic attachment. J Personality Soc Psychol 1998; 74(5):1364–1379.

29. Morokoff PJ, Heiman JR. Effects of erotic stimuli on sexually functional and dysfunctional women: multiple measures before and after sex therapy. Behav Res Ther 1980; 18:127–137.

30. Beck JG, Bozman AW. Gender differences in sexual desire: the effects of anger and anxiety. Arch Sex Behav 1995; 24(6):595–612.

31. Katz RC, Gipson MT, Turner S. Brief report: recent findings on the sexual aversion scale. J Sex Marital Ther 1992; 18(2):141–146.

32. Basson R. Rethinking low sexual desire in women. Br J Obstet Gynaecol 2002; 109:357–363.

33. Levin RJ. Sexual desire and the deconstruction and reconstruction of the human female sexual response model of Masters and Johnson. In: Everaerd W, Laan, Both S, eds. Sexual Appetite, Desire and Motivation: Energetics of the Sexual System. Amsterdam: The Royal Netherlands Academy of Arts and Sciences, 2000.

34. Ernst C, Földényi M, Angst J. The Zurich study: sexual dysfunctions and disturbances in young adults. Eur Arch Psychiatry Clin Neurosci 1993; 243:179–188.

35. Öberg K, Fugl-Meyer KS, Fugl-Meyer AR. On sexual well being in sexually abused Swedish women: epidemiological aspects. Sex Relationship Ther 2002; 17(4):229–341.

36. Mackay J. Global sex: Sexuality and sexual practices around the world. Sex Relationship Ther 2001; 16(1):71–82.

37. Sjögren Fugl-Meyer K, Fugl-Meyer AR. Sexual disabilities are not singularities. Int J Impot Res 2002; 14:487–493.

38. Cawood HH, Bancroft J. Steroid hormones, menopause, sexually and well being of women. Psychophysiol Med 1996; 26:925–936.

39. Dennerstein L, Lehert P, Burger H, Dudley E. Factors affecting sexual functioning of women in the midlife years. Climacteric 1999; 2:254–262.

40. Hill, CA. Gender, relationship stage, and sexual behaviour: the importance of partner emotional investment within specific situations. J Sex Res 2002; 39(3):228–240.

41. Fugl-Meyer AR, Sjögren Fugl-Meyer K. Sexual disabilities, problems and satisfaction in 18 to 74-year-old Swedes. Scand J Sexol 1999; 2(2):79–105.

42. Sipski M, Rosen R, Alexander CJ et al. Sildenafil effects on sexual and cardiovascular responses in women with spinal cord injury. Urology 2000; 55:812–815.

43. van Lankveld JJDM, Grotjohann Y. Psychiatric comorbidity in heterosexual couples with sexual dysfunction assessed with the composite international diagnostic interview. Arch Sex Behav 2000; 29:479–498.

44. Kristensen E. Sexual side effects induced by psychotropic drugs. Dan Med Bull 2002; 49:349–352.

45. Kennedy SH, Dickens SE, Eisfeld BS, Bagby RM. Sexual dysfunction before antidepressant therapy in major depression. J Affect Disord 1999; 56:201–208.

46. Bancroft J, Loftus J, Long JS. Distress about sex: a national survey of women in heterosexual relationships. Arch Sex Behav 2003; 32(3):193–204.

47. Garde K, Lunde I. Female sexual behaviour. The study in a random sample of 40-year-old women. Maturitas 1980; 2:225–240.

48. Basson R, Leiblum S, Brotto L, Derogatis L, Fourcroy J, Fugl-Myer K, Graziottin A, Heiman J, Laan E, Meston C, Schover L, van Lankveld J, Weijmar Schultz W. Definitions of women's sexual dysfunction reconsidered: advocating expansion and revision. J Psychosom Obstet Gynecol 2003; 24:221–229.

49. Fugl-Meyer KS. Erectile problems—the perspective of the female. Scand J Urol Nephrol 1998; 32(suppl 197):12.
50. Avis NE, Stellato R, Crawford S, Johannes C, Longcope C. Is there an association between menopause status and sexual functioning? Menopause 2000; 7:297–309.
51. Schreiner-Engel P, Schiavi RC. Lifetime psychopathology in individuals with low sexual desire. J Nerv Ment Dis 1986; 174:646–651.
52. Trudel G, Landry L, Larose Y. Low sexual desire: The role of anxiety, depression, and marital adjustment. Sex Mar Ther 1997; 12:109–113.
53. Bancroft J. The medicalization of female sexual dysfunction: the need for caution. Arch Sex Behav 2002; 31(5):451–455.
54. Pfaus JG, Phillips AG. Role of dopamine in anticipatory and consummatory aspects of sexual behavior in the male rat. Behav Neurosci 1991; 105(5):727–743.
55. Kohlert JG, Meisel RL. Sexual experience sensitizes mating related nucleus encumbens dopamine of responses of female Syrian hamsters. Behav Brain Res 1999; 99(1):45–52.
56. Karama S, Lecours AR, Leroux JN, Bourgouin P, Beaudoin G, Joubert S, Beauregard M. Areas of brain activation in males and females during viewing of erotic film excerpts. Human Brain Mapp 2002; 16:1–13.
57. Utian WH, Burrry KA, Archer DF, Gallagher JC, Boyett RL, Guy MP, Tachon GJ, Chadha-Boreham HK, Bouvet AA, The Esclim study group. Efficacy and safety of low, standard, and high dosages of an estradiol transdermal system (Esclim) compared with placebo on vasomotor symptoms in highly symptomatic menopausal patients. Am J Obstet Gynecol 1999; 181:71–79.
58. Davis S, Schneider H, Donarti-Sarti C, Rees M, Van Lunsen H, Bouchard C. Androgen levels in normal and oophorectomised women. Climacteric 2002; Proceeding of the 10th International Congress on the Menopause, Berlin.
59. Laughlin GA, Barrett-Connor E, Kritz-Silverstein D, von Muhlen D. Hysterectomy, oophorectomy and endogenous sex hormone levels in older women: the Rancho Bernardo Study. J Clin Endocrinol Metab 2000; 85(2):645–651.
60. Zumoff B, Strain GW, Miller LK, Rosner W. Twenty-four hour mean plasma testosterone concentration declines with age in normal premenopausal women. J Clin Endocrinol Metab 1995; 80:1429–1430.
61. Mushayandebvu T, Castracane VD, Gimpel T, Adel T, Santoro N. Evidence for diminished mid cycle ovarian androgen production in older reproductive aged women. Fertil Steril 1996; 65:721–723.
62. Jiroutek MR, Chen MH, Johnston CC, Longcope C. Changes in reproductive hormones in sex hormone binding globulin in a group of postmenopausal women measured over 10 years. Menopause 1998; 5:90–94.
63. Burger HG, Dudley EC, Dennerstein L, Hopper JL. A prospective longitudinal study of serum testosterone, dehydroepiandrosterone sulphate and sex hormone binding globulin levels through the menopause transition. J Clin Endocrinol Metab 2000; 85:283–288.
64. Judd HL. Hormonal dynamics associated with the menopause. Clin Obstet Gynecol 1976; 19:775.
65. Nathorst-Böös J, von Schoultz H. Psychological reactions and sexual life after hysterectomy with and without oophorectomy. Gynecol Obstet Invest 1992; 34:97–101.

66. Leiblum S, Bachmann G, Kemmann E. Vaginal atrophy in the postmenopausal woman: the importance of sexual activity and hormones. J Am Med Assoc 1983; 249:2195–2198.

67. Goldstadt R, Davis SR. Transdermal testosterone therapy improves well-being, mood and sexual function in pre-menopausal women. Menopause 2003; 10(5):390–398.

68. Arlt W, Callies F, Van Vlijmen JC, Koehler I, Reincke M, Bidlingmaier M, Huebler D, Oettel M, Ernst M, Schulte HM, Allolio B. Dehydroepiandrosterone replacement in women with adrenal insufficiency. N Eng J Med 1999; 341(14):1013–1020.

69. Lovas K, Gebre-Medhin G, Trovik T, Fougner K, Uhlving S, Nedrobo B et al. Replacement of dehydroepiandrosterone in adrenal failure: no benefit for subjective health status and sexuality in a 9-month randomized parallel group clinical trial. J Clin Endocrinol Metab 2003; 88(3):1112–1118.

70. Hunt P, Gurnell E, Huppert F. Improvement in mood and fatigue after dehydroepiandrosterone replacement in Addison's disease in a randomized, double blind trial. J Clin Endocrinol Metab 2000; 85:4650–4656.

71. Barnhart K, Freeman E, Grisso JA, Rader DJ, Sammel M, Kapoor S, Nestler JE. The effect of dehydroepiandrosterone supplementation to symptomatic perimenopausal women on serum endocrine profiles, lipid parameters, and health-related quality of life. J Clin Endocrinol Metab 1999; 84(11):3896–3902.

72. Baulieu E, Thomas G, Legrain S, Roger M, Debuire B, Faucounau V. Dehydroepiandrosterone (DHEA), DHEA sulphate, and aging: contribution to the DHEAge study to a socio-biomedical issue. Proc Nat Acad Sci 2000; 97(8):4279–4284.

73. Bachmann G, Bancroft J, Braunstein G, Burger H, Davis S, Dennerstein L, Goldstein I, Guay A, Leiblum S, Lobo R, Notelovitz M, Rosen R, Sarrel P, Sherwin B, Simon J, Simpson E, Shifren J, Spark R, Traish A. Female androgen insufficiency: the Princeton consensus statement on definition, classification, and assessment. Fertil Steril 2000; 77(4):660–665.

74. Padero MCM, Bhasin S, Friedman TC. Androgen supplementation in older women: too much hype, not enough data. Am Geriatr Soc 2002; 50:1131–1140.

75. Labrie F, Belanger A, Cusan L, Candas B. Physiological changes in dehydroepiandrosterone are not reflected by serum levels of active androgens and estrogens but of their metabolites: Intracrinology. J Clin Endocrinol Metab 1997; 82(8):2403–2409.

76. Sanders SA, Graham CM, Bass J, Bancroft J. A prospective study of the effects of oral contraceptives on sexuality and well being and their relationship to discontinuation. Contraception 2001; 64:51–58.

77. Charmandari E, Weise M, Bornstein SR, Eisenhofer G, Keil MF, Chrousos GP, Merke DP. Children with classic congenital adrenal hyperplasia have elevated serum leptin concentrations and insulin resistance: potential clinical implications. J Clin Endocrinol Metab 2002; 87(5):2114–2120.

78. Rossouw JE, Anderson GL, Prentice RL, LaCroix AZ, Kooperberg C, Stefanick ML, Jackson RD, Beresford SA, Howard BV, Johnson KC, Kotchen JM, Ockene J. Risks and benefits of estrogen plus progestin in healthy postmenopausal women: principal results from the Women's Health Initiative randomized controlled trial. J Am Med Assoc 2002; 288(3):321–333.

79. Schnarch D. Desire problems: A systemic perspective. Principles and practice of sex therapy, New York: Guilford Press, 2000.

80. Basson RJ. Using a different model for female sexual response to address women's problematic low sexual desire. J Sex Marital Ther 2001; 27:395–403.
81. Trudel G, Marchand A, Ravart M, Aubin S, Turgeon L, Fortier P. The effect of a cognitive behavioral group treatment program on hypoactive sexual desire in women. Sex Rel Therapy 2001; 16:145–164.
82. McCabe MP. Evaluation of a cognitive behaviour therapy program for people with sexual dysfunction. J Sex Marital Ther 2001; 27:259–271.
83. Hurlbert DF. A comparative study using orgasm consistency training in the treatment of women reporting hypoactive sexual desire. J Sex Marital Ther 1993; 19:41–55.
84. Sarwer DB, Durlak JA. A field trial of the effectiveness of behavioral treatment for sexual dysfunctions. J Sex Marital Ther 1997; 23:87–97.
85. Hawton K, Catalan J. Prognostic factors in sex therapy. Behav Res Ther 1986; 24:377–385.
86. Whitehead A, Mathews A. Factors related to successful outcome in the treatment of sexually unresponsive women. Psychol Med 1986; 16:373–378.
87. Hawton K, Catalan J, Fagg J. Low sexual desire: sex therapy results and prognostic factors. Behav Res Ther 1991; 29:217–224.
88. Hawton K. Treatment of sexual dysfunctions by sex therapy and other approaches. Br J Psychiatry 1995; 167:307–314.
89. Besharat MA. Management strategies of sexual dysfunctions. J Contemp Psychother 2001; 31:161–180.
90. Hirst JF, Watson JP. Therapy for sexual and relationship problems: the effects on outcome of attending as an individual or as a couple. Sex Marital Ther 1997; 12:321–337.
91. Crenshaw TL, Goldbert JP, Stern WC. Pharmacologic modification of psychosexual dysfunction. J Sex Marital Ther 1987; 13:239–252.
92. Basson RJ, Weijmar Schultz W, Binik I, Brotto L, Echenbach D, Laan E, Redmond G, Utian W, van Lankveld J, Wesselmann U, Wyatt G, Wyatt L. Womens Sexual Desire and Arousal Disorders and Sexual Pain. In. Khouri S, Giuliano F, Rosen R, Lue T, Basson, eds. The 2nd International Consultation on Sexual Dysfunctions. Health Publications, Paris, 2004.
93. Ross LA, Alder EM. Tibolone and climacteric symptoms. Maturitas 1995; 21(2):127–136.
94. Rymer J, Chapman MG. Fogelman I, Wilson POG. A study of the effect of tibolone on the vagina in postmenopausal women. Maturitas 1994; 18:127–133.
95. Beardsworth SA, Kearney CE, Purdie DW. Prevention of postmenopausal bone loss at lumbar spine and upper femur with tibolone: a 2-year randomized controlled trial. Br J Obstet Gynecol 1999; 106(7):678–683.
96. Palacios S. Tibolone: what does tissue specific activity mean? Maturitas 2001; 37:159–165.
97. The Million Women Study Collaborators. Breast cancer and hormone replacement therapy in the million women study. Lancet 2003; 362:419–427.
98. Castelo-Branco C, Casals E, Figueras F. Two-year prospective and comparative study of the effects of tibolone on lipid pattern, behaviour of apolopoproteins A1 and B. Menopause 1999; 6(2):92–97.
99. Kökçü A, Cetinkaya MB, Yanik F, Alper T, Malatyalioğlu E. The comparison of effects of tibolone and conjugated estrogen medroxy progesterone acetate therapy on sexual performance in postmenopausal women. Maturitas 2000; 36:75–80.

100. Nathorst-Böös J, Hammar M. Effects on sexual life—a comparison between tibolone and a continuous estradiol—norethisterone acetate regimen. Maturitas 1997; 26:15–20.

101. Castelo-Branco C, Vicente JJ, Figueras F, Sanjuan A, Martinez de Osaba MJ, Casals E, Pons F, Balasch J, Vanrell JA. Comparative effects of estrogens plus androgens and tibolone on bone, lipid pattern and sexuality in postmenopausal women. Maturitas 2000; 34:161–168.

102. Mendoza N, Suárez AM, Álamo F, Bartual E, Vergara F, Herruzo A. Lipid effects, effectiveness and acceptability of tibolone vs. transdermic 17 β estradiol for hormonal replacement therapy in women with surgical menopause. Maturitas 2000; 37:37–43.

103. Ganz PA, Desmond KA, Belin TR, Neyerowitz BE, Rowland JH. Predictors of sexual health in women after a breast cancer diagnosis. J Clin Oncol 1999; 70:2371–2380.

104. Segraves RT. Buproprion sustained release for the treatment of hypoactive sexual desire disorder in premenopausal women. J Clin Psychopharmacol 2004; 24(3):339–342.

4

Male Hypoactive Sexual Desire Disorder

William L. Maurice

Department of Psychiatry,
University of British Columbia, Vancouver,
British Columbia, Canada

The problem is that God gives men a brain and a penis,
and only enough blood to run one at a time.

Robin Williams

Why are men interested in sexual contact?
I find sex . . . the desire to have sex . . . a nuisance.
I'd rather read a book or listen to music.

A Patient

SEXUAL DESIRE DIFFERENCES IN MEN AND WOMEN

Men (especially young men) are often perceived as being ready to be sexual with anyone, anytime, and anyplace. This viewpoint about men and sex is held not only by women, but by most men too (including Robin Williams). However, the ease with which a man's penis becomes erect is not necessarily an accurate barometer of what is taking place in his mind. The idea that a man may be much less interested in sex compared with other men may not make sense to many. In the argot of the times, such an idea represents a "disconnect"; it does not "compute."

The notion that men are controlled by their sexual longings is puzzling and mysterious to men who simply do not feel the same way. Likewise, partners find the experience of being with a perpetually sexually disinterested man to be not only confusing, but agonizing.

Case Study

Jim, 32 years old, and Rebecca (not their real names), 31 years old, were referred to a psychiatrist because of lack of sexual desire on Jim's part. They had been married for 5 years and did not have children. Actually, Rebecca initiated the referral through their family doctor. In tears, she told the doctor of her longing to have children and hearing the ticking of the biological clock. In the course of asking detailed fertility-related questions, the doctor discovered that intercourse was taking place only about once in 2 months. No other couple-related sexual activity occurred in the interval.

In retrospect, Rebecca had always been more sexually interested than Jim prior to their marriage, and in the early days, sexual frequency seemed not to be a problem. In accord with the psychiatrists' usual pattern of practice to see partners separately as part of an assessment, and in an effort to understand Jim's point of view, he saw Jim alone. The psychiatrist discovered in the process that Jim was in fact just as disinterested in sexual matters as his wife described. He had few thoughts about sexual issues, denied having sexual fantasies or dreams, masturbated rarely, and had never had any sexual experiences with other women (or men). Although Jim understood his wife's distress, he also thought that her sexual interest was excessive. With reluctance, Jim accepted the idea of referral to another psychiatrist who had a special interest in the care of people with sexual problems.

The idea of including separate chapters on sexual desire problems in men and women in this book is unusual. The editors evidently considered that such problems in the two gender groups were not identical. However, apart from disorders, is sexual desire itself different for men and women?

In what appears to have been an effort to redress an attitudinal imbalance in much of human history in which men were perceived to be much more sexual than women, Masters and Johnson (1) attempted to make the two genders sexually symmetrical. However, in the early part of the 21st century, attitudes towards sexuality in men and women seem to have evolved (at least in some parts of the world) so as to permit the idea that they may be sexually different without at the same time implying that one is superior to the other. Apart from social attitudes and in spite of some similar determinants, science and the clinical experience of health professionals who care for people with sexual difficulties suggest that there may be major differences in sexual desire for men and women.

Levine (2) has written extensively on the subject of sexual desire generally and although recognizing differences between men and women, has focussed particularly on underpinnings that are common to both. He theorized three components to sexual desire: drive, motivation, and wish. Levine defined *drive* as "the biological component that has an anatomy and neurophysiology," *motivation* as the psychological component that is influenced by such issues as personal mental states, for example, joy or sorrow, and interpersonal states such as mutual affection or disagreement, and *wish* as the cultural component that "reflects values, meanings, and rules about sexual expression that are inculcated in childhood and may be reconsidered throughout life." He further commented that "wishes are mediated through motivation."

In the late 20th century and early 21st, one of the major themes occupying sexuality professionals has been the sexuality of women generally, and women's sexual desire in particular. This focus on women has resulted in, paradoxically, clarification of how men are different from women, particularly in the area of sexual desire.

For example, a study of couples found that lesbian pairs engaged in sexual activity considerably less often than those who were either heterosexual or gay men (3). Explanations might include the notion that sexual events in heterosexual couples often seem to occur on the initiative of men and that men are obviously omitted from consideration in a lesbian twosome. One might therefore reason that a lower level of sexual activity in lesbian couples suggests that sexual desire in women is, from a quantitative viewpoint, less than that in men. Nichols (4) also looked at lesbian couples and not only observed that they "exhibit stereo-typical female sexual behavior" but also speculated about women being "wired" differently.

Tiefer (5) has persuasively argued that the sexual *concerns* of men and women are quite different and that women's sexual voices are largely absent from the classification system for sexual dysfunctions that is commonly used, namely, DSM-IV-TR (6). She incisively argues that there is nothing in the DSM system that is addressed to issues of, for example, emotion or communication, danger, commitment, attraction, sexual knowledge, respect, feelings about bodies, pregnancy, or contraception (p. 101). Moreover, she views the DSM system as "obsessively genitally focused," having a biological emphasis, and constructed in such a way as to reflect the sexuality of men (p. 97–102).

Examining the issue of women's sexual desire from a different perspective, Basson (7) comes to a similar conclusion. She suggests four aspects of women's sexuality that speak to the need for a model that is specific to women: first, women have a lower biological urge; second, context is often crucial in determining a women's motivation (or willingness) to engage in sexual activity; third, women's sexual arousal is represented psychologically and may or may not be accompanied by genital and/or nongenital changes; fourth, orgasm is not necessary to have a feeling of satisfaction, and even when it occurs, can manifest in a variety of forms. "Thus ... sexual arousal and ... desire occur simultaneously at some point after ... women have chosen to experience sexual stimulation; this choice is based initially on needs other than a desire to experience physical sexual arousal ..."

Baumeister et al. (8) have extensively reviewed the literature comparing the strength of the "sex drive" of men and women. They report finding that men think about and fantasize about sexual matters more often than women; want to engage in sexual activity more often regardless of sexual orientation; want a greater number of sexual partners; masturbate more frequently; are less willing to forgo sexual activity; experience earlier onset of sexual desire; are drawn to a wider variety of sexual practices; and are prepared to make more material and pragmatic sacrifices in order to engage in sexual activity. They summarized their findings by saying: "we did not find a single study, on any of near a dozen different measures, that found women had a stronger sex drive than men." In reflecting on possible explanations for this difference, they considered the roles of biology as well as social, and cultural factors, and concluded that "the role of biology is moderated by social factors more for women than for men."

These studies and observations argue that there are substantial differences in sexual desire in men and women; sexual desire in men seems to be quantitatively greater; lesbian relationships represent an informative group in learning about sexual desire in both gender groups; the DSM classification system seems more relevant to men; and while sexual desire usually precedes arousal in men, the opposite may be true in women.

"NORMAL" SEXUAL DESIRE FOR MEN

If one accepts the notion that sexuality generally and sexual desire in particular may be different in men and women, another question quickly follows: "when considering sexual desire, what is 'normal' for men?" A corollary to this question is: "since there is a general understanding that sexual activity changes with age, what represents normal sexual desire for men as they get older?"

An exceptional source of information on men and sexuality (including sexual desire) is the Massachusetts Male Aging Study (MMAS), a survey that involved a random sample of men in the general population aged 40–70, and one in which questions were asked about sexual issues from the viewpoint of *both* behavior and subjective thinking (9). A total of 1709 men participated in the study. A self-administered questionnaire included 23 items on such sex-related subjects as: satisfaction; frequency of activity; frequency of desire; frequency of thoughts, fantasies, or erotic dreams; frequency of erections and erectile difficulties; orgasm difficulties; genital pain; frequency of ejaculation; and attitudes to sexual changes with age. Reports were divided into two categories: behavioral and subjective phenomena. Only the latter will receive comment here, as sexual desire is a subjective phenomenon (which, indeed, might have behavioral consequences but far from always).

Results of the survey indicated "a consistent and significant decline with age in feeling desire, in sexual thoughts and dreams, and in the desired level of sexual activity." The decline in sexual interest neither preceded nor followed a similar decline in sexual behavior or events. "They appeared to occur together. Since the data were cross-sectional, it was not possible to answer the question about which came first... there was no evidence here of a disjunction between the level of sexual activity desired and the level of activity actually reported; it is not the case that as men age they desire at a level that is different from that which they report." However, the authors also found that *satisfaction did not follow the same path* in that "... men in their sixties reported levels of satisfaction with their sex life and partners at about the same level as younger men in their forties."

The authors of the MMAS considered many factors that might be associated with the decline in sexual interest and found that "aging and its social correlates... were strongly predictive of decreased involvement with sexual activity... (and that)... good health was associated with more involvement..." The authors concluded that the MMAS study, by considering men in their middle years, goes part way towards filling the gap of "up-to-date normative data available to inform clinicians as to the usual levels of activity and interest of normally aging men."

CLASSIFICATION

General Sexual Issues

Sexual disorders in general are classified in the Text Revision of the fourth edition of the Diagnostic and Statistical Manual of Mental Disorders (DSM-IV-TR).* One of the sections in DSM-IV-TR is titled "Sexual and Gender Disorders." Sexual disorders classified in the DSM system follow the thinking of Masters and Johnson (1), and Kaplan (10). The former described a "Sex Response Cycle" (SRC) that consisted of four phases, each of which they named: "excitement," "plateau," "orgasm," and "resolution." Kaplan then added another element that had previously been missing, namely, "desire." In addition, she reconceptualized the SRC into three parts: "desire," "response," and "orgasm," each of which was associated with a different disorder. The DSM system is similarly organized.

To many, the SRC is intellectually appealing and clinically useful in organizing thoughts about patient problems. However, it is not without considerable

---

*The *International Statistical Classification of Diseases and Related Health Problems*, 10th Revision (ICD-10), is used in Canada but ICD-9 is still used in many parts of the world. The development of DSM-IV-TR was closely coordinated with Chapter V of ICD-10.

drawbacks. First, as discussed earlier, some see it as much more useful when considering the sexual sequence experienced by men compared with women (5). Second, the phases are described in such a way as to seem discrete; but, in actual fact, they flow into each other. For example, desire is not simply at the beginning of a sexual event, but under ordinary circumstances, continues the whole way through (11). Similarly (although ostensibly less common in men vs. women), desire may *follow* arousal as, for example, when a man awakens in the morning with an erection and only *then* becomes sexually interested.

Sexual Desire Disorders

The DSM-IV-TR (6) category of Sexual and Gender Disorders is divided into three parts, one of which is Sexual Dysfunctions. One of the group of sexual dysfunctions is "Sexual Desire Disorders" (SDD) of which there are two kinds: (A) hypoactive sexual desire disorder (HSDD) and (B) sexual aversion disorder (SAD). No distinction is made between SDDs that affect men and those affecting women. The assumption is evidently made that sexual desire and desire problems are the same in both gender groups—a concept that is debatable.

In the description of HSDD in DSM-IV-TR (6), three criteria are necessary to establish the diagnosis: first, a deficiency or absence of sexual fantasy and desire for sexual activity; second, the fact that it causes "marked distress or interpersonal difficulty"; and third, that the disorder is not better viewed as a result of a major psychiatric or medical condition, or of substance abuse (this third criterion being somewhat problematic—see Sections "Etiology" and "Summary and Conclusions").

According to DSM-IV-TR (6), the principal distinguishing feature of SAD is a "persistent or recurrent aversion to, and avoidance of, all (or almost all) genital sexual contact with a sexual partner." The diagnosis is somewhat controversial in that some observers think that sexual desire problems exist on a continuum, rather than in separate categories. As the diagnosis of SAD is rarely made in men, and because a Pubmed search failed to reveal any articles with this diagnosis in the title, the issue will not be discussed further.

Subtypes of HSDD

Clinicians are directed to subtype the diagnosis of HSDD, that is, to say if the pattern has been (A) "lifelong" or "acquired" (i.e., always existed since puberty or followed a period of "normal" sexual desire), (B) "situational" or "generalized" (i.e., has existed only in some sexual circumstances or all) and (C) due to psychological or combined factors. Maurice (12; pp. 54–55) considers diagnostic subtyping to be clinically useful in helping to point towards the etiology and thus assessment and treatment—for example, acquired problems would require a more diligent search for the explanation of change than those which are lifelong. Likewise, if a man has a situational difficulty, for example, not sexually active with his partner but masturbating several times each week, there is little rationale for considering some biological explanation since his SRC is obviously intact.

Maurice has described four HSDD syndromes: (i) desire discrepancy, (ii) lifelong and generalized, (iii) acquired and generalized, and (iv) acquired and situational (12; pp. 161–165). On the basis of clinical impression, the most common desire difficulties in men are those that are (A) lifelong but also situational (very unusual in women) and (B) acquired and generalized—usually resulting from a medical, psychiatric, or other sexual, disorder (Fig. 4.1).

Although clinically useful, these syndromes have not been the subject of empirical research. Nevertheless, one can sometimes extract information from survey data that seem to apply to this scheme. For example, Kinsey et al. described a small group of men (147 from approximately 12,000 interviewed) who they referred to as "low rating" [defined as under 36 years old and whose

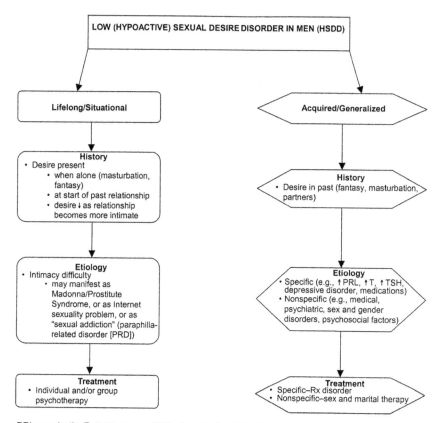

PRL = prolactin; T= testosterone; TSH = thyroid-stimulating hormone

Figure 4.1 Assessment of low sexual desire disorder in men.

rates (of sexual behavior) averaged one event in 2 weeks or less] (13; p. 207). They also described another group of men about half as large in number as "sexually apathetic" in that "they never, at any times in their histories, have given evidence that they were capable of anything except low rates of activity" (p. 209). One could conclude from Kinsey's observations that not only did these men have a lifelong and generalized disinterest in sexual matters, but also they were quite unusual.

Lifelong and Situational

"The most striking feature that differentiates a *situational* desire disorder from one that is *generalized* is the continued presence of sexual desire in some form. The sexual feelings that do exist in the present occur typically when the person is alone and are manifest either in thought and/or action (through masturbation), rather than in sexual activity with the patient's usual partner . . . the present level of sexual activity (with the partner) often represents a . . . change from the beginning of the relationship when the frequency was . . . greater." (12; p. 165) Detailed history-taking reveals that even at the start of the relationship, the woman often took the sexual initiative and even then, sexual experiences took place infrequently.

In this syndrome, the man's desire disorder represents a lifelong pattern but is also situational, because there are times when he can be quite sexual, typically when alone through masturbation, or at the beginning of a new relationship with a partner.

Case study

Alex is 35 years old and Sharon is 33 (not their real names). They have been married for 7 years and have no children. Neither have had any major health difficulties, smoke, or use street drugs. She asked her family doctor to refer both of them because of his disinterest in "sex." Three injections of testosterone did not result in any sexual change. Alex was initially reluctant to talk with someone else about this issue but eventually acceded to Sharon's strongly worded request (and that of the consultant) that they been seen together.

When a consultation took place and when they were asked for details of their sexual difficulties, she said that the last time that any sexual activity occurred was 1 week ago but before that was 3 months, and before that was 5 months.

In talking with them of the history of their premarital sexual relationship, it became apparent that she particularly appreciated the fact that she did not have to fend-off his sexual advances as she had to do with other men, and more often than not, she would take the initiative sexually. The difference in sexual interest became more apparent immediately after their marriage. To her great distress, no sexual activity occurred on their honeymoon and since then, had been only a few times each year.

When she was seen alone, she related that in the first few years of their marriage, she would make her sexual interest known to him but stopped doing so because of constant rejection. She described regularly comparing herself to women friends who would complain about the opposite, namely that they were not particularly interested themselves and frequently had to resort to subterfuge to control the sexual insistence of their husbands. She initially blamed herself for this state of affairs and wondered whether he found her attractive anymore and if he, in fact, still loved her. She also considered the idea that maybe he was interested in another woman, or that he was gay and interested in a man. She eventually satisfied herself that those worries were baseless and concluded that it was he that had some sexual difficulty. She thought that his trouble related to his strong attachment to his mother.

While finding that sexual offers from other men bolstered her opinion of herself, these were consistently declined because "that wasn't what I wanted." She wondered if she should divorce Alex and find someone else but was also concerned about giving up the life that the two of them had built together.

When he was seen alone, he explained that the same thing happened on the two occasions when he lived together with women before he married, that is, that his sexual desire for them quickly disappeared. With considerable hesitation he revealed that nowadays, he would masturbate several times each week while looking at pictures of nude women on the internet. He knew that his wife would be angry and might even leave him if she discovered his private sexual interests. Given the fact that the testosterone injections did not prove helpful, he accepted the notion that psychologically oriented care might be fruitful. He started to wonder if his sexual difficulties related to his family-of-origin and growing-up years.

Acquired and Generalized

The major differences between the acquired and generalized form of a sexual desire disorder, and the lifelong and situational form, are twofold: (a) the present status represents a considerable change from the past when the patient's sexual desire was not problematic for either him or his partner and (b) sexual desire is presently absent in any form.

Case study

Bob is a 55-year-old man who had been married for 27 years to Marie (not their real names). He works as a sales manager. They have two children, the youngest of whom moved out 1 year ago. She has had no major health problems. He has had diabetes for 5 years and the main treatment was diet, exercise (because he was greatly overweight), and an oral medication.

He described erection problems and waning sexual desire over the previous 2 years. He could not say which developed first. He reported thinking little about sexual matters in the present and only occasionally trying to engage in sexual activity with his wife—usually on her initiative. He also reported no inclination to masturbate and added that since he married, he "didn't need to", given that sexual activity with his wife was sufficient for his sexual needs. In the present, he said that pictures of women undressed did not "do anything" for him. His erections with his wife were 5/10 (on a scale of 0–10 where 0 meant no erection whatsoever, and 10 was full and stiff. He was not aware of morning erections although would sometimes wake up with some swelling of his penis (about 2–3/10). The last time he recalled a full erection under any circumstance was about 4 years prior. He did not report ejaculation difficulties now or in the past but did say that the intensity of his orgasm had lessened.

Bob was all the more distressed because his current sexual status was markedly different than in the past. Until recent years, he would have sexual thoughts regularly, took the initiative in inviting his wife to bed (several times each week), enjoyed looking at women's bodies especially in the summertime when they were less covered, and had no erection problems prior to about 4 years ago.

He wondered if the sexual changes were a result of his age. He had read an article in a newspaper about "andropause" and thought that this might be the explanation of his difficulties. He asked his family doctor about oral medications for "ED" (he had seen advertisements on television), and testosterone, and received both. Neither oral medications nor three injections of testosterone resulted in any sexual change. When he was seen in consultation by a "sex specialist" who asked about his knowledge of the connection between diabetes and sexual difficulties, he recalled hearing something in a diabetic clinic he had attended but confessed that his knowledge was only fragmentary.

Unfortunately, most of the empirical research on HSDD in men has either not subtyped the syndrome, or the report is unclear and results are embedded in a difficult-to-interpret melange of information. For example, one study separated three groups of college-age men: those with "Inhibited Sexual Desire" (ISD—a term that was used in earlier versions of the DSM for HSDD), erectile dysfunction, and controls (14). Not surprisingly, the men with ISD fantasized less about sexual matters than the other two groups. However, the ISD group masturbated more than the other two. Evidently, there were many men with a *situational* desire disorder in the ISD group. To illustrate the lack of clarity about what constituted a diagnosis of ISD as well as the absence of subtyping, two men who described no fantasy at intake were *excluded* from the study!

EPIDEMIOLOGY

The best information on the epidemiology of sexual disinterest in men comes from surveys of the general population and convenience samples. In the literature on this subject, little attempt is made to distinguish between the different diagnostic subtypes described in the "Classification" section of this chapter.

An excellent source of population-based information on sexual disinterest in men comes from the National Health and Social Life Survey (NHSLS; 15).

Laumann and his colleagues interviewed a probability sample of 3432 adults (including 1410 men) in the US between the ages of 18 and 59. Because the study is so often cited, it is worth examining the results in some detail.

In a 90 min interview on many sex-related subjects, one of the questions asked was "during the last 12 months has there ever been a period of several months or more when you lacked interest in having sex?" (No apparent attempt was made to subtype the responses.) Overall, 16% of the men said they were indeed not interested in sex (vs. 33% of the women). When the responses were assembled into 5-year groupings, the highest numbers of those who answered "yes" were from men who were in two groups: those who were 40–44 and 50–59 years old. These numbers do not quite fit with the common perception of waning sexual desire with increasing age. The figures seem to suggest a greater degree of complexity. Contrary to expectations, the *fewest* men who answered "yes" were in the group of men who were 44–49 years. Looking at the opposite end of the sexually active age spectrum, and again not quite fitting with common beliefs, 14% of the *youngest* group of men (18–24 years old) also answered positively.

Some social factors examined in the Laumann et al. study correlated with lack of sexual desire in men (15). Those who answered affirmatively included 20% of the "never married" men (vs. 12% of the married); 22% of the men whose education was "less than high school" (vs. most of the other levels of education where the range was 13–16%); and 20% of black men (vs. 15% of whites). The impact of religion was unclear with no one religious group outstanding. The relationship to poverty was striking in that 25% of poor men responded positively (vs. 13–15% of men at other income levels).

In the same survey, health and happiness were also separately correlated with sexual disinterest. The greater the impairment of health and the magnitude of unhappiness, the greater the extent of sexual disinterest.

Further analysis of the sexual dysfunction data from the NHSLS survey used multivariate techniques to estimate the relative risk (RR) for each demographic characteristic as well as for key risk factors (16). In comparing the oldest group of men (50–59) to the youngest (18–29), the former were three times as likely to experience low sexual desire. Similarly, "never married" men were almost three times as likely to experience lack of sexual desire compared to those who were "currently married."

The statistical method of latent class analysis (LCA) was also used for "analyzing risk factors and quality-of-life concomitants in relation to categories of sexual dysfunction rather than individual symptoms." Risk factors that were found to be predictors of low sexual desire in men included "daily alcohol consumption," "poor to fair health," and "emotional problems or stress." The same was true of "thinking about sex less than once weekly" (more than three times as likely vs. those who thought about sex more than once weekly), ever had any "same-sex activity" (more than twice as likely vs. those that never did), and "sexually touched before puberty" (about twice as likely vs. those that were not touched).

When considering quality-of-life concomitants, men with low sexual desire experienced a low level of physical satisfaction and a low level of general happiness, with their "primary" partner.

Another survey using a stratified probability sample was conducted in Britain and concerned the prevalence of sexual function problems in people who had at least one heterosexual partner in the past year. The study took place from 1999 to 2000 and involved 11,461 men and women aged 16–44 (17). The response rate was 65.4%. Problems were reported according to two duration periods: those which lasted at least 1 month in the past year, and those which lasted at least six months in the past year. Thirty-five percent of men reported at least one sexual problem in the past year, and "lack of interest in sex" was the most common such concern (17%) in the shorter time period. The prevalence dropped to 2% when considering the "at least 6-months" time frame.

In yet another study involving 100 "normal" volunteer couples who were well-educated and who regarded their marriages as ones that were "working," Frank et al. (18) found that a similar (to the US and UK studies) percentage of men (16%) were sexually disinterested.

Similarly, when a sample of gay men were asked about sexual concerns, including "lack of interest in or desire for sex," 16% said it was a current problem and 49% indicated that it was a problem at some time in their lives (19). Two other studies that bear on the subject of epidemiology are described elsewhere in this chapter: (a) the section on "Classification—Subtyping of HSDD Syndromes" includes the finding by Kinsey et al. (13) of a small group of men with the lifelong and generalized form of HSDD, and (b) the section on "Etiology—Presence of Another Sexual or Gender Disorder in a Patient or Partner" includes results of an investigation conducted by Segraves and Segraves (20) who reported on men and women with HSDD in a population that was recruited for a study of sexual disorders generally.

ASSESSMENT

There are three components to the evaluation of any sexual dysfunction: history, physical examination, and laboratory examination. The history is always crucial. The decision to also conduct a physical and laboratory examination (or refer the patient for this purpose if the clinician is not a physician) depends mostly on diagnostic subtyping, which in turn depends on the history.

History

Maurice (12) outlined a brief set of topics that a clinician might cover with the process of history-taking to determine the pattern of any sexual dysfunction (Table 4.1).

Table 4.1 Pattern of a Sexual Dysfunction: What to Ask

1. Duration of difficulty: lifelong or acquired
2. Circumstances in which difficulty appears: generalized or situational
3. Description of difficulty
4. Patient's sex response cycle (desire, erection, ejaculation/orgasm if male; desire, vaginal lubrication, orgasm, absence of coital pain if female)
5. Partner's sex response cycle (see #4)
6. Patient and partner's reaction to presence of difficulty
7. Motivation for treatment (when difficulty not chief complaint)

Reprinted from Maurice W. Sexual Medicine in Primary Care. St. Louis: Mosby, Inc. 1999:53.

Sexual desire in men manifests in three ways: (i) psychologically through thoughts, fantasies, and dreams; (ii) behaviorally in sexual activity with a partner; and (iii) behaviorally in sexual activity with oneself through masturbation or self-stimulation. Topics in Table 4.1 form the basis of the following *suggested* questions that one might ask when faced with a man who says that he is not sexually interested.

1. *Has a feeling of low sexual desire always been a part of your life or was there a time when you were more interested?*
   Comment: This question will help to determine if the desire problem is one that is "lifelong" or "acquired." Talking about the duration and the past might also allow the man to reflect on times when, for example, he encountered a similar pattern of initial desire followed by disinterest.

2. *What kinds of things are you thinking about when the two of you are sexual with each other? and/or What sort of sexual thoughts or fantasies do you have at other times? and/or About how often are you and she/he sexually involved with each other?*
   Comment: These questions help to determine if the problem is "situational" or "generalized." Understandably, many clinicians object to the idea of asking people about fantasies, or what is going on in a patient's mind. Our society treasures privacy and for most people, nothing is more private than their sexual fantasies. This attitude of psychological intrusion challenges a health professional to separate his/her social self from his/her work function. For example, there is simply no doubt that finding out if a man is thinking about other men or about women in an erotic situation is *essential*, not elective, in determining his sexual orientation, which may, in turn, help to clarify the reason for his apparent sexual disinterest.
   Sexual desire is a feeling which usually (but not always) manifests in sexual behavior. Extrapolating from sexual behavior to determine someone's sexual desire (the third question in #2) can be problematic since there are many reasons for someone engaging in sexual activity

apart from being sexually interested (the most common being the idea of wanting to please one's partner).

Other questions that are worth asking in this context include: *"When was the last time that any sexual activity took place?" and/or "How often has any sexual activity taken place in, say, the last 6 months?"*

3. *"Have you had sexual experiences with other women since you have been in this relationship? and "Have you ever had sexual experiences with other men?" and "How often do you have sexual thoughts about other women? and "other men?"*

   Comment: All four questions might help to clarify whether the desire problem is "situational" or "generalized." For reasons mentioned previously, thoughts can be more revealing than actions.

4. *Tell me about your masturbation experiences? How often do you masturbate? Do you look at pictures in magazines at the same time (or videos, or on the internet)? What do the pictures show? Women? Men? Couples? "What are the people doing?"*

   Comment: Again, these question will help to determine if the desire difficulty is "situational" or "generalized." If, for example, the man is masturbating and thinking about sexual matters but at the same time not sexually interested in his partner, then the desire difficulty is clearly situational. Questions about the content of pictures tell the clinician about the man's erotic focus, be it individuals belonging to the opposite or same sex, or sexual activities that are not mainstream.

5. *Some men have sexual thoughts about women in the summertime when their bodies are not so covered. What's your own experience?*

   Comment: This question can be yet another way of finding out if the man finds others to be erotically appealing and who the people might be.

Physical Examination

A physical examination is necessary when HSDD is acquired and generalized in a man. However, one might legitimately ask what to look for since HSDD can be seen as a symptom of a disorder, or, as a syndrome (i.e., as a collection of symptoms which result from a wide variety of causes). When associated with another disease, loss of sexual desire may resemble other phenomena like loss of appetite or fatigue—symptoms linked to many different medical and psychiatric disorders ranging from depression to cancer, and not having any specific physical findings.

When no specific cause of HSDD is apparent from the history, one must then consider an unrecognized disorder (like renal, cardiac, or endocrine disease) when conducting a physical examination. The principal endocrine disorders would be hypoandrogen states and hypothyroidism. Signs of the former can be subtle and in men, are often delayed. When considering hypogonadism, examination of the testes is mandatory. "Since generalized disease and endocrine disorders can coexist, the presence of the former does not necessarily mean that the explanation for sexual desire loss has been found and that a search for an accompanying endocrine disorder, is, therefore, unnecessary." (12; p. 180).

Laboratory Examination

A labaratory exam is only warranted when the sexual desire problem is clearly generalized. When a lab exam is required, the following should be considered:

1. *Testosterone (T)*: (see section on "Hormones" in this chapter).
2. *Prolactin (PRL)*: When an abnormal value is detected, it is best to repeat the test at least once and preferably twice since errors are common. When PRL is high, the T level is also often abnormal. More elaborate assessment of an abnormal PRL level involves brain imaging [magnetic resonance imaging (MRI) or computerized tomography (CT)], visual fields, and pituitary function tests. Patients who have repeatedly abnormal PRL levels, who require more elaborate testing, and where the etiology is not apparent, should be referred to an endocrinologist. Values which are higher than normal infrequently occur in a healthy man. When the PRL level is abnormal, one of the most common pathological causes is the use of an antipsychotic medication. An unusual but serious cause is a prolactin-secreting tumor.
3. Erectile dysfunction (ED) often occurs together with sexual disinterest and it may not be easy to establish which preceded the other. Under such circumstances, it is wise to investigate common causes of ED by ensuring that the patient does not have diabetes (obtaining a fasting blood sugar), or elevated lipids [assessing his total cholesterol, high density lipoprotein (HDL), low density lipoprotein (LDL), and triglycerides], or abnormal thyroid function [investigating his thyroid stimulating hormone (TSH)].

HORMONES

Two hormones influence sexual desire in men: androgens generally—of which the most consequential is T, and PRL.

Testosterone (T)

Components and Measurement (21)

There are three kinds of T: (i) free, that is, not bound to any protein (FT), (ii) bound to albumin, and (iii) bound to sex hormone binding globulin (SHBG). Only $\sim$2% of T is in the free form; about 60% of the remainder is weakly bound to albumin and other proteins; and about 40% is bound with a higher binding affinity to SHBG (Fig. 4.2).

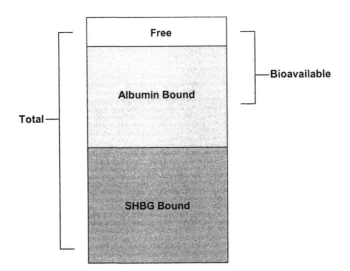

Figure 4.2   Testosterone partitions in the serum. [Reprinted with permission from (Testosterone and Aging: Clinical Research Directions) (2004) by the National Academy of Sciences, courtesy of the National Academies Press, Washington, D.C.]

Total T comprises FT with whatever is bound to protein. The part that is most easily available to tissues is referred to as bioavailable testosterone (BAT) and includes both FT and the portion that is bound to albumin.

Total T is measured by radioimmunoassay which is a validated, standardized, and reproducible assay. However, as SHBG increases with age, and therefore a greater percentage of the total T is bound to SHBG, this measure may not be so informative in older men. BAT is measured in several ways including separately calculating the total T and SHBG. Measurement of FT is more difficult and "controversial" (21; p.18).

Segraves and Balon estimate that 200–350 ng/dL of T is required for normal sexual function and that above 450 ng/dL, "it is difficult to demonstrate a relationship between testosterone and sexual activity." (22; p. 216).

Measurement of T is best performed in the morning because of the diurnal variation in blood levels.

Normal Aging Changes in the Quantity

In adult men, T increases greatly from 0.2 to 0.7 nmol/L (50–20 ng/dL) to the normal adult male level of 10–35 nmol/L (∼300–1000 mg/dL) by about age 17. The level of BAT (see later) remains balanced until men are in their 30s or 40s and then decreases slowly over the remainder of the man's life at a rate of about 1.2% per year. (The latter contrasts with women who experience a sudden drop in estrogen and progesterone when ovulation ends.) In healthy men, mean serum T levels decrease by $\sim$30% between ages 25 and 75. Mean FT levels decrease by as much as 50% over the same period. The steeper decline of FT is explained by the age-associated increase in SHBG. "At any age, the range of values observed, both for T and FT, is very wide...it is evident that...the limits of normality are rather arbitrary and that the sensitivity threshold for androgens might vary from tissue to tissue and possibly, also according to age" (23).

In addition to T, many hormones gradually change in the aging male including growth hormone (GH) and adrenal compounds [dehydroepiandrosterone (DHEA) and its sulfate (DHEAS)].

Origin, Production, and Control

Testosterone in men derives mostly from the testis but a small amount comes from the adrenal cortex. Hormonal control over the production of testicular T begins in the hypothalamus, which secretes gonadotropin-releasing hormone (GnRH) (Fig. 4.3). GnRH, in turn, stimulates the anterior part of the pituitary gland to produce both leutinizing hormone (LH) and follicle stimulating

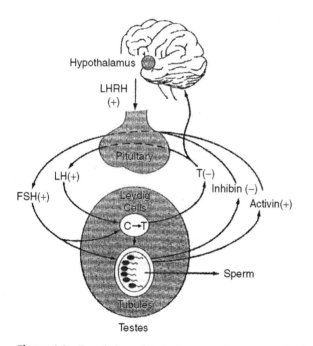

Figure 4.3 Regulation of testosterone and sperm production by LH and FSH. (C = cholesterol, T = testosterone). *Source*: Griffin JE, Wilson JD. Disorders of the testes. In: Braunwald E, Fauci AS, Kasper DL, Hauser SL, Longo DL, Jameson JL, eds. Harrison's Principles of Internal Medicine. 15th ed. New York: McGraw-Hill, 2001:2143. (Reprinted with permission.)

hormone (FSH) both of which act on cells in the testes. LH causes the Leydig cells to produce T and FSH induces the Sertoli cells to produce spermatozoa. A negative feedback mechanism results in the testes controlling the output of LH and FSH. In older men, the function of both the testes and the hypothalamic-pituitary axis are diminished and for both reasons, the output of T is less (24).

About 5–6 mg of T is secreted daily into the plasma of men, usually in a pulsatile manner every 60–90 min, and in a diurnal rhythm in which peak levels occur during the morning (although less pronounced in older men) (25). In addition to intraday fluctuations, there is a wide range of normal levels between different individuals.

Actions

Testosterone can act either (a) directly on target cells or (b) indirectly by being converted first to its principal metabolites, dihydrotestosterone (DHT), and estradiol. Although both T and DHT bind to the androgen receptor, the latter does so more strongly and is therefore more potent. Two enzymes convert T to its metabolites: *5 alpha-reductase*, which converts T to DHT and which is found especially in prostate, skin, and reproductive tissues, and *aromatase* which converts T to estradiol and is found especially in adipose tissue, liver, and some central nervous system nuclei. Thus, the actions of T are widespread throughout the body.

Effects on Sexuality

The sex-related impact of T in men has been demonstrated in two groups: (a) those who have been deprived of this hormone in a significant manner and who are hypogonadal as a result (the most extreme example of which is men who have been castrated—physically or chemically—for any reason and in varying degrees) and (b) those who are generally healthy (including their hormone levels, otherwise referred to as "eugonadal").

The influence of androgens on sexual desire is particularly prominent and was summarized by Bancroft (26; pp. 92–93). From his studies on hypogonadal men, he concluded that within 3–4 weeks of androgen withdrawl: (i) sexual interest declines as measured by the frequency of sexual thoughts (ii) sexual activity appears to diminish (as a result of decreased sexual desire) but is more difficult to assess because of the confounding effects of a sexual partner, and (iii) the capacity for ejaculation disappears. When androgen replacement is given, these phenomena are reversed within 7–10 days. As well, the impact of androgen replacement on sexual desire is dose-related.

Fantasy (or imagery)-associated erections and nocturnal erections are both androgen-dependent, and cease as a result of androgen withdrawal. The fact that only certain aspects of erectile function are affected suggests that the impact in this area is indirect, that is, on the man's central nervous system rather than directly on his genitalia. Segraves suggests that when a man experiences erectile dysfunction in the context of T deprivation, the origin of the difficulty can be described as "performance anxiety" superimposed on a biogenic desire disorder (27; p. 278).

Segraves and Balon summarize the impact of the therapeutic use of T in *eugonadal* men by saying that "a relatively low level . . . is sufficient to maintain normal sexual activity, and that there is no demonstrable relationship between sexual function and variations of testosterone above this threshold value" (22; p. 215).

Changes in Effects with Age

The mystery of what happens to T as men age is not easy to unravel and possibly involves three separate issues: changes in production, carrier proteins, and receptor sensitivity.

The decrease in normal levels of T with age (described previously) seems partly explained by a decrease in function of both testicular tissue (Leydig cells) and the pituitary-hypothalamic axis. However, a second factor explaining the diminution may be that the protein SHBG increases with age and therefore, more T is bound and less is free. A third issue is the possible decline in the level of sensitivity of T receptors (especially those in the central nervous system) which might explain both reduced sexual desire in the aging male and the need for large doses of T in treating hypogonadal states in older men.

Segraves and Balon summarized results of the changes in T that accompany aging as follows (22):

> *Decreased*: Production; the number of Leydig cells in the testis; the levels of bound and free hormone; testicular response to LH.
> *Increased*: SHBG; estradiol; FSH; LH.

DHEA and DHEAS

Dehydroepiandrosterone (DHEA) and its sulfate (DHEAS) are androgens that originate in the adrenal glands. "To date, no carefully controlled study of dehydroepiandrosterone's effect on libido has been studied" despite observations on the benefits of DHEA on erections (22).

Prolactin

PRL derives from the anterior pituitary gland and its secretion is tonically inhibited by the hypothalamus through a balance of hypothalamic prolactin-inhibiting hormone (PIH) and putative prolactin-releasing hormone (PRH) (28). PIH is actually dopamine; so, anything that interferes with dopamine production results in increased PRL (the most common pathological reason being the use of many drugs used in psychiatry, e.g., risperidone and the phenothiazines).

Elevated PRL in men (and women) results in diminished sexual desire, as well as the possibility of erection and/or ejaculatory problems in the form of diminished volume. In a very informative study of men presenting to a clinic because of sexual disorders and who were later found to be hyperprolactinemic, Schwartz et al. (29) concluded that it was generally futile to attempt to separate "psychogenic" and "organic" sexual problems, because many of the men presented with a *situational* pattern that seemed to be exacerbated by psychological factors and that improved at times of increased arousal. Even more striking (and a sobering lesson to those who are not flexible in their approach to treating sexual problems in men), sex therapy administered before the hyperprolactinemia was discovered, actually resulted in improvement!

ETIOLOGY

Theoretical Perspectives: Biological, Psychological, and Social

Not only are there multiple origins for HSDD in men, but the theoretical perspective of the observer regarding sexual issues as a whole make understanding sexual problems like HSDD even more difficult.

One might look first at differing points of view about sexuality in general. Some view sexual difficulties from primarily a biomedical perspective and regard "sex" as "natural." Kolodny et al. wrote: "to define sex as natural means just as an individual cannot be taught to sweat or how to digest food, a man cannot be taught to have an erection, nor can a woman be taught to lubricate vaginally. Because the reflex pathways of sexual functioning are inborn does not mean that they are immune from disruption due to impaired health, cultural conditioning, or interpersonal stress" (30; p. 479) "Some have reworded 'naturally' to mean 'automatically, without purpose or without effort'" (31).

Others look at sexuality and see the absence of intimacy as being crucial to understanding the psychological origins of many sexual difficulties (11,32). One can particularly appreciate (and learn from) the implications of the absence of intimacy for sexual relationships generally, and sexual desire in particular, when considering the plight of those with a serious mental illness who, by the very nature of the disorder, also have substantial intimacy difficulties (33). "The roots of intimacy difficulties are in the patient's past...this...needs to be thoroughly explored because it may well have included turmoil in his or her family-of-origin, as well as a dearth of love and nurturing connections which are so often a rehearsal for love relationships later in life. Likewise, the patient's past may not have included the experimental love and sexual relationships of adolescence in which so much learning takes place about oneself and others."

Still others look at sexual matters from a "social constructionist" point of veiw. Tiefer wrote that "the primary influences on women's sexuality are the norms of the culture, those internalized by women themselves and those enforced by institutions and enacted by significant others in women's lives" (5; p. 2)

It may well be that these viewpoints do not apply equally to men and women, and that sexuality in men is, for example, more "natural." However, even as the word "natural" is applied to men, it does not explain the contribution to sexual problems of either intimacy issues or cultural variations in sexual behavior.

"During development and growth, there is interaction with the environment that builds up experience and potentiation of 'sexual' stimuli. The social and cultural environment determines sexual expression and the meaning of sexual experience" (31).

Intimacy Difficulty

See "Theoretical Perspectives" immediately above (11,32,33).

Endocrine Abnormalities

Little endocrine research has been done on men with HSDD.

Schiavi et al. compared 17 physically healthy men with HSDD to 17 age-matched non-dysfunctional volunteers (34). All were 25–55 years old. The HSDD men were described as having a generalized and persistent lack of sexual desire. Men with HSDD who did and did not have accompanying erectile problems, were also compared. The authors found that men with HSDD had significantly lower plasma total T levels (but not FT, PRL, LH, or estradiol) measured hourly throughout the night, when compared with controls. As well, they also reported that the men with secondary erectile problems had a different nocturnal penile tumescence (NPT) pattern than those whose erections were not problematic. The authors concluded that there was a relation between the decrease in T and the diminution in sexual drive and speculated that NPT findings may reflect a central biological abnormality. In support of the latter idea, they cited another study in which they found that men with HSDD had a higher prevalence of mood disorders on a lifetime basis (but not at the time of evaluation) and wondered if both mood and sexual desire disorders might represent some neurobiologic abnormality (35).

Presence of Another Sexual or Gender Disorder in a Patient or Partner

Sexual Dysfunctions

Three studies demonstrate that it is common for HSDD to be associated (or comorbid or correlated) with another sexual dysfunction. However, correlation is not the same as causation. The same factor(s) may result in both disorders. Nevertheless, the observation is at least noteworthy, and beyond that, may be etiologically meaningful.

1. Segraves and Segraves reported on 906 subjects (including 374 men) who had been recruited for a pharmaceutical company study of sexual disorders (20). Only the men will be discussed in this chapter. They were described as age 51 (SD = 10.1), and 30% (*n* = 113) had

a primary diagnosis of HSDD. Almost half (47%) had a secondary diagnosis of erectile impairment and a few ($n = 3$) had retarded ejaculation (patients with premature ejaculation were excluded from the study).

2. Schiavi reviewed 2500 charts of individuals and couples referred between 1974 and 1991. This survey included 1775 men, of which 13.3% ($n = 236$) were 60 years old or older (range 60–84). Most of the men (66%) were diagnosed with erectile disorder but 28% had HSDD either alone [3% ($n = 8$)] or associated with another sex-related diagnosis [ED—14% ($n = 34$); PE—11% ($n = 27$)]. In some, ED was the cause while in others it was the result. In most "it was not possible to determine the primary dysfunction" (36: p. 115).

3. Together with colleagues, Schiavi also examined the psychobiology of a group of sexually healthy men aged 45–74 living in stable sexual relationships (36; pp. 41–53). Seventy-seven couples were studied. One of the issues considered was a comparison of men with and without a sexual dysfunction. Seventeen men met their criteria for erectile dysfunction and five for HSDD (22% and 6.5%, respectively, of the total group). They found a significant difference in the age of the HSDD men who did and did not have accompanying ED (70.8 and 58.6 years, respectively). They added that the number of men with HSDD was too small to do any statistical comparisons with men who were not experiencing this disorder.

Sexual Difficulties in a Partner

Sexual difficulties in a partner, for example, intercourse-related pain experienced by a woman, may result in profound change in the level of sexual desire in the other person.

Case Study

Rob and Melissa (not their real names), both 23 years old and university students, were referred because intercourse had not yet occurred in their 3-month-old marriage. With relish, they regularly engaged in other sexual activities. History from both, plus her pelvic exam, revealed a diagnosis of vaginismus uncomplicated by vaginal pathology. Conventional treatment of vaginismus was successful in a technical sense (intercourse took place), but Melissa was chagrined to find that it was not as pleasurable as she anticipated (12). From the time of Rob's initial attempt to insert even part of his penis, he was concerned over her report of intercourse-related pain, and found that his sexual desire had diminished considerably when compared with the pre-treatment level. He found that in general, he was thinking much less about sexual matters, and when he and Melissa were sexual together, his erections were less than full and he was unable to ejaculate in her vagina. Moreover, he reported that his desire to masturbate had plummeted. His sexual desire slowly returned (but not to the pre-treatment level) as he accepted her reassurance that her intercourse pain was progressively diminishing. Her continuing lack of physical pleasure in intercourse (she looked forward to the closeness) seemed to impede the recovery of his own desire.

Child Sexual Abuse (CSA)

The results of investigations on the sex-related impact of CSA on adult men are unclear. One study indicated that did not predict sexual dysfunction in a clinical sample of adult men asking for treatment of this disorder (37). However, in a different study that reviewed the sexual consequences of CSA on adolescents and adults, the authors described a wide variety of effects on adult men (although HSDD was not reported) (38).

Paraphilias (PAs) and Paraphilia-Related Disorders (PRDs)

PAs and their cousins, PRDs, usually manifest with a high level of sexual desire (39). However, from the perspective of a partner, the opposite is usually the case.

Case Study

Alan and Amy (not their real names), both 32 years old; were referred by their family physician because of Alan's low level of sexual desire which had been a problem for most of the 7 years of their marriage. They lived alone. Alan was a university professor and Amy was a primary school teacher. Their first 6 months together (they had lived in separate cities before marrying) were sexually harmonious but difficulties became apparent after that time. They explained that nowadays they would go to bed at different times, and that he would hardly touch her. Six months prior to the first visit, she discovered magazines in the back of his car which depicted men dressed as women. Alan asked Amy if he could do the same when they were sexual together, that is, be dressed as a woman. She tried on a few occasions but eventually found the idea to be repellant.

When Alan was seen alone, he explained that his low level of sexual interest was only in relation to his wife but that whenever possible, he would get dressed as a woman, found himself sexually aroused in the process, and masturbate. They were referred for care to a psychiatrist who specialized in treating couples where one partner had a paraphilia.

Medical Disorders

General Comments

Medical conditions in which all sexual dysfunctions occur, and more specifically loss of sexual desire, result from biological, psychological and/or social, or interpersonal factors, and most often from a combination of these elements (40). Examples of biological factors include: direct physiological effects of the

illness or its treatment, physical debilitation, and bowel and/or bladder inconti-
nence. Examples of psychological factors include: adopting the "patient role" as
an asexual person, altered body image, mood difficulties, and fear of death or
rejection by a partner. Examples of social and interpersonal factors include: communication difficulties regarding feelings or sexuality, difficulties initiating a
sexual encounter after a period of abstinence, lack of partner, and lack of privacy.

Cardiovascular Diseases (22)

These include disorders of the heart (myocardial infarction, angina pectoris, coronary artery disease, conduction problems), hypertension, and atherosclerosis.
Cardiac problems may cause sexual difficulties on their own or as a result of
their treatment (see later). Likewise, just experiencing the disorder may cause
mood or body image problems. Some cardiovascular diseases may result in
avoidance of sexual activity and therefore its limitation. Whenever a sexual dysfunction occurs in the context of a cardiovascular disease, the clinician should
attempt to separate the various etiological factors.

Cancers

The "general comments" made earlier are particularly applicable in any discussion of cancer.

Epilepsy

Of all types of epilepsy, that which affects the temporal lobe (TLE) has been the
most frequently studied in relation to sexual consequences. TLE is particularly
linked with low sexual desire in patients undergoing temporal lobe surgery (an
admittedly unrepresentative group afflicted with this disorder) (41). The association between other kinds of epilepsy and low sexual desire is unclear.

Genetic Disorders

Kleinfelter's syndrome (47 XXY).

Testicular Disease

Trauma; mumps orchitis, undescended testes.

Secondary Hypogonadism (Resulting from Hypothalamic-Pituitary Disorders)

Pituitary tumors (especially prolactinoma); and iron overload disorders (e.g.,
hemochromatosis and thalassemia).

Endocrine Disorders

Cushing's syndrome, diabetes.

Multisystem Disease

Chronic renal failure, chronic liver disease, AIDS.

Psychiatric Disorders

Major Depression

Sexuality is commonly affected by mood disorders. Specifically, diminished sexual desire is often seen as a feature of depression (42). Schreiner-Engel and Schiavi looked at the relationship between HSDD and depression using an unconventional strategy (35). They examined couples where one partner reported generalized HSDD (22 of the men and 24 of the women—all of whom were euthymic at the time) and compared them to a control group. Interestingly, they found that those with sexual desire difficulties had a significantly higher lifetime rate of affective disorder—almost twice as high as the control group. Furthermore, the authors theorized that there may be a common biological etiology to the two disorders, or, that affective psychopathology may contribute to the pathogenesis of the desire disorder.

Bipolar Disorder

There is little information on sexual dysfunctions in untreated euthymic patients who have a bipolar disorder. However, manic patients are often described as "hypersexual" but the meaning is often not clear. "Hypersexual" could refer either to either an increase in sexual desire, or an increase in sexual activity (which may result from factors other than sexual desire such as having an exaggerated opinion of one's desirability).

Schizophrenia

Finding an untreated population of people with this disorder is unusual as is any attempt to establish the nature of sexual desire in this condition that is separate from medications.

Anxiety Disorders

In a study of sexual dysfunctions and posttraumatic stress disorder (PTSD) in men, three groups were compared: (i) untreated patients ($n = 15$), (ii) PTSD patients treated with selective serotonin reuptake inhibitors (SSRIs) ($n = 27$), and (iii) normal controls (43). Untreated and treated PTSD patients had significantly poorer sexual functioning in all domains examined, including sexual desire.

Drugs

General Comments

Unfortunately, few double-blind placebo-controlled trials exist to guide clinicians in understanding the sexual impact of medications. As a result, much of the information that follows is based on less refined information as, for example, case reports. Caution in interpretation is therefore advisable.

Unless otherwise referenced, information in this section has been taken from Segraves and Balon (22) and Kaufman and Vermeulen (23).

In general, there is often great difficulty in differentiating the sexual consequences of a disorder from side effects of the medication used in treatment. When thinking about a sexual desire problem, attempting this separation requires care in determining that it did not exist *before* drug treatment began (i.e., making sure that it is, in fact, acquired rather than lifelong). Likewise, one would expect drug-related sexual problems to occur under all circumstances rather than some (i.e., to be generalized rather than situational), and that the desire problem would disappear if the drug is stopped but reappear if resumed. Last, one would want to determine that the diminished sexual desire would not be better explained by the onset of an illness or exposure to an environmental stress.

Antipsychotics

This group includes those which are "typical" (also called "neuroleptics" and "traditional," for example, phenothiazines, thioxanthenes, and butyrophenones), as well as "atypical" (e.g., risperidone, olanzapine, quetiapine, and clozapine). Men who are taking antipsychotic drugs generally complain of various sexual side effects including loss of sexual desire (although interference with ejaculation seems particularly common). One factor that seems especially noteworthy is that many of the typical antipsychotics, as well as risperidone in the atypical group, result in an elevation in PRL which, in turn, has significant sexual consequences including a lessening of sexual desire (see below).

Antianxiety Agents

Alprazolam (Xanax) was reported to sometimes result in diminished sexual desire in both men and women (44). In that SSRIs are often used to treat anxiety, the information on "antidepressants" immediately below is of relevance.

Antidepressants

The incidence of sexual dysfunction generally with antidepressants is estimated at 30–50%. All types of antidepressants (TCAs, MAOIs, SSRIs) are linked to decreased sexual desire. Sexual dysfunctions generally are said to be less with bupropion, mirtazapine, moclobemide, and maybe reboxetine.

Mood Stabilizers

Lithium may result in diminished sexual desire in a minority of patients.

Drugs Used in Urological Practice

Finasteride is used in the treatment of benign prostatic hypertrophy (BPH); its mode of action is to block the conversion of T to DHT by inhibiting the enzyme *5-alpha reductase*. Diminished sexual desire is commonly reported.

Several drugs are used in the treatment of prostate cancer, a disease which is often androgen-dependent. The treatment strategy is therefore to lower or eliminate the effect of androgens which, in turn, has a predictable markedly negative impact on sexual desire. Flutamide interferes with the binding of T and DHT to the androgen receptor. Flutamide is used both alone and in combination with either leutinizing-hormone releasing hormone (LHRH) or finasteride. Drugs used to treat metastatic prostate cancer include LHRH agonists (synthetic analogues of LHRH including leuprolide, flutamide, nafarelin, and nilutamide), and androgen receptor blockers. LHRH agonists act by blocking the pituitary release of gonadotropins thereby decreasing the production of androgens (Fig. 4.3).

Cardiovascular Drugs

Substances that are known to be associated with lowering of sexual desire include: chlorthalidone, clofibrate, clonidine, gemfibrozil, hydrochlorthiazide, methyldopa, propanolol, reserpine, spironolactone, and timolol.

Cancer Chemotherapy Drugs

Cytotoxic drugs often have substantial effects on the gonads. Loss of sexual desire often accompanies their use and may be, at least in part, a result of hormonal changes. The treatment of some cancers in men might involve the use of anti-androgenic drugs resulting in a substantial decrease in T. Bone marrow transplant (BMT) in men may cause a substantially lower level of sexual desire. Androgen replacement therapy is often suggested to men who have received high-dose chemotherapy with BMT.

Anticonvulsant Drugs

Carbamazepine, clonazepam, gabapentin, phenobarbital, phenytoin, and primidone have been linked to sexual dysfunction (including, but not limited to, low sexual desire). The picture is often confounded by the appearance of sexual disorders associated with epilepsy itself as well as with the paucity of published information on this entire subject. Sexual effects seem related to enzyme induction as well as changes in sex hormone levels (via SHBG), and possibly, neurotransmitters.

"Recreational" Drugs

Recreational drugs include nicotine, marijuana, alcohol, heroin, methadone, and MDMA. Given the connection between cigarette smoking and ED as well as the apparent link between ED and HSDD, nicotine can be considered as an indirect cause of sexual desire disorders in men. Many who use marijuana frequently also report low sexual desire. The sexual effects of chronic use of alcohol are legion and include ED (possibly due to peripheral neuropathy), testicular atrophy, low T, and high SHBH in those with cirrhosis, and hyperestrogenism also associated with alcohol-related liver disease. Any of these difficulties may also result in low sexual desire. Chronic use of heroin and all other opiates results in diminished sexual desire, possibly related to low T levels.

Drugs Used in Gastrointestinal Practice

Cimetidine has been reported to result in diminished libido in men and to have an antiandrogenic effect.

Madonna/Prostitute Syndrome

Freud described a man choosing one woman for love and another for sexual activity and seemingly unable to fuse the two (45). He referred to this idea as the Madonna/Prostitute Syndrome. This notion seems especially applicable today to some young men who also relate experiences consistent with a lifelong and situational form of HSDD (12; and see Case Study in the "Lifelong and Situational" section of the "Classification" section).

Ill Partner

Severe medical and psychiatric illness can alter partner-related sexual desire.

Case Study

Tanya and Phillip (not their real names) were each 27 years old and married for the first time for 3 years. They did not have children, did not smoke or use street drugs, and neither had had major health problems in the past. They described themselves as Christian and although they did not have intercourse before marriage, they "could not keep their hands off each other" during that time and enthusiastically engaged in a variety of sexual activities. Their sexual experiences in the early years of their marriage were uncomplicated and highly pleasurable to both. In the second year of their marriage Tanya developed an episode of mania. When they were initially referred (because of lack of sexual desire on Phillip's part), she had been taking maintenance medication for the previous 12 months.

When Phillip was seen alone (they were initially seen together), he professed his continuing love for Tanya but at the same time said that she was not the same person whom he married. He hoped that their active and pleasurable sexual experiences would return and was puzzled by his own diminished sexual desire. He found himself thinking about sexual matters and fantasizing about old girlfriends. He had masturbated regularly before he and Tanya met but not through their courtship and early part of their marriage. He had begun masturbating again in recent months and contrary to his expectations, the frequency had not diminished. He had no idea why his sexual desire for Tanya had seemingly disappeared.

Although little exists in the literature on the sexual impact on partners when one of them becomes ill, the syndrome of diminished sexual interest in the well partner is familiar to sexuality professionals who work with the physically ill in rehabilitation centers (B. Lawrie, personal communication, 2004). The change seems much more evident in men than women, perhaps because men are generally perceived as perpetually sexually interested and ready in a way that is ordinarily unaffected by environmental circumstances. The very fact that men are so influenced by severe illness in a partner suggests that this general perception is exaggerated. In the context of Levine's tripartite definition of sexual desire, men in this instance lose the "motive" to engage in sexual activity with their partner (even though the drive may continue to exist) (2).

Relationship Discord

From both the point of view of clinical impression as well as clinical research, anger resulting from relationship discord seems to have a different effect on sexual desire in men compared with women. An experimental study may bear this out. Twenty-four men and an equal number of women, all university students, were asked to indicate their level of sexual desire in relation to audiotapes describing different sexual events (46). When subjects were presented with a stimulus that provoked anger, the authors found that significantly fewer men (21%) than women (79%), indicated that they would have terminated the sexual encounter.

Psychosocial Issues

Examples of psychosocial issues include: religious orthodoxy, anhedonic or obsessive-compulsive personality traits (accompanied by difficulties displaying emotion as well as discomfort with close body contact), widower's syndrome (found in a man after his partner has died and resulting from attachment to his partner or the unfamiliarity of sexual activity with a new person), lack of attraction to partner, and primary sexual interest in other men (47).

AGE-RELATED HYPOGONADAL SYNDROME: (ANDROPAUSE/ADAM/PADAM)

Terminology and Definitions

"Hypogonadism" refers to the consequences of diminished function of the gonads; occurs at any age and for a variety of reasons; and is classified into two forms on the basis of the source of the problem, that is, either of testicular origin, or as a result of disorder in the hypothalamic-pituitary axis (Fig. 4.3). Sex-related phenomena associated with hypogonadism are described in the "Hormones" section of this chapter.

The term "andropause" indicates a particular type of hypogonadism that is related to aging in men and is said to consist of the following: diminished sexual desire and erectile function, decrease in intellectual activity, fatigue, depression, decrease in lean body mass, skin alterations, decrease in body hair, decrease in bone mineral density resulting in osteoporosis, and increase in visceral fat and obesity (24). The word andropause is an attempt to draw a parallel in men to the experience of menopause in women. Whereas menopause occurs abruptly, andropause is said to occur quite slowly. As well, menopause is associated with the irreversible end of reproductive life, whereas in men spermatogenesis and fertility continue into old age. In the opinion of some observers, trying to equate the two is rather questionable (23).

The existence of andropause is a subject of controversy partly because of great difficulty distinguishing this syndrome from age-related confounding variables such as nonendocrine illnesses (both acute and chronic diseases), poor nutrition (inadequate or excessive food intake), smoking, alcohol use, and medications (24,48). Some observers have less doubt about the existence of a disorder but prefer to use a different name: ADAM (androgen decline in the aging male) (49), or PADAM (partial ADAM which refers to androgen decline that is still within the normal range).

To underline the fact that many hormones decline with age, the word "adrenopause" has also been used to describe the diminution of the adrenal androgens DHEA and DHEAS (see section titled "hormones"), and "somatopause" to describe the same in the somatotrophic hormone, growth hormone (GH).

Diagnosis

Given that andropause/ADAM/PADAM is purported to be one form of hypogonadism, the phenomena described under "Assessment" above in this chapter, applies here as well.

Low sexual desire is usually seen as a symptom of andropause/ADAM/ PADAM. To explain the desire change, a great deal of emphasis has been given to laboratory values, especially alterations in T. However, the typical history has received much less attention. Only one study of aging men seems to have examined various manifestations of sexual desire. Schiavi et al. reported on 77 volunteer couples who responded to an announcement concerning a examination of factors contributing to health, well-being, and marital satisfaction in older men. Three groups of men were compared: 45–54, 55–64, and 65–74. The following were conclusions related to the issue of sexual desire: (i) sexual interest, responsiveness, and activity was noted even among the oldest men; (ii) increasing age was associated with ED, but not with HSDD or PE (premature ejaculation); (iii) the following frequencies consistently decreased with age: desire for sex, sexual thoughts, maximum time uncomfortable without sex, coitus, and masturbation; and (iv) "... the degree of satisfaction with the men's own sexual functioning or enjoyment of marital sexuality did not change with age" (36, pp. 41–53).

As far as the laboratory is concerned, measuring BAT is the preferred parameter for determining hypogonadism, although it is not always available (24). Abnormality is judged by comparing the T level with young adult men (23). "If the testosterone level is below or at the lower limit, it is prudent to confirm the results with a second determination with assessment of LH and . . . FSH."

Etiology

In addition to hormones, many other changes take place in male physiology which contribute to the aging process. One nonsexual example that is cited for the purpose of providing perspective, is the multiple factors which are associated with diminished bone mass and which include: low estradiol (E2), vitamin D deficiency, low GH, low T, poor nutrition, smoking, certain medications, excess alcohol, inactivity, lack of exercise, poor calcium intake, genetic predisposition, and certain illnesses.

TREATMENT

General Considerations

The DSM-IV-TR (6) diagnosis of any sexual dysfunction has four requirements: first, diagnostic subtyping must occur (see "Classification" section in this chapter); second, another Axis I diagnosis be excluded (except another sexual dysfunction); third, an existing medical condition could not explain the dysfunction; and fourth, substance abuse also not be present. In the absence of a thorough assessment (history, physical and laboratory exams when appropriate), the clinician is actually considering a presenting symptom rather than a diagnosis. The two should not be confused. The distinction is crucial.

Treatment follows diagnostic subtyping (Fig. 1). (A) If HSDD is acquired and generalized, the clinician must make substantial efforts towards finding the explanation(s) for the change. HSDD is sometimes (the frequency appears to be unknown) accompanied by another sexual dysfunction, especially ED, and when both occur together, it may be revealing and useful to find out which came first and to act accordingly. One might envision how a lack of sexual desire can cause erectile problems. However, the opposite is not so clear. The extent to which the presence of ED can result in a generalized lack of sexual desire appears to be entirely unknown. (B) If HSDD is lifelong but situational, a biogenic explanation is unlikely and individual psychotherapy undertaken by a mental health professional seems preferred. (C) If HSDD is acquired but situational, a biogenic explanation is, again, unlikely (with the possibly exception of hyperprolactinemia). In this circumstance, psychotherapy seems indicated but depending on the apparent etiology, could be provided individually or together with a partner. (D) If the history reveals that HSDD has been lifelong and generalized, change is unlikely and the clinician should direct therapeutic energy towards helping the person (or, more likely, the couple) to adapt. Kinsey's admonition seems relevant: "...there is a certain skepticism in the profession of the existence of people who are basically low in capacity to respond. This amounts to asserting that all people are more or less equal in their sexual endowments, and ignores the existence of individual variation. No one who knows how remarkably different individuals may be in morphology, in physiological reactions, and in other psychologic capacities, could conceive of erotic capacities (of all things) that were basically uniform throughout a population" (13).

Psychotherapy

O'Carroll surveyed the psychological and medical literature from 1970 to 1989, searching for controlled treatment studies of HSDD. He found eight such reports, two of which involved only men. (Of the other six, two included both men and women as the "identified patient" and four concerned women as the patients together with their partners) (50). His commentary was critical and reflected substantial discouragement in that he found no controlled studies with a homogeneous sample in which psychotherapy was the mainstay of treatment and none which included both drug/hormone treatment and psychotherapy.

Nevertheless, some of what does exist in the literature on the psychotherapy of HSDD in men will be reviewed. Heiman et al. considered studies on the treatment of sexual desire disorders in couples (51). None of the studies involved only men; most referred to the treatment of HSDD in women only, or included reports that referred to both men and women as the "identified patient." Of the three studies that included men with sexual desire difficulties, only one included information concerning diagnostic subtyping (52). The latter investigation reported on a 3-month follow-up of 152 couples in which at least one person had a desire difficulty as part of the presenting complaint. Fifty-eight (38%) of the men had a diagnosis of low sexual desire. Seventeen percent were lifelong and 40% were "global." Numbers of patients were not given in the report. In comparing couples in which either the man or the woman presented with a desire difficulty, the authors concluded that initially there was a lower rate of sexual activity when the man was the "identified patient," that men tended to initiate sexual activity more often, and that men were more likely to have a situational and acquired form of desire difficulty. With a behavioral form of treatment, the authors found at follow-up that significant treatment gains had been made and maintained. In addition, they also claimed that the lifetime/acquired and global/situational distinction "did not predict therapeutic outcome." This latter statement failed to distinguish between couples in which the man or the woman was the identified patient, unfortunate because it is quite conceivable that the distinction has more meaning for one gender than the other.

The review by Heiman et al. described another study involving a 3-year follow-up of 38 couples treated for sexual dysfunction (53). The group included six men identified as having HSDD with or without another sexual dysfunction diagnosis. Thirty-three percent of all the men had a "notable health problem" (it was unclear how many of the six men with HSDD were in this group). In spite of the fact that a diagnostic subtyping system was adopted, it was inexplicably not included in the report. A behavioral form of treatment was used and the results were reported separately for men and women. The authors concluded that "the diagnostically relevant items (that were measured), that is, desire for sexual contact and frequency of sexual contact, clearly demonstrate a lack of sustained success for both men and women."

The Heiman et al. report also included a study by McCarthy of (i) 20 couples in which the results for the men and women were not separately stated and (ii) eight men without partners of whom many reported improvement but the original problems were quite unclear (the example of HSDD given in the report was apparently a result of another sexual dysfunction) (54).

O'Donohue et al. surveyed the sex-related literature on the psychological treatment of male sexual dysfunctions (55). They explicitly excluded studies that relied only on medical intervention. In a clear statement concerning the treatment of sexual desire problems, the authors concluded that "no controlled treatment-outcome studies were found for the treatment of . . . sexual aversion disorder and hypoactive sexual desire disorder . . . in men."

Several studies in the O'Donohue review had a mixture of diagnoses and some included men with HSDD. In one such group the results were not reported separately for men and women. Another looked at 40 couples in which the men experienced erectile dysfunction and/or loss of sexual interest, and compared the effectiveness of three treatments: weekly couple counseling, monthly couple counseling, and T (56). Subjects were divided into two groups, with high or low levels of sexual interest. Each group was randomly allocated to (i) testosterone or placebo therapy and (ii) weekly or monthly counseling. Results indicated no statistically significant group differences in initial clinical ratings and "substantial relapse between the first and second follow-up in the erections ratings and sexual interest ratings." In addition "the frequency of sexual thoughts at the second follow-up were (statistically) significantly greater in the placebo group."

Drugs

O'Carroll's review found only one study in which a drug was used therapeutically by itself for HSDD. The investigation concerned the use of bupropion in a nondepressed population (57). The idea of using bupropion therapeutically resulted from the fact that it is a norepinephrine and dopamine reuptake inhibitor and that dopamine is thought to facilitate many aspects of sexual function including desire. As dopamine is linked to sexual stimulation and pleasure, it was thought that bupropion might be helpful for people with HSDD (58).

The study subjects involved 60 patients of which half were men. All of the patients had low desire and 14/25 men had another sexual dysfunction diagnosis as well. Significantly, more (63%) of the bupropion-treated group reported being much or very much improved (vs. 3% of the placebo group) but changes in the frequency of sexual behavior were "much less dramatic and consisted largely of trends . . .". Unfortunately, results were not reported separately for men and women (an exception being the statement that "more men (86%) than women (44%) showed . . . improvement" with the drug).

Testosterone

Follow-up Investigation

O'Carroll's survey uncovered only one study describing the therapeutic use of a hormone alone. This investigation involved a double-blind crossover comparison of T and placebo in a group of men with normal circulating T levels (59). Ten men complained principally of loss of sexual interest and 10 men complained of erectile failure. The authors found a significant increase in sexual interest produced by T in the first group but qualified this by saying that in only 3/10 of the subjects was it considered to be an "adequate form of treatment," and in the others, "the changes were either small or did not generalize to the sexual relationship." O'Carroll concluded his review by saying that T "may have a modest role to play in the treatment of some men who present with low sexual interest . . ." but he also cautioned others in the interpretation of the data to remember that this study involved a group of only 10 men (50).

Forms of T (21)

T is weakly soluble in water and is therefore poorly absorbed. In addition, T is rapidly metabolized in the liver. For both reasons, there is limited bioavailability via the oral route and so other methods of delivery have been developed: injections and transdermal (patch, and gel). An exception to comments about oral delivery is testosterone undecanoate (available in Europe and Canada at the time this is written) which is absorbed via the lymphatic system and is therefore only partially inactivated in the liver.

Testosterone enanthate and testosterone cyprionate can be given by injection, usually 150–200 mg given every 2–3 weeks (amount and frequency depends on blood level monitoring).

Patches deliver 4–6 mg/day. Scrotal skin (shaved) is highly permeable but concerns have developed over high levels of DHT and therefore nonscrotal patches have been developed. Gel formulations are applied to nongenital skin. Transdermal methods are advantageous in that one could immediately stop the drug if that seems desirable.

Age-Related Hypogonadal Syndrome (Andropause/ADAM/PADAM)

Not only has the validity of an age-related hypogonadal syndrome in men provoked controversy, but it has also raised the issue of whether or not it should be treated with T. In 2002, the National Institute on Aging and the National Cancer Institute asked the Institute of Medicine (IOM) to conduct an independent assessment of the potential benefits and adverse health effects of testosterone therapy in older men and to offer recommendations. The result was the report entitled: "Testosterone and Aging" (21).

Treatment with T is approved for the care of clearly established male hypogonadism—at any age. However, there have been few studies (especially randomized, double-blind, and placebo-controlled) on the use of T in healthy middle-aged or older men who may have a T level in the low range of a young adult but may also have one or more symptoms that are common both to hypogonadism and aging. The IOM report summarized their review of studies on the use of T in older men by cautioning that although finding 31 placebo-controlled trials, the largest sample size involved 108 subjects, the duration of treatment in 25 of the trials was 6 months or less, and only one lasted more than 1 year. In what might be interpreted as understatement, the report concluded that "...assessments of risks and benefits have been limited, and uncertainties remain about the value of this therapy for older men" (21; pp. 1–2).

One can do little better than quote from some the comments and judgements in the IOM report: "Viewed by some as an *anti-aging tonic*, the growth in testosterone's reputation and increased use by men of all ages in the United States has outpaced the scientific evidence about its potential benefits and risks" (p. 11). "Experience with the use of postmenopausal hormone therapy in women and the growing body of scientific evidence about its risks and potential benefits provides an apt and timely example of the need for sustained analysis of short- and long-term effects of new treatments and the caution that must be exercised in widely prescribing drugs as preventive measures. In the meantime, clinicians are searching for therapies, and an enthusiastic and perhaps overly optimistic citizenry is eager to not only treat diseases associated with aging but also possibly delay the timing of their initial onset" (p. 163).

Testosterone Replacement Therapy (TRT): General and Adverse Effects (24)

Sexual: (a) In hypogonadal men: Primary effect appears to be central and on sexual desire (mediated by markedly increased fantasy), rather than peripheral on the genitalia; sleep-related erections are androgen-dependent as is the rigidity of those erections; androgens have no effect on visual erotic stimuli. (b) On eugonadal men: "It is assumed that (normal) men have plasma androgens at concentrations substantially higher than the threshold levels required for behavioral activation"; desire increased without change in sexual behavior (60).

Prostate: Increase in prostate size and in prostate-specific antigen (PSA), but the prostate remains within normal size for eugonadal men and the PSA within normal levels. "The possibility cannot be excluded that promotion of precursor lesions is stimulated by androgens; therefore, androgen substitution should not lead no [sic] superphysiological [sic] plasma levels of androgenic steroids." This warning must make clinicians especially vigilant in view of the fact that incidental prostate cancer is found in 10% of men undergoing surgery for an enlarged prostate. Some believe that a biopsy should be done before initiation of hormonal treatment.

Hematopoiesis: Stimulation of renal production of erythropoietin (by both T and DHT); evidence for a direct effect of androgens on erythropoietic stem cells; androgen receptors have been found in cultured erythroblasts. However, treatment with T does not always lead to problems with polycythemia.

Sleep apnea: Exacerbation of pre-existing sleep apnea; special attention should be given to men who are overweight, heavy smokers, or who have chronic obstructive lung disease.

Gynecomastia: Especially in men with liver or kidney disease.

Body composition: Decrease in body fat; increase in lean body mass; and change in some aspects of muscle strength.

Bone: Increase in bone density and slowing of bone turnover.

Mood and cognition: Improvement in spatial cognition; improvement in sense of well-being.

Body fluid and glucose metabolism: Fluid retention (resulting in worsening hypertension); peripheral edema; congestive heart failure; decrease in fasting blood glucose; decrease in insulin resistance.

Skin: Change in regulation of sebaceous glands and hair growth.

Hyperprolactinemia

Depending on the cause, hyperprolactinemia can be treated medically or surgically.

When the etiology is a prolactin-secreting tumor of the pituitary gland (prolactinoma), then surgery becomes an option. The sooner such a diagnosis is made the better since 40% of patients already have visual field defects at the time of presentation.

Most commonly, hyperprolactinemia is treated medically by using dopamine D2 agonists such as bromocriptine initiated at 2.5 mg/day and titrated up to 25 mg/day, or cabergoline, a longer acting dopamine agonist, starting at 2.5 mg twice a week and increasing to 0.5 mg twice/week (22; p. 34–35). As psychosis is a side effect of bromocriptine it should be used with caution.

Drug-Induced Diminished Desire

- Hyperprolactinemia: (described earlier)
- Strategies for antidepressants (22; p. 60): (i) decrease dosage, (ii) drug holiday, (iii) small dose of neostigmine 7.5–15 mg before intercourse, and (iv) add dopaminergic agent [e.g., bupropion 150 mg/day or more; dextroamphetamine, methylphenidate, permoline (starting with low dose, for example, 5 mg of methylphenidate and titrate up)].
- Cancer chemotherapy: Androgen replacement therapy is often suggested to men who have received high dose chemotherapy associated with bone marrow transplantation.

SUMMARY AND CONCLUSIONS

Some may see it as a truism that men and women are sexually different, but in the latter half of the 20th century there has been a strong effort to view the two as functionally symmetrical. In spite of this attempt at equation, evidence about just how men and women differ, especially in the crucial area of sexual desire, is rapidly accumulating. Although doubtlessly unintentional, investigations of sexual desire in women have shed light on the same in men. These observations have insinuated that the pattern of sexual desire resulting in arousal is more true of men than women (where desire might *follow* arousal), and that sexual desire tends to be quantitatively greater in men.

According to several different studies, at any one time $\sim 16\%$ of men experience HSDD. However, sexual desire manifests in different ways (both psychologically and behaviorally), and it is far from clear just who is included in this 16%. Does it represent, for example, men who have sexual thoughts but do not act on them? Men who act on some occasions but not others (acquired and situational)? Men who had sexual thoughts and feelings in the past but not nowadays (acquired and generalized)? Men who do not have those feelings now and never have thought much about sexual issues (lifelong and generalized)? The tendency of sexual desire in men to decline as they become older has been repeatedly demonstrated. But does this observation mean that an elderly man who experiences diminished sexual desire has HSDD and is part of the 16% (men who are sometimes referred to as having "andropause," "ADAM" or "PADAM"? Or, conversely, should we look at the age-related decline not as pathological, but rather as a "normal" part of the process of becoming older? And who decides the answer? Is this a medical decision made by health professionals or one which is social? Lots of questions and few answers. The "bottom line" is that the definition of HSDD in men in most studies is quite unclear, so one might fairly ask (at least rhetorically): just what are the boundaries surrounding the diagnosis?

Apart from the issue of diagnostic borders, the assessment of HSDD in men is not complicated and involves a few questions in the history about sexual thoughts, fantasies, activities with a partner or oneself, a consideration of health status, and conducting a few laboratory tests. Those procedures will help in the process of subtyping, which, in turn, is essential for determining etiology and treatment.

Each of the subtypes of HSDD has many possible origins. For example, if a man finds that he is completely absorbed sexually at the beginning of a new relationship and not otherwise, or only when watching a computer screen displaying engaging women without clothes, then obviously his sexual desire is quite intact but is highly focussed. In this instance, biomedical speculation about the etiology will not (with the possibly exception of hyperprolactinemia) be fruitful and does not make clinical sense. Thinking in psychosocial ways about etiology and treatment in such an instance will be more productive and, on the basis of clinical experience, intrapersonal issues involving the capacity for intimacy loom large.

If, on the other hand, the man has desire difficulties of relatively recent origin which extend to all circumstances when he would be expected to react with sexual feelings, then a clinician might indeed think about biomedical matters. Medical and psychiatric disorders, or medications used in treatment, appear to be a frequent cause of acquired HSDD. If the man is ostensibly healthy, considering subtle problems like hormone aberrations might prove helpful. Two hormones in particular greatly influence sexual desire, namely, testosterone and prolactin, and both must be scrutinized if the problem is generalized.

Published information on the treatment of HSDD in men who do not have any obvious explanation for their difficulties, leaves clinicians with little guidance. First, diagnostic subtyping is virtually nonexistent. Second, there are no controlled studies on a homogeneous sample of men in which psychotherapy was the mainstay of treatment. As well, a review of the use of couple therapy resulted in pessimistic conclusions. Third, only one placebo-controlled drug study (bupropion in a nondepressed mixed population of men and women) has taken place but fortunately suggested improvement. Fourth, only one study of the use of a hormone (testosterone) alone has occurred but included a mere 10 patients, a fact which even one of the authors decried.

HSDD in men can be an agonizing condition, especially when sexual desire is actually present but is not expressed in a way that involves the patient's partner. The reproductive consequences can be severe. To suggest that more research is needed into this disorder would be an understatement. All aspects of HSDD in men need to be carefully examined, starting with as basic an issue as trying to clarify what is encompassed within the definition.

REFERENCES

1. Masters WH, Johnson VE. Human Sexual Response. Boston: Little, Brown and Co., 1966.
2. Levine SB. The nature of sexual desire: a clinician's perspective. Arch Sex Behav 2003; 32:279–285.
3. Blumstein P, Schwartz P. American Couples. New York: William Morrow and Company, Inc., 1983.
4. Nichols M. Low sexual desire in lesbian couples. In: Leiblum SR, Rosen RC, eds. Sexual Desire Disorders. New York: The Guilford Press, 1988:387–412.
5. Tiefer L. Sex is Not a Natural Act and Other Essays. Boulder: Westview Press, 1995.
6. American Psychiatric Association Diagnostic and Statistical Manual of Mental Disorders, 4th ed. Text Revision. Washington, DC: American Psychiatric Association, 2000:535–582.
7. Basson R. The female sexual response: a different model. J Sex Marital Ther 2000; 26:51–65.
8. Baumeister RF, Catanese KR, Vohs KD. Is there a gender difference in strength of sex drive? Theoretical views, conceptual distinctions, and a review of relevant evidence. Personality Soc Psych Rev 2001; 5:242–273.

9. McKinlay JB, Feldman HA. Age-related variation in sexual activity and interest in normal men: results from the Massachusetts Male Aging Study. In: Rossi AS, ed. Sexuality Across the Life Course. Chicago: The University of Chicago Press, 1994:261–285.

10. Kaplan H. The New Sex Therapy. New York: Brunner/Mazel Inc., 1973.

11. Schnarch D. Constructing the Sexual Crucible: An Integration of Sexual and Marital Therapy. New York: W.W. Norton & Company, Inc., 1991.

12. Maurice WL. Sexual Medicine in Primary Care. St. Louis: Mosby Inc., 1999.

13. Kinsey AC, Pomeroy WB, Martin CE. Sexual Behavior in the Human Male. Philadelphia: W.B. Saunders Company, 1949.

14. Nutter DE, Condron MK. Sexual fantasy and activity patterns of males with inhibited sexual desire and males with erectile dysfunction versus normal controls. J Sex Marital Ther 1985; 11:91–98.

15. Laumann EO, Gagnon JH, Michael RT, Michaels S. The Social Organization of Sexuality: Sexual Practices in the United States. Chicago: The University of Chicago Press, 1994.

16. Laumann EO, Paik A, Rosen RC. Sexual dysfunction in the United States. J Am Med Assoc 1999; 281:537–544.

17. Mercer CH, Fenton KA, Johnson AM, Wellings K, Macdowall W, McManus S, Nanchahal K, Erens B. Sexual function problems and help seeking behaviour in Britain: national probability sample survey. Br Med J 2003; 327:426–427.

18. Frank E, Anderson C, Rubenstein D. Frequency of sexual dysfunction in normal couples. New Engl J Med 1978; 299:111–115.

19. Rosser BRS, Metz ME, Bockting WO, Buroker T. Sexual difficulties, concerns, and satisfaction in homosexual men: an empirical study with HIV prevention implications. J Sex Marital Ther 1997; 23:61–73.

20. Segraves KB, Segraves RT. Hypoactive sexual desire disorder: prevalence and comorbidity in 906 subjects. J Sex Marital Ther 1991; 17:55–58.

21. Institute of Medicine (IOM). Testosterone and Aging: Clinical Research Directions. Washington, DC: National Academies Press, 2004.

22. Segraves RT, Balon R. Sexual Pharmacology: Fast Facts. New York: W.W. Norton & Company, 2003.

23. Kaufman JM, Vermeulen A. Declining gonadal function in elderly men. Bailliere's Clin Endo Metab 1997; 11:289–309.

24. Wespes E, Schulman CC. Male andropause myth, reality, and treatment. Int. J Impot Res 2002; 14(suppl 1):S93–S98.

25. Bremner WJ, Vitiello MV, Prinz PN. Loss of circadian rhythmicity in blood testosterone levels with aging in normal men. J Clin Endo Metab 1983; 56:1278–1281.

26. Bancroft J. Human Sexuality and Its Problems. 2nd ed. London: Churchill Livingstone, 1989.

27. Segraves RT. Hormones and libido. In: Leiblum SR, Rosen RC, eds. Sexual Desire Disorders. New York: The Guilford Press, 1988:271–312.

28. Ganong WF. Physiology of reproduction in women. In: DeCherney AH, Pernoll ML, eds. Current Obstetric and Gynecologic Diagnosis & Treatment. 8th ed. Norwalk: Appleton & Lange, 1994:124–145.

29. Schwartz MF, Bauman JE, Masters WH. Hyperprolactinemia and sexual disorders in men. Biol Psychiatry 1982; 17:861–876.

30. Kolodny RC, Masters WH, Johnson VE. Textbook of Sexual Medicine. Boston: Little Brown, 1979.
31. Everaerd W, Laan ETM, Both S, Van Der Velde J. Male sexuality. In: Szuchman LT, Muscarella F, eds. Psychological Perspectives on Human Sexuality. New York: Wiley, 2000:60–100.
32. Levine S. Sexual Life: A Clinician's Guide. New York: Plenum Press, 1992:37–48.
33. Maurice WL. Sexual potentials and limitations imposed by illness. In: Levine S, Risen C, Althof S, eds. Handbook of Clinical Sexuality for Mental Health Professionals. Boston: Brunner-Routledge, 2003:393–406.
34. Schiavi RC, Schreiner-Engel P, White D, Mandeli J. Pituitary-gonadal function during sleep in men with hypoactive sexual desire disorder and in normal controls. Psychosom Med 1988; 50:304–318.
35. Schreiner-Engel P, Schiavi RC. Lifetime psychopathology in individuals with low sexual desire. J Nerv Ment Dis 1986; 174:646–651.
36. Schiavi RC. Aging and Male Sexuality. Cambridge: Cambridge University Press, 1999.
37. Sarwer DB, Crawford I, Durlak JA. The relationship between childhood sexual abuse and adult male sexual dysfunction. Child Abuse Neglect 1997; 21(7):649–655.
38. Loeb TB, Williams JK, Carmona JV, Rivkin I, Wyatt G, Chin D, Asuan-O'Brien A. Child sexual abuse: associations with the sexual functioning of adolescents and adults. Ann Rev Sex Res 2002; 13:307–345.
39. Kafka M. Hennen J. The Paraphilia-related disorders: An empirical investigation of nonparaphilic hypersexuality disorders in outpatient males. J Sex Marital Ther 1999; 25:305–319.
40. Bullard DG. The treatment of desire disorders in the medically ill and physically disabled. In: Leiblum SR, Rosen RC, eds. Sexual Desire Disorders. New York: The Guilford Press, 1988:348–384.
41. Sorensen AS, Bolwig TG. Personality and epilepsy: new evidence for a relationship? A review. Comp Psychiatry 1987; 28(5):369–383.
42. Kennedy SH, Dickens SE, Eisfeld BS, Bagby RM. Sexual dysfunction before antidepressant therapy in major depression. J Affective Disord 1999; 56:201–208.
43. Kotler M, Cohen H, Aizenberg D, Matar M, Loewenthal U, Kaplan Z, Miodownik H, Zemishlany Z. Sexual dysfunction in male posttraumatic stress disorder patients. Psychother Psychosom 2000; 69:309–315.
44. Lydiard RB, Howell EF, Laraia MT, Ballender JC. Sexual side effects of Alprazolam. Am J Psychiatry 1987; 144:255.
45. Freud S. The transformations of puberty: (3) the libido theory. In: Freud S, ed. On Sexuality: Three Essays on the Theory of Sexuality and Other Works. Middlesex: Penguin Books, 1905/1977.
46. Beck JG, Bozman AW. Gender differences in sexual desire: the effects of anger and anxiety. Arch Sexual Behav 1995; 24:595–612.
47. LoPiccolo J, Friedman JM. Broad-spectrum treatment of low sexual desire: integration of cognitive, behavioral, and systemic therapy. In: Leiblum SR, Rosen RC, eds. Sexual Desire Disorders. New York: The Guilford Press, 1988:107–144.
48. Vermeulen A, Kaufman JM. Diagnosis of hypogonadism in the aging male. The Aging Male 2002; 5:170–176.
49. Morales A, Tenover JL. Androgen deficiency in the aging male: when, who, and how to investigate and treat. Urol Clin North Amer 2002; 29(4):975–982.

50. O'Carroll R. Sexual desire disorders: a review of controlled treatment studies. J Sex Res 1991; 28(4):607–624.
51. Heiman JR, Epps PH, Ellis B. Treating sexual desire disorders in couples. In: Jacobson NS, Gurman AS, eds. Clinical Handbook of Couple Therapy. New York: The Guilford Press, 1995:471–495.
52. Schover LR, LoPiccolo J. Treatment effectiveness for dysfunctions of sexual desire. J Sex Marital Ther 1982; 8:179–197.
53. De Amicis LA, Goldberg DC, LoPiccolo J, Friedman J, Davies L. Clinical follow-up of couples treated for sexual dysfunction. Arch Sex Behav 1985; 14(6):467–489.
54. McCarthy BW. Strategies and techniques for the treatment of inhibited sexual desire. J Sex Marital Ther 1984; 10:97–104.
55. O'Donohue WT, Swingen DN, Dopke CA, Regev LG. Psychotherapy for male sexual dysfunction: a review. Clin Psychol Rev 1999; 19(5):591–630.
56. Bancroft J, Dickerson M, Fairburn CG, Gray J, Greenwood J, Stevenson N, Warner P. Sex therapy outcome research: a reappraisal of methodology 1. A treatment study of male sexual dysfunction. Psychol Med 1986; 16:851–863.
57. Crenshaw TL, Goldberg JP, Stern WC. Pharmacologic modification of psychosexual dysfunction. J Sex Marital Ther 1987; 13(4):239–252.
58. Bartlik B, Kaplan P, Kaminetsky J, Roentsch G, Goldberg J. Medications with the potential to enhance sexual responsivity in women. Psychiatric Annal 1999; 29:46–52.
59. O'Carroll R, Bancroft J. Testosterone therapy for low sexual interest and erectile dysfunction in men: a controlled study. Br J Psychiatry 1984; 145:146–151.
60. Schiavi R. Androgens and sexual function in men. In: Oddens BJ, A Vermeulen A, eds. Androgens and the Aging Male. New York: The Parthenon Publishing Group, 1996:111–125.

5

Sexual Aversion Disorder

Jeffrey W. Janata and Sheryl A. Kingsberg

*Case Western Reserve University School of Medicine,
University Hospitals of Cleveland, Cleveland, Ohio, USA*

INTRODUCTION

Crenshaw (1) has been credited for first describing the sexual aversion syndrome. Her description, published in 1985, remains one of two comprehensive manuscripts describing this disorder, joined only by Kaplan's 1987 book (2), Sexual Aversion, Sexual Phobias and Panic Disorder. Kaplan suggested that sexual aversion is best conceptualized as encompassing a dual diagnosis, sexual anxiety and panic disorder. Kaplan believed that one must treat the underlying organic panic disorder with medication before addressing the sexual aversion. Her model served to de-emphasize the aversion elements of the diagnosis in favor of the panic component. Seen in historical context, however, she had identified the biological underpinnings of the sexual disorders in ways that current conceptual formulations take for granted. Recently, others have again underscored the relationship between sexual aversion and panic disorder (3).

Despite this early work, sexual aversion disorder is often overlooked in the spectrum of sexual disorders. Although it was first recognized as a diagnosis in 1984, with the publication of DSM-III-R (4), relatively little has been written about the etiology and treatment of sexual aversion. Often considered a variant of an anxiety disorder, sexual aversion was not included in any of the earlier DSM editions. Although it finally achieved diagnostic status as a sexual disorder in 1984, it is often ignored or pushed to a secondary status within the field of sex therapy. A review of the most widely used sex therapy handbooks rarely finds any text that devote a chapter solely to sexual aversion. Most include some explanation of aversion in the context of understanding hypoactive desire, the impact of sexual abuse, or vaginismus and dyspareunia.

Sexual aversion disorder is sometimes referred to as sexual phobia. Gold and Gold (5) argued against the latter descriptor, noting that aversion implies an element of abhorrence and disgust, while phobia does not. In our experience, sexual aversion routinely is clinically characterized by revulsion and disgust in ways that phobias only rarely are. Nonetheless, according to DSM-IV-TR (6) criteria, sexual aversion does not require the physiologic responses that we often associate with aversion. While sexual aversion typically encompasses these responses (e.g., nausea, revulsion, shortness of breath), aversion by these criteria can also be expressed as simple avoidance of partnered sexual behavior and a panic response to engaging in partnered sexual activity.

Aversion is a conditioned response that applies to many behaviors. Aversion may be best recognized as the conditioned response that develops in response to cancer chemotherapeutic agents. In this context, aversion implies more than phobic avoidance; aversion is characterized by nausea and vomiting. In contrast, however, others writing on sexual aversion (7) maintain that sexual aversion is equivalent to sexual phobia—the essential diagnostic feature is persistent fear and avoidance.

From our perspective, conditioned aversion is perhaps best understood using Mowrer's two-factor theory (8). Mowrer theorized that two separate learning processes contribute to avoidance conditioning. A conditioned emotional response results from pairing a previously neutral or positive stimulus (sexual behavior) with a painful or traumatic event (and thus is classically conditioned). Having been paired with discomfort, the sexual stimuli now produce aversive emotional reactions (e.g., anxiety, revulsion, disgust) in the absence of the original painful stimulation. The later conditioned avoidance response is operantly conditioned (negatively reinforced) in that avoidance of sexual stimulation eliminates or reduces the aversive response. Sexual aversion, from the two-factor avoidance perspective, can be conceptualized as maintained by this avoidance response.

Sexual aversions can be general or quite specific (2). Aversions can develop in response to any sexual stimulus, overt or covert, such that a patient may present with a circumscribed aversion to a highly specific sexual thought or behavior, or may exhibit more global revulsion to sexuality in any form.

Incidence and prevalence of sexual aversion disorder are not known, despite being considered widespread by several overviews (1,5). In addition, diagnostic criteria do not address gender differences in prevalence. Gold and Gold (5) describe the typical etiologic model for the development of aversion in women to be sexual abuse, while the etiologic model for men in their view is performance anxiety. Our clinical experience is that significantly more women than men meet the criteria for sexual aversion disorder. Ponticas (9) hypothesizes that this gender distinction may be an artifact. Men with sexual aversion disorder are likely to resist entering relationships and thereby avoid the resulting relationship conflict that might lead them into therapy. Moreover, more women with sexual aversion disorder may present clinically due to the overlap in etiology and diagnostic criteria with hypoactive sexual desire disorder which has a much greater prevalence in women than in men.

Since the criteria for sexual aversion disorder overlap with symptoms of both panic disorder and hypoactive sexual desire disorder, even experts in treating sexual disorders remain somewhat unclear regarding how and when to diagnose sexual aversion.

Diagnostic Criteria

DSM-IV-TR (6) includes sexual aversion disorder in its Sexual and Gender Identity Disorders classification (Table 5.1).

In response to these criteria, The Sexual Function Health Council of the American Foundation for Urologic Disease convened the Consensus Development Panel on Female Sexual Dysfunction (10). Their stated belief was that DSM-IV is limited to mental disorders and thus too narrow to provide a useful, broad diagnostic classification for female sexual dysfunction.

Two of the panel's proposed amendments to the DSM-IV criteria are relevant to sexual aversion. While the DSM-IV criteria emphasize "interpersonal distress," the panel preferred to emphasize "personal distress" as critical to the

Table 5.1 DSM-IV-TR Criteria for Sexual Aversion Disorder (302.79)

A. Persistent or recurrent extreme aversion to, and avoidance of, all (or almost all) genital sexual contact with a sexual partner
B. The disturbance causes marked distress or interpersonal difficulty
C. The sexual dysfunction is not better accounted for by another Axis I disorder (except another sexual dysfunction)

diagnosis. Second, the panel specifically distinguished between psychogenic and organically based disorders. This revised classification system includes sexual aversion under the category of sexual desire disorders along with hypoactive sexual desire disorders (Table 5.2).

The consensus panel developed a very detailed document to describe and justify their new classification system. Sexual aversion disorder, however, was given little attention and by virtue of being placed in the category of sexual desire disorders, is likely to be overlooked.

DSM-IV-TR distinguishes between lifelong (primary) and acquired (secondary) sexual aversion. This is a distinction that, in light of Mowrer's two-factor theory (8), is difficult to defend. From the perspective of learning theory, aversion must, by definition, be acquired. Lifelong sexual aversion must still have been acquired at some point along the way. Crenshaw (1) defines lifelong aversion as a negative or unenthusiastic response to sexual interactions from earliest memories to present. However, no matter how absent the memory of life before the aversion, the aversion was certainly learned, either directly or vicariously. Crenshaw observes that patients presenting with primary aversion often were raised in strict religious and moral environments, which supports our contention that the aversion was learned, albeit vicariously. She also suggests that there may have been some history of psychosexual trauma, which again would have been learned and not lifelong.

We suggest that these early authors may have intended that "primary" refers to aversion developed so early in life that the individual did not have the opportunity to experience normal partnered sexual behavior before acquiring the aversion. Cases in the literature described as examples of primary aversion [e.g., case history of Bridgitte and Ms. C (2) and case histories 1 and 2 (1)] typically involve early, presexual negative conditioning of sex in childhood, mediated by environmental learning but specifically not by sexual abuse. Secondary aversion, in contrast, would be diagnosed in cases of specific recollection of childhood abuse or later negative sexual experience that is the proximate cause of current sexual aversion.

Table 5.2 1999 Consensus Classification of Female Sexual Dysfunction

I. Sexual desire disorders
A. Hypoactive sexual desire disorder
B. Sexual aversion disorder
II. Sexual arousal disorder
III. Orgasmic disorder
IV. Sexual pain disorders
A. Dyspareunia
B. Vaginismus
C. Other sexual pain disorders

It is further possible that this "secondary" descriptor has been maintained in the taxonomies because sexual aversion has been confounded with hypoactive sexual desire. Hypoactive sexual desire may legitimately be either a biologic or a learned condition. The biologic contribution could well have been present since birth or early in life and thereby represent a "primary" or lifelong condition. Moreover, a patient with hypoactive sexual desire may become avoidant of sexual activity. Sexual disinterest in the context of the demands of a relationship could evolve into irritation or anger and appear clinically very much like aversion. This presentation, however, would be absent in the fear and anxiety response to sexual behavior, which is critical for the aversion diagnosis.

PROPOSED SEXUAL AVERSION CRITERIA REVISION

Given the difficulties inherent in the current classification systems for sexual aversion disorder (DSM-IV-TR and the 1999 Consensus Classification), we have proposed (11) a revised classification system that is based on a modification of these taxonomies. This proposed classification maintains the distinction between primary and secondary sexual aversion. However, this distinction will only be useful for the diagnostic differentiation of the acquisition of aversion early in life and the lifelong presence of hypoactive sexual desire (Table 5.3).

With this modified taxonomy in mind, we will describe a case of primary sexual aversion.

Case Example: Joyce

Joyce is a 38-year-old woman who has been married for 8 years. She presents with a long, intermittent history of bulimia and other features consistent with

Table 5.3 Elements of the Current Classification System (DSM-IV-TR) for Sexual Aversion Disorder and a Proposed Revision to the Classification System

Diagnosis	
	Current DSM-IV-TR criteria
Lifelong (primary sexual aversion)	Lifelong anxiety, fear, or disgust to sexual stimuli
Acquired (secondary sexual aversion)	Acquired anxiety, fear, or disgust to sexual stimuli
	Proposed revised criteria
Primary sexual aversion	Acquisition of fear, anxiety, or disgust *before* the development of healthy sexual interactions with a partner
Secondary sexual aversion	Acquisition of fear, anxiety, or disgust *after* the development of healthy sexual interactions with a partner

obsessive–compulsive spectrum disorder. Her bulimic symptoms responded rather readily to an exposure-based cognitive behavioral treatment strategy. Over the course of therapy she gradually was able both to cease purging and to expose herself to foods she had previously restricted and to situations she had avoided.

During the course of treatment she eventually acknowledged a history of sexual abuse as an early adolescent. She had denied any abuse history during the initial evaluation, but was able to reveal her history as she became more trusting of and comfortable with her therapist. She reported that she had never revealed her abuse to anyone other than a cousin and that her immediate family, including her husband, were unaware of her history of abuse.

Joyce is the second child in a close family that includes her and two siblings. She describes her parents as caring and involved, yet not particularly emotionally disclosing. She categorizes her family as supportive and celebrative of personal successes while tending to avoid discussion of emotionally difficult issues. Joyce reports feeling that if she had revealed her abuse, her parents would be devastated and retrospectively guilty over not having protected her better as a child.

Joyce reports that her abuse represented her first sexual experiences. When she was 12 a 17-year-old neighbor began seeking her out during neighborhood games and activities, encouraging her to spend increasing amounts of time with him. Joyce was friendly with his siblings and naturally trusting of him. He became increasingly sexually aggressive, progressing from touching her relatively quickly to forced fellatio and intercourse, and she recalls feeling that she did not want to resist him for fear that he would be disappointed or angry with her. The abuse continued for about 2 years until, at age 14, she threatened to inform his parents of his actions and he ceased his abuse of her. He left for college shortly thereafter.

Joyce began dating at age 15 and was sexually active "fairly quickly" in each of a succession of relationships. She describes herself as promiscuous throughout high school and college. The majority of her relationships are characterized by relatively early onset of physical intimacy, which included intercourse and oral sex (both fellatio and cunnilingus). Sexual behavior always began as pleasurable for her but fairly rapidly became unpleasant. She reports that she felt very sexually attracted to her male partners initially, but at the point in the relationship that sex became routine or expected, her responsiveness declined and sexual behavior became aversive to her. Intercourse became painful and disgusting to her and she experienced revulsion at even the idea of sex with her current partner. Importantly, she maintained sexual drive such that she masturbated to orgasm on a regular (once a week) basis and she also continued to experience sexual attraction and desire for men other than her partner.

She met her future husband, Bill, when she was 28. As in other relationships, she was attracted to him and initially had a pleasurable and fulfilling sexual relationship with him. She experienced desire arousal and orgasm when they were sexual. She was frustrated when their sex became aversive to her but decided to "tough it out," assuming, she supposes in retrospect, that her sexual response would improve given enough time and love. Joyce also hoped that the state of being married would also help her response since she had some guilt over nonmarital sex and expected to feel a postmarital reduction in the anxiety she associated with sexual behavior. She married Bill after dating for 2 years.

Joyce reports that at no point during marriage did her sexual aversion dissipate. On the contrary, Bill became increasingly frustrated with her avoidance of sex and demanded more frequent intercourse. Joyce's attempts to explain her aversive response to him were not helpful and he became irritated and verbally abusive of her. At the point that she disclosed her history of sexual abuse in therapy, she and Bill were in considerable marital distress. Their frequency of intercourse had declined to roughly monthly, and then only with considerable endurance of distress from Joyce and verbal intimidation from Bill.

Case Discussion

Joyce's symptoms meet the DSM-IV-TR criteria for sexual aversion, evidencing persistent and recurrent avoidance of sexual genital contact with her husband, which causes marked personal and interpersonal distress and which is not better accounted for by another psychiatric disorder. Joyce also meets the Consensus Panel criteria that emphasize personal rather than partner distress as the relevant feature. Her symptoms are clearly related to the acquisition of fear and subsequent avoidance. Joyce did not evidence or report particular fear or avoidance of sexual interactions until sexual behavior was paired with abuse and victimization. She retained sexual drive and desire even while she felt pressured into sex in each of her relationships after her childhood sexual abuse. In each case, including her marriage, sexual interactions after the early relationship phase (limerance) became negatively conditioned. Joyce acquired an aversion response which then was maintained by sexual avoidance.

General Treatment Considerations

In Joyce's case, effective treatment first required relating her history of sexual abuse to her husband, Bill, so that we could begin to interpret her aversion to him in the context of her adolescent experience. This revelation evoked some sensitivity to Joyce's response from Bill and temporarily tempered his insistence on intercourse. We used this period to assess more fully their sexual history, to describe her sexual disorder to them both, and to develop a treatment plan. The theory and methods that characterize systematic desensitization were reviewed and the couple agreed to the treatment plan.

Cognitive Behavioral Treatment

The literature on treatment of sexual aversion emphasizes the usefulness of cognitive behavioral treatment approaches (9,12) and there is support for the practical and relatively brief use of systematic desensitization (13). In this case, treatment consisted first of the creation of a hierarchy of aversion- and anxiety-provoking images, ranging from masturbation, which evoked the least anxiety, to intercourse, which evoked the greatest anxiety. In addition, Joyce was taught diaphragmatic deep breathing and an autogenic relaxation technique. The least anxiety-provoking stimuli were addressed first, with Joyce imagining each situation and reporting being able to remain relaxed and anxiety-free before each stimulus was subsequently approached *in vivo*. Importantly, sexual situations were designed to remain fully in her control; Bill had agreed to allow Joyce to determine the rate at which each of the items on the hierarchy was engaged. Fifteen sessions conducted over a period of 5 months were needed to help Joyce and Bill resume the healthier sexual life that had characterized their early history.

The persistence of avoidance behavior was first articulated by Freud (14); Mowrer (15) subsequently described this phenomenon as the neurotic paradox. The common observation that avoidance is remarkably difficult to extinguish has been explained by the theory of conservation of anxiety. The theory suggests that individuals learn rapid avoidance over time, which prevents the elicitation of fear. It is further suggested that if fear is not elicited it will not extinguish.

The theory of conservation of anxiety explains why sexual aversion rarely abates on its own and can be so treatment resistant. Crenshaw (1) posits that the sexual aversion syndrome is progressive and rarely reverses spontaneously. Patients like Joyce are treatable in so far as they are willing to purposefully expose themselves to the anxiety accompanying sexual behavior. We have found (11) that this exposure process can be facilitated by the following:

1. the clinician's conceptualizion of the patient's sexual aversion in clear behavioral terms, emphasizing how aversion is acquired and maintained;
2. the patient's ability to verbalize an understanding of the ways in which aversion is acquired and maintained. This understanding should allow her to generate specific examples of the process of exposure;
3. the patient maintaining records of anxiety and aversion symptoms during the treatment process and the clinician referring to those records frequently during sessions. We have found that patients are likely to adhere to record-keeping instructions to the degree that clinicians make those records integral to the process of psychotherapy;
4. emphasis on maintenance and generalization as the therapy draws to a close to address relapse issues.

Insight-Oriented Treatment

Psychodynamic psychotherapy, with its emphasis on deeper conflicts, defense mechanisms, and transference, is considered to be the treatment of choice for those patients who report psychic pain as a component of their sexual aversion or who conceptualize their problems as symptomatic of early childhood issues (16). Patients who desire insight and express psychological curiosity about themselves are particularly likely to benefit from insight-oriented treatment.

There is evidence that sexual aversion may be predicted by a history of childhood sexual abuse. Noll et al. (17), utilizing a prospective design, demonstrated a relationship between childhood sexual behavior problems and subsequent sexual aversion, and found evidence that abuse by the biological father particularly predicted later sexual aversion. In clinical practice, patients with such a history may well benefit from desensitization approaches in conjunction with more traditional, uncovering psychotherapy.

The literature on psychodynamic approaches to sexual aversion emphasizes the integration of behavioral strategies and insight-oriented approaches (2). In clinical practice, this combined approach typically takes one of two forms. First, psychodynamic therapists recognize the utility of behavioral strategies and integrate them into their treatment regimens. Second, interestingly, it is often the case that patients who embark on a behavioral treatment will find that the process of behavior change itself begins to stimulate internal exploration. "Behavior change leads to insight" is at least as commonly observed in practice as the more familiar notion that "insight leads to behavior change." These patients are likely to pursue psychodynamic psychotherapy after completion of a course of cognitive behavioral psychotherapy.

In the case example above, the aversion response was gradually desensitized and she was able to resume and maintain a healthy sexual relationship with her husband. This psychotherapeutic process stimulated her desire to better understand her history of abuse and the psychological trauma that followed. As the behavioral treatment of her sexual aversion neared its completion, the therapeutic strategy moved to the development of insight into the effects of her childhood and adolescent trauma.

Pharmacology

Unfortunately, the usefulness of pharmacotherpay in the treatment of sexual aversion has not been adequately explored in the literature. Kaplan (2) describes the use of monoamine oxidase inhibitors (MAOIs) and tricyclic antidepressants for treating sexual aversion disorder, commenting on the well-established efficacy of these medications in the treatment of panic. Subsequently, of course, selective serotonin reuptake inhibitors (SSRIs) have also been demonstrated to be effective in treating panic and may, therefore, have a role in the treatment of sexual aversions. Importantly, anorgasmia is a potential side-effect of SSRIs, but patients will sometimes find it preferable to aversion.

In our case example, Sertraline was an important adjunct to Joyce's treatment. She reported that the medication helped decrease her distress as she engaged in the exposure process. She felt that her use of relaxation strategies to modulate anxiety was aided somewhat when the SSRI was added, and she attributed a general improvement in her mood to the medication as well.

In practice, as illustrated in this case, cognitive behavioral, psychodynamic, and pharmacotherapeutic strategies are often integrated very effectively as each approach serves to enhance and augment the others.

CONCLUSION

Sexual aversion disorder clearly represents an overlooked topic in the sexual disorders literature. Our concern is that the diagnostic criteria have been sufficiently vague and overlapping with hypoactive sexual desire, to leave clinicians and researchers confused about how and when to make an accurate diagnosis. We have proposed a revision to the diagnostic criteria, which may help both to better define sexual aversion disorder and to distinguish it more clearly from hypoactive sexual desire.

In our proposed revision, primary aversion would be diagnosed when an individual's initial sexual experience, either directly or vicariously, is negative. Secondary aversion is to be diagnosed when the patient has had normal, pleasurable sexual development and experiences until a traumatic or painful experience, either direct or vicarious, negatively reconditions sexual interactions with a partner.

With advances in diagnostic clarity, better estimates of incidence and prevalence can be obtained. Anecdotal evidence suggests that this disorder is more prevalent than many clinicians may be aware, particularly in men, who may not be as likely to present for treatment as are women.

REFERENCES

1. Crenshaw TL. The sexual aversion syndrome. Journal of Sex and Marital Therapy 1985; 11:285–292.
2. Kaplan HS. Sexual Aversion, Sexual Phobias, and Panic Disorder. New York: Brunner/Mazel, 1987.
3. Figueira I, Possidente E, Marques C, Hayes K. Sexual dysfunction: a neglected complication of panic disorder and social phobia. Archives of Sexual Behavior 2001; 30:369–377.
4. American Psychiatric Association. DSM-III-R: Diagnostic and Statistical Manual of Mental Disorders. 3rd ed. Washington, DC: American Psychiatric Press, 1987.
5. Gold SR, Gold RG. Sexual aversions: a hidden disorder. In: O'Donohue W, Greer JH, eds. Handbook of Sexual Dysfunctions: Assessment and Treatment. Needham Heights, MA: Allyn & Bacon, 1993.
6. American Psychiatric Association. DSM-IV-TR: Diagnostic and Statistical Manual of Mental Disorders. 4th ed. Washington, DC: American Psychiatric Press, 2000.
7. Katz RC, Jardine D. The relationship between worry, sexual aversion, and low sexual desire. Journal of Sex and Marital Therapy 1999; 25:293–296.

8. Mowrer OH. On the dual nature of learning—a reinterpretation of "conditioning" and "problem-solving." Harvard Educational Review 1947; 17:102–148.

9. Ponticas Y. Sexual aversion versus hypoactive sexual desire: a diagnostic challenge. Psychiatric Medicine 1992; 10(2):273–281.

10. Basson R, Berman J, Bernett A, Derogatis L, Ferguson D, Fourcroy F, Goldstein I, Graziottin A, Heiman J, Laan E, Leiblum S, Padma-Nathan H, Rosen R, Seagraves K, Seagraves R, Shabsigh R, Sipski M, Wagnor G, Whipple B. Report of the international consensus development conference on female sexual dysfunction: definitions and classifications. Journal of Urology 2000; 163:888–893.

11. Kingsberg SA, Janata JW. Sexual aversions. In: Levine SB, Althof SE, Risen CB, eds. Handbook of Clinical Sexuality for Mental Health Professionals. Philadelphia/London: Brunner/Routledge, 2003.

12. Crenshaw TL, Goldberg JP, Stern WC. Pharmacological modification of psycho-sexual dysfunction. Journal of Sex and Marital Therapy 1987; 13:239–252.

13. Finch S. Sexual aversion disorder treated with behavioral desensitization (letter). Canadian Journal of Psychiatry 2001; 46(6):563–564.

14. Freud S. The problem of anxiety. New York: The Psychoanalytic Quarterly Press, W.W. Norton & Co, 1936.

15. Mowrer OH. Learning theory and the neurotic paradox. American Journal of Orthopsychiatry 1948; 18:571–610.

16. Roth S. Psychotherapy: The art of wooing nature. Northvale, NJ: Jason Aronson Inc., 1990.

17. Noll JG, Trickett PK, Putnam FW. A prospective investigation of the impact of child-hood sexual abuse on the development of sexuality. Journal of Consulting and Clinical Psychology 2003; 71(3):575–586.

6

Female Sexual Arousal Disorder*

Ellen Laan and Walter Everaerd

University of Amsterdam, Amsterdam, The Netherlands

Stephanie Both

*Leiden University Medical Centre, Leiden, The Netherlands
and University of Amsterdam, Amsterdam, The Netherlands*

---

*The part on the history of women's sexuality has previously been published in Everaerd W, Laan E, Both S, van der Velde J. Female Sexuality. In: Szuchman LT, Muscarella F, eds. Psychological Perspectives on Human Sexuality. New York: John Wiley & Sons, 2000:101–146.

"THE MAIDEN MUST BE KISSED INTO A WOMAN"

Most pharmacological treatments that are currently being developed for women with sexual arousal disorder are aimed at remedying a vasculogenic deficit. In a study we did in the late 1990s we compared pre- and postmenopausal women with and without sexual arousal disorder, diagnosed according to strict DSM-IV criteria (1). Women with any somatic or mental comorbidity were excluded. This study investigated whether pre- and postmenopausal women with sexual arousal disorder were less genitally responsive to visual sexual stimuli than pre- and postmenopausal women without sexual problems. From the findings of this study we concluded that in such women, sexual arousal disorder is unrelated to organic etiology. In other words, we are convinced, from this and other studies to be reviewed, that in women without any somatic or mental comorbidity, impaired genital responsiveness is not a valid diagnostic criterion. The sexual problems of women with sexual arousal disorder are not related to their potential to become genitally aroused. We propose that in healthy women with sexual arousal disorder, lack of adequate sexual stimulation, with or without concurrent negative effect, underlies sexual arousal problems. This view is at odds with the dominant view on male sexual arousal problems.

In the history of sexological science, the study of women's sexuality has been neglected, or has been obscured by comparisons with sexuality of men. In textbooks, descriptions of women and men's sexuality were often aimed at increasing awareness of similarities in physiological and psychological mechanisms (2). Even today, as will be shown later in this chapter, clear conceptualizations of women's sexual problems and dysfunctions seem hindered by dominance of the "male model."

For a long time, the general idea in western culture has been that although women may have a disposition for sexual feelings, in decent and healthy women these feelings will only be aroused by a loving husband. "In women . . . , especially in those who live a natural and healthy life, sexual excitement also tends to occur spontaneously, but by no means so frequently as in men. (...) In a very large number of women the sexual impulse remains latent until aroused by a lover's caresses. The youth spontaneously becomes a man; but the maiden—as it has been said—'must be kissed into a woman'" (3, p. 241). Stekel believed that it was a man's task to awaken sexual feelings in a woman, a responsibility that should not be taken lightly. "As a matter of fact it is the duty of every man whose wife is unfortunately anaesthetic to investigate for himself his marital partner's erogenous zones, adroitly, carefully until he discovers the areas or positions which are capable of rousing his wife's libido and of bringing on her orgasm during intercourse" (4, p. 133). He disapprovingly remarked: "There are men so brutally blunt and so selfish that they take no trouble to study their wives so as to become acquainted with their erogenous zones and learn to meet their particular desires" (p. 130). About half a century earlier, a book entitled *The Functions and Disorder of the Reproductive Organs* by W. Acton, a surgeon (5), passed through many editions and was popularly regarded as a standard authority on the subjects with which it dealt. The book was almost solely concerned with men; the author evidently regarded the function of reproduction as exclusively appertaining to men. He claimed that women, if "well brought up," are, and should be, absolutely ignorant of all matters concerning it. "I should say," this author remarked, "that the majority of women (happily for society) are not very much troubled with sexual feeling of any kind." The supposition that women do possess sexual feelings he considered "a vile aspersion."

It was not until the late 18th century, however, that the above view had become the dominant one. For thousands of years prior to this, scholars had assumed that conception could not take place without the woman becoming sexually aroused and having an orgasm (6, pp. 2–3). Thus, sexual pleasure for women was not only accepted, but also essential. Yet, although sexual feelings in women were acknowledged, they were not always considered to be unproblematic. Shorter summarized the prevalent view of women's sexuality in the Middle Ages as follows: "Women are furnaces of carnality, who time and again will lead men to perdition, if given a chance. (...) Because the flame of female sexuality could snuff out a man's spirit, women had sexually to be broken and controlled" (7, pp. 12–13).

Ellis had distinctive opinions about differences between women and men concerning the physiological mechanisms involved in sexuality (3). In men, the process of tumescence and detumescence was considered to be simple. In women "we have in the clitoris a corresponding apparatus on a small scale, but behind this has developed a much more extensive mechanism, which also demands satisfaction, and requires for that satisfaction the presence of various conditions that are almost antagonistic.... It is the difference, roughly speaking, between a lock and a key.... We have to imagine a lock that not only requires a key to fit it, but should only be entered at the right moment, and, under the best conditions, may only become adjusted to the key by considerable use" (p. 235). It seems that phrases such as "an extensive mechanism behind the clitoris" served to conceal ignorance about physiological facts. Even today, scholars acknowledge that "it is glaringly obvious that we know so little about sexual arousal that we cannot answer some of the most elementary questions about the . . . human genital function" (8, p. 3).

In his excellent book on the role of the body in female sexuality, Laqueur (6) demonstrated that conceptions about human sexuality were not the result of scientific progress. Instead, he argued, they were part of social and political changes, "explicable only within the context of battles over gender and power" (p. 11). Feminists have long criticized the notion that the behavior and abilities of women are uniquely determined by their biology. This criticism led to an almost total rejection of the role of biology in the construction of gender (9). It also contributed to an image of female sexuality devoid of the body. Masters and Johnson (10) were the first to carefully study and describe the genital and extragenital changes that occurred in sexually aroused women. Tiefer critiqued the suggestion of the human sexual response cycle as a universal model for sexual response, not in the least because the concept of sexual desire was not included in the model, therewith eliminating "an element which is notoriously variable within populations" (11, p. 4). She argued that the human sexual response cycle, with its genital focus, neglects women's sexual priorities and experiences. Indeed, Masters and Johnson did not assess the subjective sexual experience of the 694 men and women who were studied. Their emphasis on peripheral physiology, particularly the genital vasocongestive processes associated with sexual response, may reflect the influence of primarily male-dominated theorizing and research in sexology, with its inevitable emphasis on penile–vaginal sexual contact. Tiefer wondered why problems such as "too little tenderness" or "partner has no sense of romance" were excluded (11). These problems have been frequently reported by women (12). The sexual response cycle model assumes men and women have and like the same kind of sexuality. Yet, various studies show that women care more about affection and intimacy, and men care more about sexual gratification in sexual relationships (13). There seems to be support for the cliché "Men give love to get sex, and women give sex to get love." Men and women are raised with different sets of sexual values. Tiefer concludes that focusing on the physical aspects of sexuality and ignoring other aspects of the sexual response cycle favors men's value training over women's.

Recently, there has been a growing awareness of the limitations of the "male model" for understanding women's sexuality (14–16). In this chapter, we will review the current definitions of female sexual arousal disorder (FSAD) and the prevailing difficulties in pinpointing the etiology of the problems clients present. We will then present our view on the activation and regulation of women's sexual responses, which is derived from modern emotion and motivation theories, underlining differences with men's sexual responses. We will briefly discuss treatment options, and we will end with a few recommendations for clinical practice that follow from our analysis.

REVIEW OF CURRENT STATUS OF KNOWLEDGE

Epidemiology

Little research has been conducted on the prevalence of FSAD. A recent review by Simons and Carey (17) estimated the prevalence of sexual dysfunction in the population based on all prevalence studies that have appeared in the 1990s. Although 52 studies have been conducted in that decade, most studies lack sufficient methodological rigor. Only a handful of studies have used unambiguous criteria for assessing female sexual dysfunction. The frequently cited study by Laumann et al. (18) for instance, yielded an overall female sexual dysfunction prevalence figure of 43%. The study was done in a large, representative sample, but the prevalence figure was based on an affirmative response to one of seven sexual complaints. On the basis of simple yes/no answers to a problem area it cannot be established whether one is suffering from a sexual dysfunction or whether one is experiencing common sexual difficulties (19). Besides, recent studies show that even when psychometrically sound assessment techniques are used, prevalence figures of the occurrence of sexual dysfunctions are much higher than prevalence figures of the occurrence of sexual dysfunctions that cause personal or interpersonal distress (20–22). Simons and Carey therefore conclude that for most female sexual dysfunctions, stable community estimates of the current prevalence are unavailable. Only for female orgasmic disorder reliable community prevalence estimates were obtained, ranging from 7 to 10%. Given the difficulties in differentiating between FSAD and female orgasmic disorder (FOD), as will be discussed subsequently, this may be a reasonable estimate for FSAD as well.

Anatomy and Physiology

Clitoris and Surrounding Erectile Tissue

There is a considerable density of tactile receptors in the clitoris. The anterior vaginal wall is also rich in tactile receptors. Freud (23) entertained a developmental idea about excitability to explain how "a little girl turns into a woman." He argued that from the onset of puberty, libido increases in boys; at the same time, in girls, "a fresh wave of repression" occurs that affects "clitoridal sexuality." This finite period of "anasthesia," Freud thought, was necessary to enable successful transferrence of a girl's erotogenic susceptibility to stimulation from the clitoris to the vaginal orifice. Even though his suggestion that there are also tactile receptors in the anterior vaginal wall is correct, there is no evidence that the anterior wall becomes excitable at the expense of clitoral sensitivity. Contrary to Freud's belief, there is ample evidence that women who learned to know their own sexuality through masturbation are able to transfer this knowledge (or skill) to coital stimulation with a partner (12). For a long time, ideas similar to those of Freud have been used to suppress masturbation in girls and women. Even today there are many women with a partner, who feel guilty when masturbating.

The clitoris contains two stripes of erectile tissue (corpora cavernosum) that diverge into the crura inside the labia majora. On the basis of recent anatomical studies, O'Connell et al. (24) proposed to rename these structures as bulbs of the clitoris. They found that there is erectile tissue connected to the clitoris and extending backwards, surrounding the perineal part of the urethra. However, most anatomical facts have been known for a long time (25). The clitoris' parasympathethic innervation comes from lumbosacral segments L2–S2, while its sympathetic supply is from the hypogastric superior plexus. The pudendal and hypogastric nerves serve its sensory innervation. It responds with increased blood flow and tumescence on being stimulated through sexual arousal. Nitric oxide synthase (NOS), among many other neuropeptides, has been identified in the complex network of nerves in the clitoral tissue (26).

The Anterior Vaginal Wall

When Masters and Johnson (10) published their account of the physiology of the sexual response, they opposed Freud's theory of the transition of erogeneous zones in women. According to these famous sexologists, nerve endings in the vagina are extremely sparse. Therefore, during coital stimulation the clitoris is stimulated indirectly, possibly through the movement or friction of the labia. Hite's data supported this point of view. Almost all women who reached orgasm through stimulation from coitus alone had experienced orgasm through masturbation. Many women needed additional manual stimulation to orgasm during coitus, and an even larger number was unable to orgasm during coitus at all (12).

Apparently, coitus alone is not a very effective stimulus for orgasm in women. In 1950, Grafenberg (25) provided an alternative to Masters and Johnson's explanation for the relative ineffectiveness of coitus to induce orgasm. He described an area of erectile tissue on the anterior wall of the vagina along the course of the urethra, about a third of the way in from the introitus and below the base of the bladder. Strong digital stimulation of this zone would activate a rapid and high level of sexual arousal which, if maintained, induced orgasm. This paper was ignored until 1982, at which time this area was renamed as the G-spot (27). According to Levin (28), however, there is no convincing scientific evidence for the presence of either a unique G-spot with its own plexus of nerve fibers or for the fluid that is often expelled when orgasm is reached from stimulation of this area being anything other than urine. Because it is difficult to see how strong stimulation of this "G-spot" would not also stimulate other erogeneous structures such as the urethra and clitoral tissue, Levin argues that the whole area should be regarded as the "anterior wall erogeneous complex." Grafenberg pointed out that coitus in the so-called missionary position (ventral–ventral) prevents stimulation of the anterior vaginal wall and would therefore not be optimally sexually arousing for women. Instead, contact with the anterior wall is "very close, when the intercourse is performed more bestiarum or a la vache that is, a posteriori"

(25, p. 148). Thus, Grafenberg's suggestion was not that coitus itself is an ineffective sexual stimulus for women, but only coitus in the missionary position.

Sensitivity of the entire vaginal wall has been explored in several studies. Weijmar Schultz et al. (29) used an electrical stimulus for exploration under non-erotic conditions. This study confirms sensitivity of the anterior vaginal wall, even though sensitivity of this area was much lower than that of the clitoris.

Central Nervous System and Spinal Chord Pathways

Neural and spinal components of female sexual arousal anatomy have been examined in animals and spinal cord-injured (SCI) women only. There is strong evidence for the occurrence of sexual arousal and orgasm in women with SCI who have an intact S5–S5 reflex arc. Not only were genital and extra-genital responses to vibrotactile stimulation similar between able-bodied and SCI subjects in a recent study of Sipski et al. (30), subjective descriptions of sensations were indistinguishable between groups. SCI subjects did take longer than able-bodied subjects to achieve orgasm. Whipple and Komisaruk (31) suggested that, on the basis of their studies in SCI women in whom cervical stimulation was applied, the vagus nerve conveys a sensory pathway from the cervix to the brain, bypassing the spinal cord, which is responsible for the preservation of sexual arousal and orgasm in these women.

There remain large gaps in our understanding of the central nervous control of female sexual function. Most of the animal work relates to receptive behavior in female rats and very little to the control of genital responses. According to McKenna (32), the autonomic and somatic innervation of the genitals is based upon spinal mechanisms, modulated by supraspinal sites. Sensory information from the genitals project to interneurons in the lower spinal cord, which possibly generate the coordinated activity of sexual responses. The spinal reflex mechanisms are under inhibitory (through serotonergic activity) and excitatory (through adrenergic activity) control from supraspinal nuclei. These nuclei are highly interconnected. Many of them also receive genital sensory information. It is likely that during sexual activity, sensory activation of supraspinal sites causes a decrease in the inhibition, and an increase in the excitation of the spinal reflex-ive mechanisms by the supraspinal sites. Higher order sensory and cognitive processes may modulate the activity of supraspinal nuclei controlling sexual function.

Diagnosing FSAD

FSAD refers to inhibition of the "vasocongestion–lubrication response" to sexual stimulation (1). In the most recent edition of the Diagnostic and Statistical Manual of Mental Disorders (DSM-IV-TR), FSAD (302.72) is defined as the pervasive or recurrent inability to attain, or to maintain until completion of the sexual activity, an adequate lubrication–swelling response of sexual excitement, coupled with marked distress or interpersonal difficulty (1). The DSM classification of sexual disorders has been derived from phases of the sexual response cycle, on the basis of the work of Masters and Johnson (10) and Kaplan (33). This model depicts a sexual desire phase and a subsequent sexual arousal phase, characterized by genital vasocongestion, followed by a plateau phase of higher arousal, resulting in orgasm and subsequent resolution. It is assumed in this model that women's sexual response is similar to men's, such that women's sexual dysfunction in DSM-IV mirrors categories of men's sexual dysfunction. In contrast to the third edition of the DSM manual, subjective sexual experience is no longer part of the definition, possibly in a further attempt to match norms and criteria for men's and women's sexual dysfunctions (34).

There are a number of serious problems with the current DSM-IV classification criteria. Firstly, although the DSM-IV explicitly requires the clinician to assess the adequacy of sexual stimulation only when considering the diagnosis of FOD, adequacy of sexual stimulation is a critical variable in evaluating each of the female sexual dysfunctions, and FSAD in particular. Exactly what is adequate sexual stimulation? Some sort of physical (genital) stimulation is a necessary, but not necessarily sufficient, prerequisite for arousal. For many women, adequate sexual arousal involves physical as well as "psychological" and "situational" stimulation, such as intimacy with a partner, the exchange of confidences, the sharing of hopes and dreams and fears, and not only directly prior to the sexual event (35). What if certain types of sexual stimulation have been adequate in the past, but not anymore? Is it evidence of FSAD, or could it be explained in terms of habituation or an adaptation to changing life circumstances? (16) And what is meant by "completion of the sexual activity?" Is it masturbation to orgasm, sexual contact with a partner, sexual contact including coitus? These are very different activities that are known to differ in their sexually arousing qualities (12).

Secondly, the description of the first problem demonstrates that clinical judgements are required about sexual stimulation and the severity of the problem, the validity of which is questionable. The clinician has to evaluate what is normal, based on age, life circumstances, and sexual experience. Research on the basis of which clear criteria can be formulated, is lacking. There is a great variety in the ease with which women can become sexually aroused and which types of stimulation are required (36).

Thirdly, due to the lack of clear diagnostic criteria, it is often unclear in which cases an FSAD diagnosis or one of the other three main DSM-IV diagnoses is appropriate. The four primary DSM-IV diagnoses pertaining to lack of desire, arousal, orgasm problems or sexual pain, are not independent. Only very infrequently do women present with sexual arousal problems when seeking help for their sexual difficulties, but that does not mean that insufficient sexual arousal is an unimportant factor in the etiology of these difficulties. In actual clinical practice, classification is often done on the basis of the way in which complaints are presented (36). If the woman is complaining of lack of sexual desire, the diagnosis of hypoactive sexual desire disorder is easily given. If she reports trouble reaching orgasm or cannot climax at all, FOD is the most likely diagnosis. If she reports pain during intercourse, or if penetration is difficult or impossible, the clinician may conclude that dyspareunia or vaginismus is the most accurate diagnostic label. In general, women have difficulty perceiving genital changes associated with sexual arousal (37). However, women who report little or no desire for sexual activity, lack of orgasm, or sexual pain, may in fact be insufficiently sexually aroused during sexual activity. It is particularly difficult to differentiate between FSAD and FOD. FOD is defined as the persistent or recurrent delay in, or absence of, orgasm following a normal sexual excitement phase (1). In cases where the clinician does not have access to a psychophysiological test in which a woman is presented with (visual and/or tactile) sexual stimuli, while genital responses are being measured, it cannot be established that her deficient orgasmic response occurs despite a normal sexual excitement phase, *unless* she reports feelings of sexual arousal. Ironically, this subjective criterion has been removed in the DSM-IV.

Studies investigating the efficacy of psychological treatments for sexual dysfunction have demonstrated that directed masturbation training combined with sensate focus techniques (38) is very effective for women with primary anorgasmia to become orgasmic. In fact, this is the only psychological treatment of sexual dysfunctions that deserves the label "well established," and is probably efficacious in secondary orgasmic disorder (39). The success of this treatment suggests that lack of adequate sexual stimulation is an important etiological factor underlying primary, and probably also secundary, anorgasmia. Consequently, if the clinician would strictly adhere to the DSM-IV criteria, the diagnosis of neither FSAD nor FOD would be appropriate, because the problem can be reversed by adequate sexual stimulation. In any case, primary orgasmic problems may not justify a separate diagnostic category. Perhaps the diagnosis of FOD should be restricted to those women who are strongly sexually aroused but have difficulty surrendering to orgasm (40). There are no clinical or epidemiological studies that differentiate between women with primary or secondary anorgasmia and other orgasm problems, so we do not know how prevalent this is. Segraves (41) argued that FSAD hardly exists as a distinct entity, whereas we, in contrast, argue that in a classification system based on the etiology of sexual complaints, FSAD should be considered to be the most important female sexual dysfunction, with complaints of lack of desire and orgasm, and pain, frequently being consequences of FSAD.

Finally, there is a good deal of evidence that, especially for women, physiological response does not coincide with subjective experience. Women's subjective experience of sexual arousal appears to be based more on their appraisal of the situation than on their bodily responses (37). We will address this issue extensively later in this chapter. Thus, in the DSM-IV definition of FSAD, probably the most important aspect of women's experience of sexual arousal is neglected, given that absent or impaired genital responsiveness to sexual stimuli is the sole diagnostic criterion for an FSAD diagnosis.

Is Absent or Impaired Genital Responsiveness a Valid Diagnostic Criterion?

In a recent study we investigated whether pre- and postmenopausal women with sexual arousal disorder are less genitally responsive to visual sexual stimuli than pre- and postmenopausal women without sexual problems (42). Twenty-nine women with sexual arousal disorder (15 premenopausal and 14 postmenopausal), without any somatic or mental comorbidity, diagnosed using strict DSM-IV criteria, and 30 age-matched women without sexual problems (16 premenopausal and 14 postmenopausal) were shown sexual stimuli depicting cunnilingus and intercourse. Genital arousal was assessed as vaginal pulse amplitude (VPA) using vaginal photoplethysmography. We found no significant differences in mean and maximum genital response between the women with and without sexual arousal disorder, nor in latency of genital response. The women with sexual arousal disorder were no less genitally responsive to visual sexual stimuli than age- and menopausal status-matched women without such problems, even though they had been carefully diagnosed, using strict and unambiguous criteria of impaired genital responsiveness. These findings are in line with previous studies (43–45). The sexual problems these women report were clearly not related to their potential to become genitally aroused. In medically healthy women absent or impaired genital responsiveness is not a valid diagnostic criterion.

It is clear that the sexual stimuli used in this laboratory study (even though these stimuli were merely visual) were effective in evoking genital response. In an ecologically more valid environment (e.g., at home), sexual stimuli may not always be present or effective. Sexual stimulation must have been effective at one point in the participants' lives, because primary anorgasmia was an exclusion criterion. Even though a serious attempt was made to rule out lack of adequate sexual stimulation as a factor explaining the sexual arousal problems, data on sexual responsiveness collected in the anamnestic interview suggested that the women diagnosed with sexual arousal disorder are unable, in their present situation, to provide themselves with adequate sexual stimulation. The exclusion, halfway through the study, of a participant who no longer met the criteria for sexual arousal disorder after having met a new sexual partner, also illustrates that inadequate sexual stimulation may be one of the most important reasons for sexual arousal problems.

In this study, genital responses did not differ between the groups with and without sexual arousal disorder, but sexual feelings and affect did. The women with FSAD reported weaker feelings of sexual arousal, weaker genital sensations, weaker sensuous feelings and positive affect, and stronger negative affect in response to sexual stimulation than the women without sexual problems. Two explanations may account for this. Firstly, women with sexual arousal disorder may differ from women without sexual problems in their appreciation of sexual stimuli. These stimuli, even though they were effective in generating genital response, evoked feelings of anxiety, disgust, and worry. These negative feelings may have downplayed reports of sexual feelings, and were probably evoked by the sexual stimuli and not by the participants becoming aware of their genital response, because reports of genital response were unrelated to actual genital response. Negative appreciation of sexual stimuli may extend to, and perhaps even be amplified in, real-life sexual situations, because in such situations, any negative affect (i.e., towards the partner or the sexual interaction) may be more salient. Negative affect may, therefore, be partly responsible for the sexual arousal problems in the women diagnosed with sexual arousal disorder.

Secondly, women with sexual arousal disorder may be less aware of their own genital changes, with which they lack adequate proprioceptive feedback that may further increase their arousal. The general absence of meaningful correlations between VPA and sexual feelings in this and other studies (see next section) supports this notion. Perhaps women with sexual arousal disorder have less intense feedback from the genitals to the brain; there are no data, at present, to substantiate this idea. It is impossible to decide which of these explanations is more likely, because in real-life situations it can never be established with certainty that sexual stimulation is adequate, and awareness of genital response is dependent upon the intensity of the sexual stimulation. In addition, these explanations are not mutually exclusive. We can conclude, however, that the sexual problems of the women with sexual arousal disorder are not related to their potential to become genitally aroused. We propose that in healthy women with sexual arousal disorder, lack of adequate sexual stimulation, with or without concurrent negative affect, underlies the sexual arousal problems.

Organic etiology may underlie sexual disorders in women with a medical condition. There are only a handful of studies that have employed VPA measurements in women with a medical condition. The only psychophysiological study to date that found a significant effect of sildenafil on VPA in women with sexual arousal disorder was done in women with SCI (46), suggesting that in this group there was an impaired genital response that can be improved with sildenafil. Another study compared genital response during visual sexual stimulation of women with diabetes mellitus and healthy women, showing that VPA was significantly lower in the first group (47). A very recent study measured VPA in medically healthy women, in women who had undergone a simple hysterectomy, and in women with a history of radical hysterectomy for cervical cancer (48). Only in the last group was VPA during visual sexual stimuli impaired, whereas the women with simple hysterectomies reported to experience more sexual problems than the other two groups. Not presence of sexual arousal problems but presence of a medical condition that influences sexual response may therefore be the most important determinant of impaired genital responsiveness (49).

Medical conditions that have been associated with sexual arousal disorder, other than SCI and diabetes, are pelvic and breast cancer, multiple sclerosis, brain injury, and cardiac disease (50). Mental disorders such as depression may also interfere with sexual function. It is important to consider the direct biological influence of disease on sexual pathways and function, but equally important is the impact of the experience of illness. Disease may change body presentation and body esteem; ideal sexual scenarios may be disturbed by constraints that accompany illness. In many patients, sexual arousal and desire may decrease in connection with grief about the loss of normal health and uncertainty about illness outcome (51). Damage to the autonomic pelvic nerves, which are not always easily identified in surgery to the rectum, uterus, or vagina, is associated with sexual dysfunction in women (52,53). Medications such as antihypertensives, selective serotonine reuptake inhibitors, and benzodiazepines, as well as chemotherapy, most likely due to chemotherapy-induced ovarian failure, impair sexual response (50). In addition, the incidence of women complaining of lack of sexual arousal increases in the years around the natural menopausal transition. According to Park et al. (54), postmenopausal women with sexual complaints, who are not on estrogen replacement therapy, are particularly vulnerable to what they call a vasculogenic sexual dysfunction. However, psychophysiological and preliminary functional magnetic resonance imaging studies of increases in genital congestion in response to erotic stimulation, fail to identify differences between pre- and postmenopausal women (55–57). This would suggest that although urogenital aging results in changes in anatomy and physiology of the genitals, postmenopausal women preserve their genital responsiveness when sufficiently sexually stimulated. The vaginal dryness and dyspareunia experienced by some postmenopausal women may result from longstanding lack of sexual arousal/protection from pain previously afforded by estrogen related relatively high blood flow in the unaroused state (58).

Diagnostic Procedures

An ideal protocol for the assessment of FSAD should be constructed following theoretical and factual knowledge of the physiological, psychophysiological, and psychological mechanisms involved. The protocol then describes the most parsimonious route from presentation of complaints to effective therapy. Unfortunately, we are at present far from a consensus on the most probable causes of FSAD. Despite this disagreement, at least two diagnostic procedures should be considered. Firstly, assessment of sexual dysfunction in a biopsychosocial context should start with a verification of the chief complaints in a clinical interview. The aim of the clinical interview is to gather information concerning current sexual functioning, onset of the sexual complaint, the context in which the difficulties occur, and psychological issues that may serve as etiological or maintaining factors for the sexal problems, such as depression, anxiety, personality factors, negative self- and body image, and feelings of shame or guilt that may result from religious taboos. Sexual problems are common complications of anxiety disorders and impaired sexual desire, arousal and satisfaction. Laboratory studies suggest potential enhancement of genital arousal by some types of anxiety, but the precise cognitive, affective, or physiological processes by which anxiety and women's sexual function are related have as yet to be identified (50). The ongoing work of Bancroft and Janssen (59) exploring a dual control model of sexual excitation and inhibition in men as well as in women, may clarify any role of anxiety in women's predisposition to sexual inhibition and to sexual excitement. One of the most important but difficult tasks is to assess whether inadequate sexual stimulation is underlying the sexual problems, which requires detailed probing of (variety in) sexual activities, conditions under which sexual activity takes place, prior sexual functioning, and sexual and emotional feelings for the partner. Several studies have shown that negative sexual and emotional feelings for the partner are among the best predictors for sexual problems (16,60). The clinician should always ask if the woman has ever experienced sexual abuse, as this may seriously affect sexual functioning (61). Some women do not feel sufficiently safe during the initial interview to reveal such experiences; nevertheless, it is necessary to inquire about sexual abuse to make clear that traumatic sexual experiences can be discussed. The initial clinical interview should help the clinician in formulating the problem and in deciding what treatment is indicated. An important issue is the agreement between therapist and patient about the formulation of the problem and the nature of the treatment. To reach a decision to accept treatment, the patient needs to be properly informed about what the diagnosis and the treatment involve.

Ideally, in the case of suspected FSAD, the initial interviews is followed by a psychophysiological assessment. In assessment of the physical aspects of sexual arousal, the main question to be answered is whether, with adequate stimulation by means of audiovisual, cognitive (fantasy), and/or vibrotactile stimuli, a lubrication–swelling response is possible. Although psychophysiological testing to date is not a routine assessment, we feel that such a test is crucial in establishing the etiology of FSAD for two reasons. The study that was discussed extensively in the previous paragraph (42) demonstrated how difficult it is to rule out that sexual arousal problems are not caused by a lack of adequate sexual stimulation. Secondly, it showed that impaired genital response cannot be assessed on the basis of an anamnestic interview. Women with sexual arousal disorder may be less aware of their own genital changes, with which they lack adequate proprioceptive feedback that may further increase their arousal. If a genital response is possible, even when other investigations indicate the existence of a variable that might compromise physical responses, an organic contribution to the arousal problem of the individual women is clinically irrelevant. As was shown before, sexual arousal problems in medically healthy women are most likely more often related to inadequate sexual stimulation due to contextual and relational variables than to somatic causes. For estrogen deplete women, care must be taken not to simply facilitate painless intercourse in the nonaroused state with a lubricant but to consider the possibility that estrogen lack has unmasked long-term lack of sexual arousal that is of contextual etiology. Of note, nonresponse in the psychophysiological assessment does not automatically imply organicity. The woman may have been too nervous or distracted for the stimuli to be effective, or the stimuli offered may not have matched her sexual preferences. This problem of suboptimal sensitivity is not unique to this test, many other well established diagnostic tests of this nature have a similar disadvantage (62).

Two other procedures could be used to corroborate findings from the clinical interview and the psychophysiological assessment. The first is the use of self-report measures supplementary to the clinical interview. The Female Sexual Function Index (FSFI) is a brief, multidimensional scale for assessing sexual function in women, and is currently the most often used measure. Recently, diagnostic cutoff scores were developed by means of sophisticated statistical procedures (63). Self-report measures are not very useful for clinical purposes because they lack sensitivity and specificity with regard to causes of the individual patient's dysfunction.

Secondly, a careful focused pelvic exam in medically healthy women may be in order when lack of arousal is accompanied by complaints of pain or vaginistic response during sexual activity, or when a psychophysiological assessment has yielded nonresponse. In the latter case, rare diseases such as connective tissue disorder, can be identified. In the former cases the purpose of the exam may be more educational than medical, for instance to observe the consequences of pelvic floor muscle activity (50). An examination that found no abnormalities may also be of therapeutic value. Sometimes a general physical examination, including central nervous system or hormone levels is necessary (64), but in most of the cases only genital examination is required. In women with neurological disease affecting pelvic nerves or with a history of pelvic trauma, a detailed neurological genital exam may be necessary, clarifying light touch, pressure, pain, temperature sensation, anal and vaginal tone, voluntary tightening of anus, and vaginal and bulbocavernosal reflexes (50). The clinician should be aware of the emotional impact of a physical examination and the importance of timing. When a woman is very anxious about being examined it may be appropriate to wait until she feels more secure. In the case of women who are not familiar with self-examination of their genitalia, it is preferable to advice self-examination at home before a doctor carries out an examination. It is recommended that the procedure is explained in detail, what will and what will not take place, and the woman's understanding and consent obtained. It is important to realize that any medical exam is not able to examine *function*, because the genitalia are examined in a nonaroused state. As such, a medical exam can never replace a psychophysiological assessment.

ACTIVATION AND REGULATION OF SEXUAL RESPONSE

Processing of Sexual Information

In a series of studies we conducted in the 1990s [see Ref. (14) for a review], we consistently found that women's genital response and sexual feelings are not strongly correlated, and that affect influences sexual feelings. Other studies had similar findings (43–45,47–49,65). In men, correlations between genital response and sexual feelings are usually significantly positive, suggesting that for men's sexual feelings awareness of their genital response is the most important source.

A surprising finding from our studies was the ease with which healthy women become genitally aroused in response to erotic film stimuli. When watching an erotic film depicting explicit sexual activity, most women respond with increased vaginal vasocongestion. This increase occurs within seconds after the onset of the stimulus, which suggests a relatively automatized response mechanism for which conscious cognitive processes are not necessary. Even when these explicit sexual stimuli are negatively evaluated, or induce little or no feelings of sexual arousal, genital responses are elicited. Genital arousal intensity was found to covary consistently with stimulus explicitness, defined as the extent to which sexual organs and sexual behaviors are exposed (66). This automatized response occurs not only in young women without sexual problems, but also in women with a testosterone deficiency (67), in postmenopausal women (68,69), and in women with sexual arousal disorder (42). Such responses are also found during unconsensual sexual activity (70).

Such a highly automatized mechanism is adaptive from a strictly evolutionary perspective. If genital responding to sexual stimuli did not occur, our species would not survive. For women, an increase in vasocongestion produces vaginal lubrication, which obviously facilitates sexual interaction. One might be tempted to assume that, for adaptive reasons, the explicit visual sexual stimuli used in our studies represent a class of unlearned stimuli, to which we are innately prepared to respond. These stimuli seem to override the effects of various attempts at voluntary control (71).

Emotional stimuli can evoke emotional responses without the involvement of conscious cognitive processes (72). For instance, subliminal presentation of slides with phobic objects results in fear responses in phobic subjects (73). Before stimuli are consciously recognized and processed, they are evaluated, for instance as being good or bad, attractive or dangerous. According to Öhman (74), the evolutionary relevance of stimuli is the most important prerequisite for such a quick, preattentive analysis. Perhaps sexual stimuli fall within this category and can they be unconsciously evaluated and processed. A number of experiments in which sexual stimuli were presented subliminally to male subjects showed that this is indeed possible [see Ref. (72) for a review]. Preattentive processing of sexual stimuli occurs in women as well, but appears to be dependent upon the type of prime. Explicit sexual primes do not lead to priming-effects, but romantic sexual primes do (75). This seems to contradict Öhman's notion that evolutionary relevant primes can be unconsciously processed. Likely, preattentive processing is not entirely governed by evolution, but partly the result of overlearning or conditioning.

A prerequisite of automatic processing seems to be that sexual meaning resulting from visual sexual stimuli is easily accessible in memory. On the basis of a series of priming experiments Janssen et al. (76) presented an information processing model of sexual response. Two information processing pathways are distinguished (cf. 77). The first pathway is about appraisal of sexual stimuli and response generation. This pathway is thought to depend largely on automatic or unconscious processes. The second pathway concerns attention and regulation. In this model, sexual arousal is assumed to begin with the activation of sexual meanings that are stored in explicit memory. Sexual stimuli may elicit different memory traces depending upon the subject's prior experience. This in turn activates physiological responses. It directs attention to the stimulus and ensures that attention remains focused on the sexual meaning of the stimulus. This harmonic cooperation between the automatic pathway and attentional processes eventually results in genital responses and sexual feelings. Disagreement between sexual response components would occur, according to this model, when the sexual stimulus elicits sexual meanings but also nonsexual, and more specifically, negative emotional meanings. The sexual meanings activate genital response, but the balancing of sexual and nonsexual meanings determine to what extent sexual feelings are experienced.

The fact that disagreement between genital and subjective sexual arousal occurs more often in women might suggest that for women sexual stimuli have, more often than for men, sexual but also nonsexual or even negative meanings. There is some evidence that sexual stimuli generate negative sexual meanings in women more often than in men (78,79). Sexual stimuli evoke mostly positive sexual emotions in men, but a host of other nonsexual meanings, both positive and negative, in women.

Sexual Feelings

Emotions are not determined by distinctive stimuli, but by the meaning the stimulus has aquired over time. Recently, Damasio (80) introduced in this context the term "emotionally competent stimulus," referring to the object or event whose presence, actual or in mental recall, triggers emotion. While there are biologically relevant stimuli that are innately pleasurable or aversive, most stimuli will acquire meaning through classical conditioning. As a consequence, meanings of stimuli depend on the individual's past experience, and may differ from one individual to another. Stimuli may have conveyed several meanings, and meanings relevant for different emotions may be present at the same time. Moreover, the value of a stimulus may differ over time since it will be influenced by the current internal state of the organism. Thus, the rewarding value of a stimulus is dependent on the current internal state, and on prior experience with that stimulus.

There is an increasing notion that emotional responses are automatic and precede feelings (80,81). Damasio stresses that all living organisms are born with devices designed to solve automatically, without proper reasoning required, the basic problems of life. He calls this equipment of life governance the "homeostasis machine." At the basis of the organization of that machine are simple responses like approach or withdrawal of the organism relative to some object, and increases or decreases in activity. Higher up in the organization there are competitive or cooperative responses. The simpler reactions are incorporated as components of the more elaborated and complex ones. Emotion is high in the organization, with more complexity of appraisal and response. According to Damasio, an emotion is a complex collection of chemical and neural responses forming a distinctive pattern. When the brain detects an emotionally competent stimulus, the emotional responses are produced automatically. The result of the responses is a temporary change in the state of the body, and in the brain structures that map the body and support thinking. Damasio (80) and LeDoux (81), and a long time before them James (82), stress that the conscious experience of emotion, what we call feelings, is the result of the perception of these changes. In this view, feelings are based on the feedback of the emotional bodily and brain responses to the brain; they are the end result of the whole "machinery of emotion."

Recently, functional imaging studies showed that the subjective experience of various emotions such as anger, disgust, anxiety, and sexual arousal is associated with activation of the insula and the orbitofrontal cortex (83–86). It has been suggested that the insula is involved in the representation of peripheral autonomic and somatic arousal that provides input to conscious awareness of emotional states. It appears that the feedback of autonomic and somatic responses are integrated in a so-called meta-representation in the right anterior insula, and this meta-representation seems to provide the basis for "the subjective image of the material self as a feeling entity, that is emotional awareness" (83).

In men and women alike, meanings of a sexually competent stimulus will automatically generate a genital response, granted the genital response system is intact. The difference between men and women in experienced sexual feelings have to do with the relative contribution of two sources. The first source is the awareness of this automatic genital response (peripheral feedback), which will be a more important source for men's sexual feelings than for women's sexual feelings (87). For women, a stronger contribution to sexual feelings will come from a second source, the meanings generated by the sexual stimulus. In other words, women's sexual feelings will be determined to a greater extent by all kinds of (positive and negative) meanings of the sexual stimulus than by actual genital response.

Canli et al. (88) found support for the idea that emotional stimuli activate explicit memory more readily in women than in men. They asked 12 women and 12 men, during functional MRI, to rate the intensity of their emotional arousal to 96 pictures ranging from neutral to negative. After 3 weeks, they were given an unexpected memory task. It was found that women rated more pictures as highly negatively arousing than did men. The memory task revealed that women had better memory for the most intensely negative pictures. Exposure to the emotional stimuli resulted in left amygdala activation in both sexes, the central brain structure for implicit memory (77). In women only, the left amygdala and right hippocampus were activated during the most emotionally arousing stimuli that were also recognized 3 weeks later. Explicit memory is situated in the neocortex and is mediated by the hippocampus (89). These findings may suggest that in processing emotional stimuli, explicit memory is more readily accessible in women. If these findings would hold for sexual stimuli, we may have a neural basis for our suggestion that sexual stimuli activate explicit memory in women, and that the different meanings sexual stimuli may have, influence sexual feelings.

Gender Differences in Sexual Feelings

Our hypothesis is that in women other (stimulus or situational) information beyond stimulus explicitness determines sexual feelings, whereas for men peripheral feedback from genital arousal (and thus stimulus explicitness) is the most important determinant of experience of sexual arousal. This hypothesis fits well with the observed gender difference in response concordance. It coincides with Baumeister's assertion that women evidence greater erotic plasticity than men (90). After reviewing the available evidence on sexual behavior and attitudinal data of men and women, he concluded that women's sexual responses and sexual behaviors are shaped by cultural, social, and situational factors to a greater extent than men's.

Both women's and men's sexuality are likely to be driven by an interaction of biological and sociocultural factors. Evolutionary arguments often invoke differential reproductive goals for men and women (91). The minimal reproductive investment for females is higher than for males. Given these reproductive differences, it would have been particularly adaptive for the female, who has a substantial reproductive investment and a clearer relationship to her offspring, not only to manifest strong attachments to her infants but also to be selective in choosing mates who can provide needed resources. This selectivity mandates a complex, careful decision process that attends to subtle cues and contextual factors. Consistent with men's and women's reproductive differences, Bjorklund and Kipp proposed that cognitive inhibition mechanisms evolved from a necessity to control social and emotional responses (92). Women are better at delaying gratification and in regulating their emotional responses. Beauregard et al. (93) showed the involvement of the prefrontal cortex in the regulation of sexual arousal. They induced sexual arousal by sexual film and imaged brain activity. Subjects were asked to inhibit their emotional responses to the film. The fMRI data show that confrontation with a sexual stimulus resulted in activation of the emotional circuit in the brain, while inhibition of the response was coupled with activation of prefrontal areas.

The emotional significance of events or situations, in addition to the evolutionary point of view, can be put in perspective by looking at the sorts of actions that are instigated by the emotional valence of "sexual" events or situations. These actions, as is predicted by motivation theories, are connected with the satisfaction of concerns, which need not necessarily be sexual, such as satisfaction from orgasm, but may also involve intimacy or bonding. Sexual stimuli, through negative experience, may be associated with aversion and thus turn off any possibility for positive arousal (94). Sustained sexual arousal, which may increase in intensity, must be satisfying in itself or predict the satisfaction of other concerns. This idea also implies that, depending on the circumstances, there may be nonsexual concerns that attract attention with greater intensity, and thus detract attention from sexual stimuli.

What is a Sexual Dysfunction?

The experimental evidence and theoretical notions presented earlier strongly suggest that for women, sexual dysfunction is not about genital response. The women in our study who were diagnosed with FSAD according to strict DSM-IV criteria (42) turned out not to be sexually dysfunctional according to these same criteria because their genital response was not impaired. This study demonstrated that it is difficult to be sure that sexual arousal problems are not caused by a lack of adequate sexual stimulation, and that impaired genital response cannot be assessed on the basis of an anamnestic interview. This implies that the current DSM-IV criteria for sexual arousal disorder, which states that genital (lubrication/swelling) response is strongly impaired or absent, is unworkable. For most women, even those without sexual problems, it is difficult to accurately assess genital cues of sexual arousal, but this is exactly what the DSM-IV definition of sexual arousal disorder requires. The group of women the DSM-IV refers to may even be virtually nonexistent. Medically healthy women who have complaints of absent or low arousal but are genitally responsive, given adequate sexual stimulation, do not qualify for a sexual arousal diagnosis according to DSM-IV. Women with a somatic condition explaining the sexual arousal difficulties do not qualify for one of the four primary diagnoses, including FSAD, either, even though, as we have argued, the presence of a somatic condition that affects sexual response may be the most important predictor for impaired genital responsiveness. In medically healthy women impaired genital responsiveness is not a valid diagnostic criterion. Consequently, we believe that the DSM-IV criteria for sexual arousal disorder are in need of revision.

A first consensus meeting on the definitions and classifications of female sexual problems in 1998 did not generate a significantly different classification system but did propose to replace the "marked distress and interpersonal difficulty" criterion of DSM-IV with a "personal sexual distress" criterion (95). Bancroft, Loftus and Long subsequently investigated which sexual problems predicted sexual distress in a randomly selected sample of 815 North American heterosexual women aged 20–65, who were sexually active (16). The best predictors were markers of general emotional and physical well being and the emotional relationship with their partner during sexual activity. Sexual distress was not related to physical aspects of sexual response, including arousal, vaginal lubrication, and orgasm. The study provided data supporting the possibility that relationship disharmony may cause impaired sexual response rather than the opposite. The authors concluded that the predictors of sexual distress do not fit well with the DSM-IV criteria for the diagnosis of sexual dysfunction in women. These findings are in line with the problems with DSM-IV that were discussed in this chapter. When one believes, as we do, that the problems that generate most sexual distress deserve most of our research and clinical attention, the current focus of DSM-IV on genital response is unjustified. The choice of DSM-IV to exclude women with a somatic condition from the four primary diagnoses of sexual disfunction seems unwarranted as well, because women with such a condition reported highest levels of sexual distress. On the other hand, a high sexual distress score does not automatically implicate sexual dysfunction.

When should we consider a sexual problem to be a sexual dysfunction? The objective and medical connotation of the word "dysfunction" has probably promoted the choice for impaired genital responsiveness as the criterion for an arousal disorder in DSM-IV. In this chapter, we have argued that many women with a medical condition have sexual problems that may or may not be caused by the disease directly, but that the sexual problems of healthy women are better explained by lack of adequate sexual stimulation and sexual and emotional closeness to their partner. Similarly, Tiefer (96) has presented a "New View of Women's Sexual Problems" that strives to de-emphasize the more medicalized aspects of sexual problems that currently prevail, and that looks at "problems" rather than at dysfunctions [see also Refs. (19,97)]. Bancroft (98) argues that a substantial part of the sexual problems of women are a logical, adaptive response to life circumstances, and should not be considered as a sign of a dysfunctional sexual response system, which would explain why prevalence figures based on frequencies yield much higher dysfunction rates (19) than actual distress figures.

The latest classification proposal also embraces the personal distress criterion and has reintroduced a subjective criterion, but avoids an answer to the question of when a sexual problem is a dysfunction. In this proposal the word "dysfunction" is used to mean simply lack of healthy/expected/"normal" response/interest, and is not meant to imply any pathology within the woman (15). This does again suggest, however, that we have clear criteria for healthy and normal response.

The answer to the question of what is *not* a sexual dysfunction is more easy than generating clear cut criteria for sexual dysfunction. As long as lack of adequate sexual stimulation—whether this is the result of absence of sexual stimulation or of lack of knowledge about, bad technique of, a lack of attention for, or negative emotions to sexual stimuli—explains the absence of sexual feelings and genital response, the label "dysfunction" is inappropriate. Problems that are situational do not deserve the label dysfunctional, as is now possible in DSM-IV.

The study of Bancroft and colleagues might be taken to imply that only medical and somatic problems that generate sexual unresponsiveness, which cannot be understood as adaptations to life circumstances and which cause sexual distress, should be considered a dysfunction. This is a view that we can endorse. Without completely resolving this issue, we might at best suggest that a differentiation between genital and subjective unresponsiveness in all circumstances ("dysfunction") and not being able to create the right conditions for sexual arousal ("problem") is the most theoretically and clinically meaningful.

TREATMENT

Psychological Treatments

Currently, we are in a climate that overlooks and dismisses psychological treatments (99). One of the reasons for this may be that due to sociocultural pressure in the medical and larger culture, physiological treatments are seen as superior (100). The emphasis on impaired genital unresponsiveness in the DSM-IV and the success of pharmacological treatments for men's erectile dysfunction have undoubtedly contributed as well.

Prior to publication of Masters and Johnson's seminal book on sex therapy (101), sexual problems were seen as consequences of (nonsexual) psychological conflicts, immaturity, and relational conflicts. Masters and Johnson proposed to directly attempt to reverse the sexual dysfunction by a kind of graded practice and focus on sexual feelings (sensate focus). If sexual arousal depends directly on sexual stimulation, that very stimulation should be the topic of discussion (masturbation training). A sexual dysfunction was no longer something pertaining to the individual, rather, it was regarded as a dysfunction of the couple. It was assumed that the couple did not communicate in a way that allowed sexual arousal to occur when they intended to "produce" it. Treatment goals were associated with the couple concept: the treatment goal was for orgasm through coital stimulation. This connection between treatment format and goals was lost once Masters and Johnson's concept was used in common therapeutic practice. People came in for treatment as individuals. Intercourse frequency became the gold-standard indicator of sexual function. Male orgasm through coitus adequately fulfills reproductive goals, but it is not very satisfactory for many women because they do not easily reach orgasm through coitus. What has remained over the years since 1970 is a direct focus on dysfunctional sex and a focus on sexual sensations and feelings as a vehicle for reversal of the dysfunction.

Psychological treatment of sexual arousal problems generally consists of sensate focus excercises and masturbation training, with the emphasis on becoming more self-focussed and assertive (38). A lack of meaningful treatment goals for women, the difficulty in obtaining adequate control groups, and a lack of clear treatment protocols, may explain the paucity of well-controlled randomized trials of psychological therapy (50).

In the mid-1990s, a number of reviews of treatments for sexual dysfunctions following the criteria for validated or evidence based practice were published (39,102,103). Almost all of the data on psychological treatments were collected in the mid-1980s or earlier. The high success rates published by Masters and Johnson (101) have never been replicated. In their 1997 review, Heiman and Meston concluded that only the directed-masturbation treatments for primary anorgasmia fulfil the criteria of "well-established," and directed-masturbation treatment studies for secondary anorgasmia fall within the "probably efficacious" group. This conclusion is still valid up to date. There are no psychological treatments for FSAD that can be considered "evidence-based" treatments, but as we have argued earlier, directed-masturbation or comparable treatments may be as effective for FSAD as they are for FOD.

Recently, a new nonpharmacological approach to treatment was developed. The EROS Clitoral Therapy Device consists of a small cup that can be placed over the clitoris, and a pump that creates a vacuum over the clitoris. A study in 20 women with sexual arousal complaints and 12 women without sexual problems found improvements in genital sensation, vaginal lubrication, ability to reach orgasm, and sexual satisfaction relative to pretreatment (104). The authors speculate that "the increased vaginal lubrication resulting from clitoral engorgement with the EROS-CTD is due to activation of an autonomic reflex that triggers arterial vasodilatation with subsequent increases in transudate and lubrication." The EROS-CTD is marketed as an effective medical device for female sexual dysfunction (105), even though there was no control treatment such as clitoral vibration (cf. 106). For us, this "medical" device again demonstrates that, if proven effective in larger groups of women with sexual arousal difficulties, many if not most sexual arousal problems are due to a lack of adequate sexual stimulation.

Despite our support for evidence-based practice, care for people with sexual problems, according to the rules of "good clinical practice," must continue, even without solid proof of efficacy. There clearly is a great need for controlled efficacy studies in this area. From our analysis that the majority of sexual arousal problems in healthy women are not related to impaired genital responsiveness, it follows that we expect more benefit for FSAD from psychological treatments than from pharmacological treatments.

Pharmacotherapy

In the relatively short time span, compared to psychologic treatments, that pharmacological treatments have become available for men, since 1998, the effect of pharmacological treatments in women with sexual arousal problems has been investigated in several controlled and uncontrolled studies. To date, none of the treatments listed here have been approved.

Phosphodiesterase Inhibitors

Sildenafil is the first pharmacological treatment that has been investigated on a reasonable scale in controlled studies with female subjects. In the very first laboratory study, 12 healthy premenopausal women without sexual dysfunction were randomized to receive a single oral 50 mg dose of sildenafil or matching placebo in the first session and alternate medication in a second session (107). Although sildenafil was found effective in enhancing vaginal engorgement (VPA) during erotic stimulus conditions, these changes were not associated with an effect on subjective sexual arousal. The first large controlled at home study in 557 estrogenized and 204 estrogen-deficient pre- and postmenopausal women with sexual problems that included, but were not limited to, sexual arousal disorders, found no improvement with 10–100 mg of sildenafil on subjective sexual arousal and subjective perception of genital arousal, as assessed by several different measures (108). Women identified as having DSM-IV arousal disorder without concomitant hypoactive sexual desire disorder did show benefit of sildenafil beyond placebo (109). Also, an Italian study found improvement on subjective sexual arousal, pleasure, orgasm, and even on frequency of orgasm, in premenopausal women with sexual arousal complaints, although these results were obtained with unvalidated questionnaires (110). A second study from the same group in sexually functional women showed benefit of sildenafil over placebo on arousal, orgasm, and enjoyment, now with a validated questionnaire (111). A small, recent placebo-controlled laboratory study of women diagnosed with genital arousal disorder suggested only a small minority of them might benefit from sildenafil (112). The controlled laboratory study of Sipski et al. (113) in women with SCI found an enhancing effect of sildenafil on genital (VPA) and subjective sexual arousal. The beneficial effects of sildenafil over placebo were most evident in the strongest stimulus condition of both visual and manual stimulation. Several, yet unpublished, controlled studies in women with FSAD found no improvement of sildenafil.

These conflicting findings have probably led to Pfizer's recent decision to end their program of testing efficacy of sildenafil in women (114). It would be theoretically and clinically meaningful to investigate which factors may have been responsible for these inconsistent findings. Possible candidates are: inadequate sexual stimulation (sildenafil will not be effective without sexual stimulation); inadequate outcome measures; wrong patient group (e.g., women with sexual problems unrelated to genital responsiveness); estrogen depletion. In most studies, women with a medical condition were excluded from the trials. This may have been an unfortunate choice. We have argued that women with various medical conditions may have an impaired genital response and may therefore have more to gain from a genital arousal enhancing agent such as sildenafil than medically healthy women.

Prostaglandines

One placebo-controlled, single-blind, dose response study has been published investigating the effect of a local application of alprostadil in women with arousal difficulties (115). No significant differences with placebo were found. A comparison of the lowest with the highest dose did show some effects in the expected direction, but these effects were estimated by visual inspection by an MD. It is unknown whether that MD was also blinded to treatment. Apparently a larger, as yet unpublished study, in postmenopausal women did find significant improvement over placebo on genital sensation, subjective sexual arousal, and sexual satisfaction (116).

Phentolamine

Two controlled studies have investigated the effect of the alpha-1 and alpha-2 adrenergic receptor antagonist phentolamine on the basis of the hypothesis that, as in men, the smooth muscle surrounding the vaginal arterial vascular bed is mainly alpha adrenergically innervated. In the first study, an oral application was used that showed a positive effect on subjective and genital sexual arousal (VPA) in postmenopausal women with sexual arousal difficulties (117). A second placebo-controlled study studied both oral and vaginal applications in estrogenized and nonestrogenized postmenopausal women (118). Genital response was higher with the highest dose of vaginally applied phentolamine than with placebo, in estrogenized postmenopausal women only. Subjective sexual arousal was higher with the highest doses of both applications of phentolamine than with placebo, again in the estrogenized women only.

Dopamine Agonists

Dopaminergic drugs might be interesting because unlike the previously discussed drugs, they have a direct effect on the brain and may therefore have a positive influence on sexual arousal and desire. The only controlled study published to date found an enhancing effect of levodopa on an index of somatic motor preparation, the Achilles tendon reflex, in men, but not in women (119). Sumanirole is a dopamine agonist that specifically targets D2-receptors. We investigated the effect of this drug in women with complaints of sexual arousal and desire in a placebo-controlled laboratory study, but found no effects on genital or subjective sexual arousal (data not published). Buproprion was used in one uncontrolled study to counteract the sexual side-effects of selective serotonine reuptake inhibitors. Keeping in mind that no adequate control was used, the authors conclude that the results point to relief of the sexual complaints (120).

Androgens

Several companies have begun to study the effects of various androgen products and androgen–estrogen combinations. The relationship between declining androgens and sexual response has not been clarified. Sexual problems related to androgen deficiency are to be expected only when there is a real deficiency of biologically available testosterone. Recently, a consensus conference has tried to establish clear criteria for such an androgen insufficiency syndrome (64). Fourcroy (116) recently published a detailed overview of androgen treatments that are being developed, and concluded that it remains to be seen whether these products will show promise in female sexual dysfunction. Besides efficacy, there are increasing concerns about safety. For an overview of a small number of other treatments and a listing of pharmaceutical companies that are involved in these treatments, see Ref. (116).

RECOMMENDATIONS FOR CLINICAL PRACTICE

We would like to end with five questions that may help establish the heart of the problem in women with complaints about reduced or absent arousal and desire.

The first question is whether the client wants to be sexual at all. This question may refer to people that were excluded from Masters and Johnson's studies. These may be people so deeply involved in relational conflict, that they, as Masters and Johnson put it, need legal advice instead of sex and relationship therapy (101). The prognosis for a rewarding sexual relationship, even if all the relational discord was to be resolved, seems to be poor (121). Learning to stop arguing or learning to do that more effectively does not necessarily improve the sexual relationship. For that, as we have argued, situations with positive sexual meanings are a first prerequisite.

The second question refers to the sensitivity of the sexual system. As we have seen, in healthy women problems related to genital unresponsiveness are unlikely. For clinicians who need to rule out that organic etiology is underlying sexual arousal difficulties, or who question genital responsiveness for other reasons, a psychophysiological assessment will provide indispensable additional information.

Next, are there, on the basis of sexual history, positive expectations regarding sex? Are there any sexual rewards? And are these expectations activated in the given sexual situation, and which new sexual stimuli are likely to be sexually rewarding? When there are no or only a few positive experiences, one can try to help women find these experiences. A confrontation with sexual stimuli will probably only be rewarding by the sexually rewarding experience. Our disposition to respond positively to tactile stimulation must become associated with sexual stimuli.

If all these conditions are satisfied and the sexual system is activated, there will be a cascade of events that occur partly automatic and partly on the basis of conscious decisions. Whether we will be sexually active will depend, ultimately, on decisions about the partner, the circumstances, and on ideas about how we want to shape our sexual lives.

REFERENCES

1. American Psychiatric Association. Diagnostic and Statistical Manual of Mental Disorders. 4th ed. Text Revision. Washington, DC: American Psychiatric Association, 2000.
2. Kolodny RC, Masters WH, Johnson VE. Textbook of Sexual Medicine. Boston: Little, Brown, 1979.

3. Ellis A. Studies in the Psychology of Sex. Philadelphia: F.A. Davis, 1903/1920.
4. Stekel W. Frigidity in Women. New York: Washington Square Press, 1926/1967.
5. Acton W. The Functions and Disorders of the Reproductive Organs in Childhood, Youth, Adult Age, and Advanced Life. 6th ed. Philadelphia: Presley Balckstone, 1875/1957.
6. Laqueur T. Making Sex: Body and Gender from the Greeks to Freud. Cambridge: Harvard University Press, 1990.
7. Shorter E. A History of Women's Bodies. London: Penguin Books, 1984.
8. Levin RJ. The mechanisms of female sexual arousal. Annual Review of Sex Research 1992; 3:1–48.
9. Birke LIA, Vines G. Beyond nature versus nurture: process and biology in the development of gender. Women's Studies International Forum 1987; 10:555–570.
10. Masters WH, Johnson VE. Human Sexual Response. Boston: Little, Brown, 1966.
11. Tiefer L. Historical, scientific, clinical and feminist criticisms of "The Human Sexual Response Cycle" model. Annual Review of Sex Research 1991; 2:1–23.
12. Hite S. The Hite Report. New York: Dell, 1976.
13. Leiblum SR. Definition and classification of female sexual disorders. International Journal of Impotence Research 1998; 10:S104–S106.
14. Laan E, Everaerd W. Determinants of female sexual arousal: psychophysiological theory and data. Annual Review of Sex Research 1995; 6:32–76.
15. Basson R, Leiblum S, Brotto L, Derogatis L, Fourcroy J, Fugl-Meyer K, Graziottin A, Heiman JR, Laan E, Meston C, Schover L, van Lankveld J, Weijmar Schultz W. Definitions of women's sexual dysfunctions reconsidered: advocating expansion and revision. Journal of Psychosomatic Obstetrics and Gynecology 2003; 24:221–229.
16. Bancroft J, Loftus J, Long JS. Distress about sex: a national survey of women in heterosexual relationships. Archives of Sexual Behavior 2003; 32:193–208.
17. Simons J, Carey MP. Prevalence of sexual dysfunctions: results from a decade of research. Archives of Sexual Behavior 2001; 30:177–219.
18. Laumann EO, Paik A, Rosen RC. Sexual dysfunction in the United States: prevalence and predictors. Journal of the American Medical Association 1999; 281:537–544.
19. Frank E, Anderson C, Rubinstein DN. Frequency of sexual dysfunction in normal couples. New England Journal of Medicine 1978; 299:111–115.
20. Blanker MH, Bohnen AM, Groeneveld FPMJ, Bernsen RMD, Prins A, Thomas S, Bosch JLHR. Erectiestoornissen bij mannen van 50 jaar en ouder: prevalentie, risicofactoren en ervaren hinder [Erectile disorder in men of 50 years and older: Prevalence, risk factors, and experienced distress]. Nederlands Tijdschrift voor Geneeskunde 2001; 145:1404–1409.
21. Meuleman EJH, Donkers LHC, Robertson C, Keech M, Boyle P, Kiemeney LALM. Erectiestoornis: Prevalentie en invloed op de kwaliteit van leven; het Boxmeer-onderzoek [Erectile disorder: prevalence and influence on quality of life; the Boxmeer-study]. Nederlands Tijdschrift voor Geneeskunde 2001; 145:581–586.
22. Mercer CH, Fenton KA, Johnson AM, Wellings K, Macdowall W, McManus S, Nanchahal K, Erens B. Sexual function problems and help seeking behaviour in Britain: national probability sample survey. Br Med J 2003; 227:426–427.
23. Freud S. The standard edition of the complete psychological works of Sigmund Freud. London: Hogarth Press, 1953.

24. O'Connell HE, Hutson JM, Anderson CR, Plenter RJ. Anatomical relationship between urethra and clitoris. Journal of Anatomy 1998; 159:1892–1897.
25. Grafenberg E. The role of the urethra in female orgasm. International Journal of Sexology 1950; 3:145–148.
26. Levin RJ. The mechanisms of human female sexual arousal. Annual Review of Sex Research 1992; 3:1–48.
27. Ladas AK, Whipple B, Perry JD. The G-spot and other discoveries about human sexuality. New York: Holt, Rinehart & Winston, 1982.
28. Levin RJ. The G-spot: Reality or illusion? Sexual and Relationship Therapy 2003; 18:117–119.
29. Weijmar Schultz WCM, van de Wiel HBM, Klatter JA, Sturm BE, Nauta J. Vaginal sensitivity to electric stimuli: theoretical and practical implications. Archives of Sexual Behavior 1989; 18:87–95.
30. Sipski ML, Alexander CJ, Rosen R. Sexual arousal and orgasm in women: effects of spinal cord injury. Annals of Neurology 2001; 49:35–44.
31. Whipple B, Komisaruk BR. Beyond the G-spot: recent research on female sexuality. Medical Aspects of Human Sexuality 1998; 1:19–23.
32. McKenna KE. The neurophysiology of female sexual function. World Journal of Urology 2002; 20:93–100.
33. Kaplan HS. Hypoactive sexual desire. Journal of Sex and Marital Therapy 1977; 3:3–9.
34. American Psychiatric Association. Diagnostic and Statistical Manual of Mental Disorders. 3rd ed. Text Revision. Washington, DC: American Psychiatric Association, 1980.
35. Nathan SG. When do we say a woman's sexuality is dysfunctional? In: Levine SB, Risen CB, Althof SE, eds. Handbook of Clinical Sexuality for Mental Health Professionals. New York: Brunner-Routledge, 2003:95–110.
36. Leiblum S. Definition and classification of female disorders. International Journal of Impotence Research 1998; 10(suppl 2): S104–S106.
37. Laan E, Everaerd W. Determinants of female sexual arousal: psychophysiological theory and data. Annual Review of Sex Research 1995; 6:32–76.
38. Both S, Laan E. Directed masturbation. In: O'Donohue W, Fisher JE, Hayes SC, eds. Cognitive Behavior Therapy: Applying Empirically Supported Techniques in your Practice. New York: John Wiley & Sons, 2003:144–151.
39. Heiman JR, Meston CM. Empirically validated treatment for sexual dysfunction. Annual Review of Sex Research 1997; 8:148–194.
40. Heiman JR. Orgasmic disorders in women. In: Leiblum SR, Rosen RC, eds. Principles and Practices of Sex Therapy. 3d ed. New York: Guilford Press, 2000:118–153.
41. Segraves RT. Female sexual arousal disorder. In: Widiger TA, Frances AJ, Pincus H, Ross R, First M, Davis W, eds. DSM-IV Sourcebook. Washington, DC: American Psychiatric Association, 1996:1103–1108.
42. Laan E, van Driel EM, van Lunsen RHW. Seksuele reakties van vrouwen met een seksuele opwindingsstoornis op visuele seksuele stimuli [Sexual responses of women with sexual arousal disorder to visual sexual stimuli]. Tijdschrift voor Seksuologie 2003; 27:1–13.
43. Meston CM, Gorzalka BB. Differential effects of sympathetic activation on sexual arousal in sexually dysfunctional and functional women. Journal of Abnormal 1996; 105:582–591.

44. Morokoff PJ, Heiman JR. Effects of erotic stimuli on sexually functional and dysfunctional women: multiple measures before and after sex therapy. Behaviour Research and Therapy 1980; 18:127–137.

45. Wouda JC, Hartman PM, Bakker RM, Bakker IO, van de Wiel HBM, Weijmar Schultz WCM. Vaginal plethysmography in women with dyspareunia. The Journal of Sex Research 1998; 35:141–147.

46. Sipski ML, Rosen RC, Alexander CJ, Hamer R. Sildenafil effects on sexual and cardiovascular responses in women with spinal cord injury. Urology 2000; 55:812–815.

47. Wincze JP, Albert A, Bansal S. Sexual arousal in diabetic females: physiological and self-report measures. Archives of Sexual Behaviour 1993; 22:587–601.

48. Maas CP, ter Kuile MM, Laan E, Tuynman CC, Weyenborg, PhThM, Trimbos JB, Kenter GG. Objective assessment of disturbed vaginal blood flow reponse during sexual arousal in women with a history of hysterectomy. British Journal of Obstetrics and Gynaecology 2004; 111:456–462.

49. Basson R. Are our definitions of women's desire, arousal and sexual pain disorders too broad and our definition of orgasmic disorder too narrow? Journal of Sex and Marital Therapy 2002; 28:289–300.

50. Basson R, Weijmar Schultz WCM, Binik YM, Brotto LA, Eschenback DA, Laan E, Utian WH, Wesselmann U, van Lankveld J, Wyatt G, Wyatt L. Women's sexual desire and arousal disorders and sexual pain. In: Lue TF, Basson R, Rosen R, Guiliano F, Khoury S, Montorsi F, eds. Sexual medicine: sexual dysfunctions in men and women. Paris: Health Publications Limited, 2004:851–974.

51. Shover L, Jensen SB. Sexuality and chronic illness: a comprehensive approach. New York: Guilford Press, 1988.

52. Havenga K, Maas CP, DeRuiter MC, Welvaart K, Trimbos JB. Avoiding long-term disturbance to bladder and sexual dysfunction in pelvic surgery, particularly with rectal cancer. Seminars in Surgical Oncology 2000; 26:751–757.

53. Maas CP, Moriya Y, Kenter G, Trimbos B, van de Velde C. A plea for preservation of the pelvic autonomic nerves. Lancet 1999; 354:772–773.

54. Park K, Goldstein I, Andry C, Siroky MB, Krane RJ, Azadzoi KM. Vasculogenic female sexual dysfunction: the hemodynamic basis for vaginal engorgement insufficiency and clitoral erectile insufficiency. International Journal of Impotence Research 1997; 9:27–37.

55. Laan E, van Lunsen R. Hormones and sexuality in postmenopausal women: a psychophysiological study. Journal of Psychosomatic Obstetrics and Gynecology 1997; 18:126–133.

56. Maravilla KR, Cao Y, Heiman JR, Garland PA, Peterson BT, Carter WO, Weisskoff RM. Serial MR Imaging with MS-325 for evaluating female sexual arousal response: determination of intrasubject reproducibility. Journal of Magnetic Resonance Imaging 2003; 18:216–224.

57. Suh DD, Yang CC, Cao Y, Garland PA, Maravilla KR. Magnetic resonance imaging anatomy of the female genitalia in premenopausal and postmenopausal women. Journal of Urology 2003; 170:138–144.

58. Lunsen RHW van, Laan E. Genital vascular responsiveness and sexual feelings in mid life women: psychophysiological, brain, and genital imaging studies. Menopause 2004; 11:741–748.

59. Bancroft J, Janssen E. The dual control model of male sexual response: a theoretical approach to centrally mediated erectile dysfunction. Neuroscience and Biobehavioural Review 2000; 24:571–579.

60. Dennerstein L, Lehert P. Modeling mid-aged women's sexual functioning: a prospective, population-based study. Journal of Sex and Marital Therapy 2004; 30:173–183.

61. Berlo W van, Ensink B. Problems with sexuality after sexual assault. Annual Review of Sex Research 2000; 11:235–258.

62. Janssen E, Everaerd W, van Lunsen H, Oerlemans S. Validation of a psychophysiological Waking Erectile Assessment (WEA) for the diagnosis of male erectile disorder. Urology 1994; 43:686–695.

63. Wiegel M, Meston C, Rosen R. The female sexual function index (FSFI): cross-validation and development of clinical cutoff scores. Archives of Sexual Behavior. In press.

64. Bachmann G, Braunstein G, Burger H, Davis S, Dennerstein L, Goldstein I, Guay A, Leiblum S, Lobo R, Notelovitz M, Rosen R, Sarrel P, Sherwin B, Simon J, Simpson E, Shifren J, Spark R, Traish A. Female androgen insufficiency: the Princeton consensus statement on definition, classification, and assessment. Fertility and Sterility 2002; 77:660–665.

65. Meston C. The psychophysiological assessment of female sexual function. Journal of Sex Education and Therapy 2000; 25:6–16.

66. Laan E, Everaerd W, van der Velde J, Geer JH. Determinants of subjective experience of sexual arousal in women: feedback from genital arousal and erotic stimulus content. Psychophysiology 1995; 32:444–451.

67. Tuiten A, Laan E, Everaerd W, Panhuysen G, de Haan E, Koppeschaar H, Vroon P. Discrepancies between genital responses and subjective sexual function during testosterone substitution in women with hypothalamic amenorrhea. Psychosomatic Medicine 1996; 58:234–241.

68. Laan E, van Lunsen RHW. Hormones and sexuality in postmenopausal women: a psychophysiological study. Journal of Psychosomatic Obstetrics and Gynaecology 1997; 18:126–133.

69. Laan E, van Lunsen RHW, Everaerd W. The effects of tibolone on vaginal blood flow, sexual desire and arousability in postmenopausal women. Climacteric 2001; 4:28–41.

70. Levin RJ, van Berlo W. Sexual arousal and orgasm in subjects who experience forced or non-consensual sexual stimulation: a review. Journal of Clinical Forensic Medicine 2004; 11:82–88.

71. Laan E, Everaerd W, van Aanhold M, Rebel M. Performance demand and sexual arousal in women. Behaviour Research and Therapy 1993; 31:25–35.

72. Spiering M, Everaerd W. The sexual unconscious. In: Janssen E, ed. The Psychophysiology of Sex. Bloomington, IN: Indiana University Press. In press.

73. Öhman A, Soares JJF. "Unconscious anxiety": phobic responses to masked stimuli. Journal of Abnormal Psychology 1994; 103:231–240.

74. Öhman A. Fear and anxiety as emotional phenomena: Clinical phenomenology, evolutionary perspectives, and information-processing mechanisms. In: Lewis M, Haviland JM, eds. Handbook of Emotions. New York: The Guilford Press, 1993:511–526.

75. Spiering M, Everaerd W, Karsdorp P, Both S, Brauer M. Unconscious processing of sexual information: a generalization to women. Submitted for publication.

76. Janssen E, Everaerd W, Spiering M, Janssen J. Automatic processes and the appraisal of sexual stimuli: toward an information processing model of sexual arousal. The Journal of Sex Research 2000; 37:8–23.
77. LeDoux J. The Emotional Brain. New York: Simon and Schuster, 1996.
78. Dekker J. Voluntary Control of Sexual Arousal. Ph.D. dissertation, Utrecht University, The Netherlands, 1988.
79. Everaerd W. Seksuele opwinding [Sexual arousal]. Nederlands Tijdschrift voor de Psychologie 1993; 48:99–109.
80. Damasio A. Looking for Spinoza: Joy, Sorrow, and the Feeling Brain. Orlando: Harcourt Inc, 2003.
81. LeDoux J. The Synaptic Self. New York: Viking Penguin, 2001.
82. James W. What is an emotion? Mind 1884; 9:188–205.
83. Craig AD. How do you feel? Interoception: the sense of the psysiological condition of the body. Nature Reviews 2002; 3:655–666.
84. Morris JS. How do you feel? Trends in Cognitive Sciences 2002; 6:317–319.
85. Sumich AL, Kumari V, Sharma T. Neuroimaging of sexual arousal: research and clinical utility. Hospital Medicine 2003; 64:28–33.
86. Critchley HD, Wiens S, Rotshtein P, Öhman A, Dolan RJ. Neural systems supporting interoceptive awareness. Nature Neuroscience 2004; 7:189–195.
87. Laan E, Janssen E. How do men and women feel? Determinants of subjective experience of sexual arousal. In: Janssen E, ed. The Psychophysiology of Sex. Bloomington, IN: Indiana University press. In press.
88. Canli T, Desmond JE, Zhao Z, Gabrieli JDE. Sex differences in the neural basis of emotional memories. Proceedings of the National Academy of Sciences 2002; 99:10789–10794.
89. Squire LR. Memory and the hippocampus: a synthesis from findings with rats, monkey's, and humans. Psychological Review 1992; 99:195–231.
90. Baumeister RF. Gender differences in erotic plasticity: the female sex drive as socially flexible and responsive. Psychological Bulletin 2000; 126:347–374.
91. Buss DM, Schmidt DP. Sexual strategies theory: an evolutionary perspective on human mating. Psychological Review 1993; 100:204–232.
92. Bjorklund DF, Kipp K. Parental investment theory and gender differences in the evolution of inhibition mechanisms. Psychological Bulletin 1996; 120:163–188.
93. Beauregard M, Levesque J, Bourgouin P. Neural correlates of conscious self-regulation of emotion. Journal of Neuroscience 2001; 21:RC165:1–6.
94. Ungless MA, Magill PJ, Bolarn JP. Uniform inhibition of dopamine neurons in the ventral tegmental area by aversive stimuli. Science 2004; 303:2040–2042.
95. Basson R, Berman J, Burnett A, Derogatis L, Ferguson D, Fourcroy J, Goldstein I, Graziottin A, Heiman J, Laan E, Leiblum S, Padma-Nathan H, Rosen R, Segraves K, Segraves RT, Shabsigh R, Sipski M, Wagner G, Whipple B. Report of the international consensus development conference on female sexual dysfunction: definitions and classifications. Journal of Urology 2000; 163:888–893.
96. Tiefer L. A new view of women's sexual problems: why new? Why now? Journal of Sex Research 2001; 38:89–96.
97. Nathan SG. When do we say a woman's sexuality is dysfunctional? In: Levine SB, Risen CB, Althof SE, eds. Handbook of Clinical Sexuality for Mental Health Professionals. New York: Brunner-Routledge, 2003.

98. Bancroft J. The medicalization of female sexual dysfunction: the need for caution. Archives of Sexual Behavior 2002; 31:451–455.

99. Heiman JR. Psychologic treatments for female sexual dysfunction: are they effective and do we need them? Archives of Sexual Behavior 2002; 31:445–450.

100. Tiefer L. Sex is not a natural act and other essays. Boulder, CO: Westview Press, 1995.

101. Masters WH, Johnson VE. Human Sexual Inadequacy. Boston: Little, Brown, 1970.

102. O'Donohue W, Dopke CA, Swingen DN. Psychotherapy for female sexual dysfunction: a review. Clinical Psychology Review 1997; 17:537–566.

103. Baucom DH, Shoham V, Mueser KT, Daiuto AD, Stickle TR. Empirically supported couple and family interventions for marital distress and adult mental health problems. Journal of Consulting and Clinical Psychology 1998; 66:53–88.

104. Billups KL, Berman L, Berman J, Metz ME, Glennon MW, Goldstein I. A new non-pharmacological vacuum therapy for female sexual dysfunction. Journal of Sex and Marital Therapy 2001; 27:435–441.

105. About EROS therapy™, http://www.urometrics.com/products/eros/index.cfin, accessed May 9, 2004.

106. Laan E, van Lunsen RHW. Orgasm latency, duration and quality in women: validation of a laboratory sexual stimulation technique. Poster presented at 28th Conference of the International Academy of Sex Research, Hamburg, Germany, June 2002.

107. Laan E, van Lunsen RHW, Everaerd W, Boolell M, Riley A. The enhancement of vaginal vasocongestion by sildenafil in healthy premenopausal women. Journal of Women's Health and Gender-based Medicine 2002; 11:357–365.

108. Basson R, McInnes R, Smith M, Hodgson G, Koppiker N. Efficacy and safety of sildenafil citrate (Viagra®) in women with sexual dysfunction associated with female sexual arousal disorder. Journal of Women's Health and Gender-Based Medicine 2002; 11:339–349.

109. Berman JR, Berman LA, Toler SM, Gill J, Haughie S. Safety and efficacy of sildenafil citrate for the treatment of female sexual arousal disorder: a double-blind, placebo controlled study. Journal of Urology 2003; 170:2333–2338.

110. Caruso S, Intelisano G, Lupo L, Agnello C. Premenopausal women affected by sexual arousal disorder treated with sildenafil: a double-blind, cross-over, placebo-controlled study. British Journal of Obstetrics and Gynaecology 2001; 108:623–628.

111. Caruso S, Intelisano G, Farina M, Di Mari L, Agnello C. The function of sildenafil on female sexual pathways: a double-blind, cross-over, placebo-controlled study. European Journal of Obstetrics and Gynecology and Reproductive Biology 2003; 110:201–206.

112. Basson R, Brotto L. Sexual psychophysiology and effects of sildenafil citrate in estrogenized women with acquired genital arousal disorder and impaired orgasm. British Journal of Obstetrics and Gynaecology 2003; 110:1–11.

113. Sipski ML, Rosen RC, Alexander CJ, Hamer RM. Sildenafil effects on sexual and cardiovascular responses in women with spinal cord injury. Urology 2000; 55:812–815.

114. Pfizer to end tests of Viagra for women, The Associated Press, http://www.cnn.com/2004/HEALTH/02/28/viagra.women.ap/, February 28, 2004, accessed March 9, 2004.

115. Islam A, Mitchel JT, Rosen R, Phillips N, Ayers C, Ferguson D, Yeager J. Topical alprostadil in the treatment of female sexual arousal disorder: a pilot study. Journal of Sex and Marital Therapy 2001; 27:531–540.
116. Fourcroy JL. Female sexual dysfunction: potential for pharmacotherapy. Drugs 2003; 63:1445–1457.
117. Rosen RC, Phillips NA, Gendrano NC, Ferguson DM. Oral phentolamine and female sexual arousal disorder: a pilot study. Journal of Sex and Marital Therapy 1999; 25:137–144.
118. Rubio-Aurioles E, Lopez M, Lipexker M, Lara C, Ramirez A, Rampazzo C, Hurtado de Mendoza MT, Lowrey F, Loehr LA, Lammers P. Phentolamine mesylate in post-menopausal women with female sexual arousal disorder: a psychophysiological study. Journal of Sex and Marital Therapy 2002; 28 (suppl 1):205–215.
119. Both S, Everaerd W, Laan E, Gooren L. Effect of a single dose of levodopa on sexual response in men and women. Neuropsychopharmacology 2005; 30:173–183.
120. Gitlin MJ, Suri R, Altshuler L, Zuckerbrow-Miller J, Fairbanks L. Bupropion-sustained release as a treatment for SSRI-induced sexual side effects. Journal of Sex and Marital Therapy 2002; 28:131–138.
121. Everaerd W, Laan E. Desire for passion: energetics of sexual response. Journal of Sex and Marital Therapy 1995; 21:255–263.

7

Erectile Dysfunction

Kevan Wylie

Royal Hallamshire Hospital, Sheffield, UK

Porterbrook Clinic, Sheffield, UK

University of Sheffield, Sheffield, UK

Ian MacInnes

University of Sheffield, Sheffield, UK

INTRODUCTION

Erectile dysfunction (ED) is a more specific term for impotence and is useful as it has fewer stigmas attached, and distinguishes ED from orgasmic and ejaculatory dysfunction (1–4). Impotence was defined as "the persistent inability to attain and maintain an erection adequate to permit satisfactory sexual performance" (5). This indicates that the erection is either too short lived or not firm enough for the man to penetrate his partner. In extreme cases, there may be no erectile response at all, this is termed "severe" or "complete" ED. Two large-scale studies have examined the prevalence and etiology of ED. In the late 1980s, Feldman's team gathered complete information from 1290 men between the ages of 40 and 70 (6). Several of their characteristics were compared, including physical measures (e.g., height, serum cholesterol, etc.), medical conditions, medications, sociodemographics, race, and education. Erectile function was assessed using a nine-item sexual activity questionnaire. In the entire sample, the mean probability of some degree of impotence in this age group was $52.0 \pm 1.3\%$. In total, 17.2% had minimal ED, 25.2% had moderate ED, and 9.6% had complete ED. The severity of ED had some relation to increasing age even after adjusting for other factors; nevertheless, the other factors are of great importance. It was found that some diseases were strongly associated with changes in erectile function. Diabetes, heart disease, and hypertension, even when treated, were predictive of ED (after adjustment for age), and the pharmacological agents used in the treatment of these conditions seemed to relate to the group with no erectile response. Cigarette smoking was shown to be a strong risk factor for ED, especially amongst those who were still smokers at the time (56% complete impotence for current smokers compared with 21% for current nonsmokers). A Welsh study undertaken more recently has shown similar results but used a different methodology that was less discriminatory [e.g., it did not exclude men with no regular sexual partner (7)]. Both studies are weakened by the fact that >96% of the men were white, and therefore can only really reflect what is going on in their respective demographic areas.

It is all too easy to dismiss ED as a benign condition and therefore unimportant. It should be realized that ED can cause a great deal of unnecessary suffering including low self-esteem and depression. ED often occurs together with relationship difficulties. Both the man and his partner may have a variety of issues that, if left unchecked, can adversely affect his family's relationship dynamics. Other relationships outside the home may also be adversely affected. Because of the link between ED and depression (8) there is the probability of an economic impact as time off from work may be required. In addition to the psychological difficulties, there may be underlying pathology such as cardiovascular disease, diabetes, or hypertension. ED is sometimes the presenting factor in such chronic conditions (9).

There are many risk factors that cause or contribute to ED. Age is undoubtedly the greatest predictor of ED but ED is not necessarily a direct consequence of the aging process. It is simply that older men are more likely to have comorbidities. Shortness of breath, angina, pain (e.g., associated with arthritis), muscle weakness, and age associated disability can all contribute to the problem.

Other causes of ED can be classified as physical, psychological, or psychiatric, with approximately two-thirds of men having a physical cause as the major contributing factor. The physical causes are mostly due to vascular or neurological damage, but the endocrine system can also be involved. Hypertension, hyperlipidaemia, vascular disease, and diabetes can all alter the blood supply to the penis, and a problem with the venous system can cause leakage so that the erection cannot be maintained. Diabetes, alcohol misuse, multiple sclerosis, spinal cord injury (SCI), and Parkinson's disease are conditions in which neurological damage affects the transmission of erectogenic nerve signals from the brain. Altered testosterone and prolactin levels are of particular interest when exploring a hormonal cause. While thyroid function is not directly responsible for ED, it can affect sex drive, which may indirectly present as ED.

Substance misuse, schizophrenia, bipolar disorder, and personality disorders (e.g., obsessive-compulsive type) are all psychiatric risk factors for ED. Paraphilias, such as fetishism, may cause ED when the object of desire is absent. By far, the most common psychiatric cause of ED is depression. Inversely, depression is also a major consequence of ED, and it can be difficult to distinguish which occurred first (10). Ironically, some of the antidepressant treatments contribute to the long list of causative factors for ED (Table 7.1).

Table 7.1 Antidepressant Drugs Implicated as a Cause of Erectile Dysfunction

All tricyclics including
Amitryptyline
Clomipramine
Imipramine
All mono-amine oxidase inhibitors including
Phenelzine
Isocarboxazid
Tranylcypramine
All selective serotonin re-uptake inhibitors
Fluoxetine
Paroxetine
Other antidepressant drugs may NOT cause sexual dysfunction. These include:
Mirtazapine
Flupentixol
Nefadozone
Reboxetine
Tryptophan
Venlafaxine

Source: Information from British National Formulary.

Whereas the organic causes of ED are most often associated with the older age group, psychological problems can be a primary cause of ED more often seen in younger men. The young man may present as being anxious about the reliability of his erections. He may need reassurance that few men are able to achieve an erection at will, in all situations, and at all times. Secondary psychological problems may occur when the man loses the ability to enjoy satisfactory sexual activity due to a physical disorder. Anxiety, stress, loss of self-confidence and self-esteem are all common psychological problems that present in any clinic (11). Guilt about sexual thoughts or feelings, and negative cognitions may also result in ED. Although they act on physiological systems, erectogenic medications may rectify a psychological problem by helping the individual to achieve an erection. In some cases it is enough for him to break out of a psychological "vicious circle." In other cases, the underlying psychology may remain, and the person may become reliant on the medication (and therefore the prescriber) to help him achieve an erection with his partner.

Other organic causes of ED include chronic conditions such as renal disease. Surgery (e.g., prostate surgery), trauma (particularly to the pelvic region), and structural abnormalities such as Peyronie's disease are other factors that should be considered. Drugs, either prescribed or recreational, can be a source of ED. The most important groups of pharmacological agents to consider are antidepressants, the centrally acting antihypertensive drugs; central nervous system depressants; beta-adrenoceptor antagonists; and any drugs that have an anticholinergic action. A major factor that contributes both directly and indirectly to ED is smoking! Simply by giving up smoking, a man's ability to achieve an erection can improve (4,12). Additionally, nicotine is a vasoconstrictor when present in the blood. Unfortunately, the long term consequences of smoking, such as vascular disease, are not so easily rectified (12).

ANATOMY AND PHYSIOLOGY OF ERECTION

In its flaccid state, the penis acts as a tube through which urine is passed directly from the bladder via the urethra (13,14). The urethra is also a conduit for the ejaculate, which can be expelled by the penis in both its flaccid and erect state. The penile urethra is encased by a sleeve of erectile tissue called the corpus spongiosum, which expands at the tip of the penis forming the glans and at the base forming the bulb. The function of the spongiosum is to maintain the patency of the urethra during sexual activity so that the ejaculate is not prevented from being expelled by a collapsed structure. The main erectile components of the penis are the left and right corpora cavernosa that communicate via perforations to affect a single erectile chamber. These two connecting bodies attach to the rami of the pelvis after turning through a surprisingly sharp angle to become the deep erectile crura.

Through the core of both cavernosa run the cavernosal arteries, which are branches of the internal pudendal artery, itself a branch of the internal iliac artery. The cavernosal arteries give rise to numerous helicine (spiral) artery branches. These channel blood into the trabeculae of smooth muscle that makes up the walls of the tiny sinusoids of the cavernosa. The walls of the artery and the sinusoids are lined by nitric oxide (NO) producing endothelial cells. The sinusoids drain into subtunical veins that lie on the inside of the tunica albuginea, which forms a tough, noncompliant layer around each of the erectile bodies. Blood escapes this boundary by passing through emissary veins that pierce it. Blood continues its journey through circumflex veins that surround the outside of the tunica albuginea and are sandwiched between it and the "Buck's fascia." They then drain into the deep dorsal vein on the upper surface of the penis. The other major arteries, veins, and nerves of the penis lie dorsally. The complexities of the penile machinery are encased in the thin superficial "Colles' facia," which in turn is surrounded by the subcutaneous cellular tissue and skin.

The nervous system of the penis is in three parts. The parasympathetic nerves are branches of spinal nerves S2–S4, which give rise to the so-called pelvic splanchnic nerves that pass around the posterior aspect of the prostate gland, forming the prostatic plexus. Passing forward, they form the cavernous nerves, which branch into the body of the penis. It is this parasympathetic system that is able to elicit an erection. The sympathetic nerves are branches of the sympathetic chain at levels T11–L2. These pass through the inferior mesenteric plexus, the superior hypogastric plexus, and the pelvic plexus and branch off to the organs involved in ejaculation. Overactivity of the sympathetic system (e.g., in the stressed individual) maintains a persistent state of detumescence, although not all sympathetic activity is inhibitory. The sensory nerves of the penis and scrotum are all branches of the pudendal nerve, which can be traced back to branches of S2–S4. With these systems in mind, it can be seen that an erection can be initiated by two independent mechanisms. The first requires tactile stimulation of the penis. The nerve impulses synapse in the spinal cord and form a reflex arc with nerves of the parasympathetic system responsible for the erectile response. The other mechanism involves the higher centers of the brain that interpret sensory and fantasy stimuli triggering an erotic response resulting in an erection. The erection starts with the stimulation of one or both of these systems in a neuronally modulated hemodynamic response.

The exact mechanism of neurotransmission in the erectile response is not yet fully understood. It appears, however, that a few neurotransmitters are of key importance. Nerve endings of the parasympathetic system release acetylcholine (ACh), which appears to have a modulatory effect but no direct action; vasoactive intestinal peptide (VIP) is also released, causing tumescence but not erection; release of NO does cause erection. These neurotransmitters have all been isolated in penile erectile tissue, and the NO system is the one exploited by some of the current erectogenic oral preparations. NO is a potent smooth muscle relaxant and vasodilator produced by neurons and endothelial cells that contain the enzyme nitric oxide synthase (NOS). The effect of NO is to increase the amount of cyclic guanosine monophosphate (cGMP) available in the smooth muscle. cGMP is a second messenger that is utilized in a cascade system in which the intracellular concentration of calcium ions is diminished so that the calcium dependent muscle relaxes. It has previously been noted that the erectile response can be very rapid and synchronized, and it has been found that individual smooth muscle cells are able to communicate directly with each other via gap junctions.

There is another similar second messenger system that utilizes cyclic adenosine monophosphate (cAMP). In cavernosal tissue, the controlling factors for levels of cAMP are prostaglandins. PGE1 activates prostanoid receptors, which stimulate adenylate cyclase to produce cAMP. Here again, the effect is to reduce the levels of intracellular calcium and produce smooth muscle relaxation. There are other pharmacological agents that employ this alternative mechanism to elicit an erection.

In order for a sustained erection to occur, there must be: dilatation of the arteries to allow more blood to enter the penis; engorgement of the sinusoids to establish rigidity; narrowing of the venous system to prevent blood leaking back out. The simple relaxation of smooth muscle is able to achieve this. The smooth muscle in the artery wall relaxes and the artery vasodilates. At the same time, the trabecular smooth muscle relaxes and blood is allowed to fill the enlarged sinusoids. As the pressure rises, the penis becomes more tumescent and the subtunical venules become compressed between the collagenated smooth muscle and the tunica albuginea, so that outflow is diminished. Hydraulic pressure within the cavernosa increases to ~ 100 mmHg so that the penis hardens and becomes fully erect. Further reflex contraction of the ischiocavernous muscles during sexual intercourse or masturbation produces a rigid erection with internal pressures of several hundred millimeters of mercury. The activation of the sympathetic nervous system, which occurs at ejaculation, releases the neurotransmitters norepinephrine, endothelin, and neuropeptide Y. These have an opposing action to that described earlier so that smooth muscle contracts once more. Blood flow into the penis diminishes and the subtunical veins are opened, allowing blood to escape again. The penis becomes flaccid.

PATHOPHYSIOLOGY

It is the failure of the smooth muscle to relax, either partially or completely, that results in ED of differing severities. Partial relaxation is termed veno-occlusive dysfunction.

There are several etiological factors that need to be assessed in the history and examination of the affected man.

Does He have a Psychogenic Basis to His ED?

In the anxious individual, there can be overactivity of the sympathetic system leading to increased smooth muscle tone. Alternatively, signals from the brain of an individual with a psychogenic issue can override the erectogenic parasympathetic output from the sacral spinal cord. Psychosexual therapy can help the individual to deal with issues such as performance anxiety, reduced attraction to his partner (which may or may not be linked to a relationship problem), past sexual trauma, misconceptions about normal sexual function, suppressed feelings about sexuality, fear of sexually transmitted diseases or pregnancy. By enquiring about early morning and spontaneous erections, which all healthy men get, one can eliminate a physical cause for ED. Asking about the sort of situations in which the ED manifests itself can also help. For instance, if he is able to masturbate with an erection while alone, but is unable to perform with a partner suggests a "situational" response. There may be more than one partner with whom the man has sexual contact. Gay and bisexual men in "straight" relationships may have difficulty achieving an erection with a female partner due to feelings of guilt about their true sexual preference.

Does He have an Endocrinological Cause to His ED?

Androgen and prolactin levels are of particular concern. Hyperprolactinaemia occurs secondary to stress, drugs (such as neuroleptics and infertility treatments), cirrhosis, breast manipulation, or pituitary adenoma tumour. A high level of circulating prolactin causes inhibition of gonadotrophin releasing hormone which lowers levels of testosterone. Men with low testosterone levels may exhibit a decrease in sexual interest. Causes of low testosterone include renal failure, hypogonadism, bilateral cryptorchidism, other hypothalamic–pituitary–gonadal axis dysfunctions, Addison's disease, adrenalectomy, Kleinfelter's syndrome, cytotoxic therapies, mumps orchitis, and age related testicular degeneration as well as antiandrogen medications (e.g., cyproterone acetate, spironolactone, etc.). Androgens have also been shown to influence the activity of NOS in the corporal smooth muscle, which suggests a more direct effect of low levels of testosterone on erectile function. Approximately 52% of circulating testosterone is bound to albumin, 46% is bound to sex hormone binding globulin (SHBG), and 2% is unbound. Determination of free testosterone is preferred as it represents the most accurate parameter to reflect a real testosterone deficiency in the respective target cells. However, because the methods used most widely for determination of these parameters (e.g., equilibrium dialysis method) have shown poor reliability and high cost, the standard for evaluating testosterone deficiency remains determination of total testosterone, the free androgen index (free $T/SHBG \times 100\%$), LH level, and clinical symptoms.

Does He have Diabetes (a Major Cause of ED)?

Diabetes is a very common condition affecting men of all ages. In the Massachusetts Male Aging Study (6), men with treated diabetes had an age-adjusted prevalence of complete ED of 28%! The sequelae of diabetes are well documented and include vascular and neurological damage, both of which are major causes of ED, as they result in vascular insufficiency and diabetic neuropathy, respectively. Standard clinical investigations can eliminate diabetes as a causative factor.

Does He have a Neurogenic Basis to His ED?

There may be a physical problem with the nervous system. A history of SCI, pelvic trauma, pelvic surgery (especially to the prostate), multiple sclerosis, peripheral neuropathy due to, for example, diabetes or excessive alcohol consumption, can all contribute to the presentation of ED.

Does He have a Vascular Basis to His ED?

Diabetes, smoking, hypertension, hyperlipidaemia, and so on, are all underlying causative factors for vascular impairment. Since the erectile response is a hemodynamic event, it is hardly surprising that damage to the vessels will result in partial or complete loss of the ability to not only achieve but also maintain an erection long enough for it to be useful to its owner and his partner. A standard vascular examination can reveal important clues that may not only indicate a vascular reason for loss of the ability to have an erection, but may also point to major undetected pathology.

Does He have Drug Related Issues?

Drugs, whether prescribed or taken recreationally, may be a source of the problem. Commonly prescribed medications are known to affect erectile function

Table 7.2   Causes of Hyperprolactinaemia in Men

Physiological	Sleep (REM phase)
	Nipple stimulation
	Stress
	Coitus
Pathological	Production by tumours
	• Prolactinomas
	• Occurs in some acromegalics
	Interference with stalk
	• Any hypothalamic or pituitary tumour
	Idiopathic
	• Hyperprolactinaemia
	Polycystic ovary syndrome
	Primary hypothyroidism
	Chest wall injury
	Renal failure
	Liver failure
Drug-induced	Dopamine antagonists
	Oestrogens
	Opiates
	Cimetidine
	Methyldopa
	Reserpine

Source: Adapted from Kumar and Clark.

(see Table 7.2). In addition, street drugs such as cannabis, cocaine, amphetamines, and heroin have all been linked to decreased erectile function. Alcohol in excess is a well-recognized cause of ED.

HISTORY AND CLINICAL EXAMINATION

The History

A complete and accurate history of ED is essential for a reliable diagnosis. Communication about this issue can be loaded with cultural, religious, secular, and personal connotations and therefore the problem of ED must be approached with the right attitude. The clinician should at least appear to be open, sensitive, respectful, confident, and nonjudgemental. Questions should be unambiguous. Language must be clear and uninhibited by complex medical terminology. Never make an assumption about what the patient is trying to say. Use open questions to elicit the bulk of the information, and clarify issues by asking closed questions and by reflecting ideas back to ensure that you have understood what the patient means. It is also important to understand the patient's perspective and expectations. The media in particular can distort someone's point of view and myths and misunderstandings may need to be undone (only if you are sure yourself!). Keep in mind the pathophysiology of ED, and ask relevant questions about each system.

Start with general information about the man's life and work. Employment related stress and relationship difficulties are often involved in the etiology. Ask about the problem, its duration, frequency, and specifics such as whether the erection can be elicited but not maintained (suggestive of a veno-occlusive disorder). Ask about his past medical history and current treatments. As we have already seen, an elderly diabetic is in the highest risk group for ED. What is the patient's motivation for seeking help, and why now? There is sometimes a mismatch of expectation between the patient and his sexual partner. ED is often situational, occurring only in the presence of a partner, but the man may enjoy satisfactory masturbation and have spontaneous/nocturnal erections. Note that loss of nocturnal erections is a strong indicator of a physical problem, but can also be as a result of a major depressive disorder. Ask specific questions about other cardiovascular, neurological, and endocrinological symptoms. [For a more detailed description of neurological factors affecting ED refer to Lundberg et al. (15); for endocrinological factors refer to Heaton and Morales (16); for cardiological factors refer to Jackson et al. (17).] Does the man smoke or drink alcohol to excess or use recreational drugs? Some questions may be asked if the clinician suspects a specific etiology. For instance, is there a psychological reason, such as hidden guilt, about having sex outside the relationship, whether it be with a woman or another man? Gay sex is still a taboo subject for many, and the apparent inability of the society to come to terms with it can leave an individual feeling guilty or anxious about his sexual preference. Alternatively, there may be a fear of getting a woman pregnant, or contracting/passing on a sexually transmitted infection?

On occasion, a man may alter his history over time and reveal more information. He may have several issues that have prevented him from being totally frank. Being nonjudgemental will smoothen the doctor–patient relationship and result in a better consultation for both the professional and the patient.

Use of Questionnaires

The use of questionnaires, such as the International Inventory of Erectile Function (IIEF), are sometimes of relevance, and are a useful way of measuring improvement over time (18). The IIEF is a self-report tool that has been used in the clinical trials to assess the response of a subject to oral treatments for ED. It comprises 15 questions which cover five key areas of sexual function in men: erectile function; intercourse satisfaction; orgasmic function; sexual desire; and overall satisfaction. The two key questions in relation to the studies on ED are question 3 which asks about the ability to achieve an erection sufficient for penetration—"When you attempted intercourse, how often were you able to penetrate (enter) your partner?"—and question 4 which asks about the ability to maintain the erection long enough for satisfactory intercourse—"During sexual intercourse, how often were you able to maintain your erection after you had penetrated (entered) your partner?" Other questionnaires have been used in research. Some, like the IIEF, have been validated and found to have a high degree of sensitivity and specificity (19).

Physical Examination

Physical examination is often of great importance in clarifying suspected etiologies. Start with a general examination, and keep in mind some of the vascular, endocrinological, and neurological causes of ED. Assess the degree of androgenization checking for body hair and any evidence of gynecomastia. Examine the genitalia carefully for any abnormalities. Check whether the foreskin can be retracted, and look for conditions such as phimosis or balanitis. Deep palpation of the penis can reveal fibrotic thickening (Peyronie's plaques) in a proportion of men presenting to sexual dysfunction clinics. Cremasteric and bulbocavernous reflexes should be elicited as well as saddle sensation and deep tendon reflexes of the legs. The size and consistency of the testicles should be assessed. If urinary symptoms are present, rectal sphincter tone and prostatic examination are necessary. Cardiovascular risk assessment should be undertaken [see Appendix and Jackson et al. (17)].

Blood Investigations

Order blood investigations depending on your findings. In our clinic, men are offered tests for fasting glucose; prolactin levels; high density lipoprotein ratio and triglycerides; a 9 am testosterone, SHBG and free androgen index. Other specific tests may be appropriate (e.g., LH and free testosterone; TSH).

Some centers are able to offer further investigations. To assess erectile function, nocturnal penile tumescence (NPT) can be assessed using strain gauges. However, rigidity is seen as an important factor for assessment and tumescence and rigidity can be assessed using the Rigiscan monitor. This device is involved in both provocative testing of erectile response in the clinic or laboratory as well as home nocturnal testing. The patient can take the device home for nocturnal testing after receiving some tuition on its use. Rigiscan can be used to investigate suspected cases of neurological or psychological causes (20). Another device, the NEVA (nocturnal electronic volumetric assessment) is worn while asleep at home and is of particular use in the investigation of vascular disorders.

Erectile capacity can be undertaken by observing the response to an intracavernous injection of alprostadil or papaverine. This can be quantified by the use of Doppler ultrasound and undertaken in the hospital setting. Other stimuli such as vibration and erotic videotape material may be helpful to augment the response, particularly in the clinical setting. The MIDUS (Male Impotence Diagnostic Ultrasound System) is a Doppler machine that is used in clinics to measure penile blood flow. Unlike Duplex Doppler Ultrasonography performed in the hospital, the Knoll/MIDUS Ultrasound System is designed as an office-based system. Doppler Duplex sonography will allow for visualization of the vasculature in patients eligible for reconstructive surgery.

Electrophysiological testing may be indicated in specific cases [e.g., nerve conduction studies, GSA (genital sensory analyzer)].

A consensus statement of recommendations has been published following the second international consultation on sexual dysfunction (21).

TREATMENT OPTIONS FOR ED IN MEN

Guidelines for treatment have changed considerably over the past decade, and will continue to do so as new drugs and treatment options become available and are evaluated. Treatment can be subdivided into first, second and third line therapies, and includes drug therapies as well as psychotherapies and surgery. All patients should be provided with some general information about ED, which will include normalizing the condition, which can be reassuring for the man and his partner. The role of organic and psychological factors should be described and unbiased information provided on all suitable treatment options.

Pharmacotherapy for Men with ED

Few licensed drugs are currently available for the treatment of men with ED. Those that are available elicit their effect by one of two mechanisms. The agent boosts either the neuronal control mechanism or the local control mechanism (13). As we shall see, oral therapies can have their effect on either system, whereas the intracavernosal and intraurethral systems act locally to produce an erection.

First Line (Oral) Therapies

Oral agents used to treat ED should be reliable, have minimal side effects, and be simple to use (22). The oral therapies currently licensed for ED are the phosphodiesterase 5 inhibitors (PDE5 inhibitors), which have a peripheral mechanism of action, and apomorphine, which acts centrally. These agents require sexual stimulation to initiate the neuronal activation required to start the hemodynamic erectile response. This is in contrast to the PGE mediated response initiated by intracavernosal and intraurethral alprostadil administration that "forces" an erection (see later). Yohimbine is another oral agent that has been shown to have some efficacy, but this is currently unlicensed in the UK although available on prescription in the UK and US. There are several advantages of the oral agents. Because they are administered orally, they are noninvasive, unlike intracavernosal and intraurethral medications and surgery. Taking a tablet is also more discreet, which is an important characteristic because it restores some of the spontaneity of sexual activity and removes the need for interruptions. In addition, oral methods of drug delivery are not associated with fibrosis (a potential adverse effect when using intracavernosal injections), neither is there any penile or urethral pain that can occur with alprostadil use when given by injection or as the intraurethral pellet. As a consequence, oral therapies are now considered to be first line therapy.

Inhibitors of phosphodiesterase 5:   As we have already seen, NO is required for normal erectile function (13). NO is a gas and is derived from L-arginine (an amino acid) and oxygen in the presence of the enzyme NOS. NO, interacts with soluble guanylate cyclase, which then dephosphorylates guanosine tri-phosphate (GTP) to produce the second messenger cyclic guanosine mono-phosphate (cGMP). It is the amount of cGMP present that determines the extent of relaxation in corporal smooth muscle by stimulating the reduction of intracellular calcium (23,24).

Phosphodiesterase (PDE) is a molecule that has many different isoforms, and is found in most mammalian tissue (24). PDE5 is the predominant isoenzyme found in the corpus cavernosum and is a cGMP-binding, cGMP specific PDE (24,25). Its role in the reversal of the penile erection is to decrease the levels of cGMP so that vasoconstriction and trabecular smooth muscle contraction take place. Theoretically, by blocking the action of PDE5, the erection should be maintained. This is the proposed mechanism of action of the PDE5 inhibitors.

PDE5 inhibitors are not suitable for all patients, and it may take several attempts at taking them before they have the desired effect (26). All PDE5 inhibitors are absolutely contraindicated for patients who are taking any form of nitrate, including sublingual sprays and nitrates used recreationally (e.g., amyl nitrate). There are currently three licensed PDE5 blocking drugs available in the UK and US: sildenafil (Viagra), vardenafil (Levitra), and tadalafil (Cialis).

Sildenafil (Viagra).   Since its introduction in 1998, sildenafil has been the subject of many clinical trials on men within the age range of 19–87 years. It the most studied of the PDE5 inhibitors and currently the most widely used treatment for ED. Sildenafil has been shown to be effective and well tolerated by patients with various etiologies (22,27,28). Sildenafil has a molecular structure similar to that of cGMP [see Fig. 7.1 (24)] and is highly selective for PDE5, with some selectivity for PDE6 found in the retina, which would reasonably account for the transient [usually minutes (24)] visual disturbance that some men experience. In a complex interaction between the molecules, sildenafil increases its own binding affinity by a positive feedback mechanism, making more cGMP available (24). More cGMP means more NO available to relax smooth muscle, which results in improved erections.

Sildenafil is rapidly absorbed, and has a plasma half-life of $\sim$4 h (25). Of the circulating sildenafil, 96% is bound to plasma proteins and therefore is not excreted in urine (24). When correctly taken just once daily, there is no significant accumulation of the drug in the body, as it takes just over 24 h to achieve total clearance. Clinical experience since its introduction has shown sildenafil

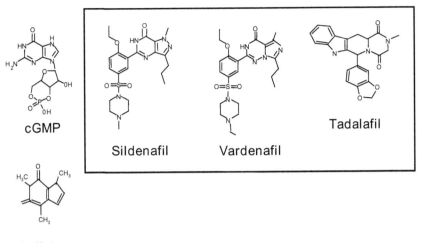

cGMP

Sildenafil

Vardenafil

Tadalafil

Caffeine

Figure 7.1 Structure of sildenafil and other molecular structures.

to be a safe agent in most groups of patients (29). Sildenafil is an oral medication, licensed for clinical use in three doses: 25, 50, and 100 mg. It should be taken ~1 h before sexual activity, after which time plasma levels should be at a peak. Further time may be required if taken with a high-fat meal as this increases transit time in the gut, but no dose adjustment is necessary (24). After starting on 50 mg per day, the dose can be titrated up or down, depending on tolerance and efficacy, and should not normally exceed 100 mg, as adverse events are more likely to occur at higher doses with no proven increase in efficacy (30).

Sildenafil is cleared chiefly by the cytochrome P450 enzyme CYP3A4 with minor involvement by CYP2C9 (30). Reduced function of these enzymes results in higher plasma levels and so for certain groups of patients, a lower dose is recommended. Reduced clearance occurs in elderly patients over the age of 65: patients with severe renal impairment (creatinine clearance <30 mL/min) and hepatic impairment (e.g., due to cirrhosis). For patients in these groups, sildenafil should not be prescribed >25 mg. Some pharmacological agents inhibit CYP3A4, and for this reason the lowest dose of sildenafil should also be prescribed for patients taking ketoconazole and itraconazole (antifungal agents), saquinavir, erythromycin, cimetidine, and diltiazem. Coadministration of ritonavir and sildenafil is not recommended as ritonavir inhibits both CYP3A4 and CYP2C9, causing a drastic increase in the plasma concentration of sildenafil (24). Grapefruit juice is a weak inhibitor of CYP3A4 in the gut wall, and may result in modest increases in plasma concentration (30). Concomitant use with alpha adrenoceptor antagonists should also be avoided (discussed subsequently).

Sildenafil is mostly well tolerated (22). In the more recent clinical trials, only ~2–3% of men discontinued treatment due to adverse effects, which is a similar proportion to those taking placebo (31). Most men who discontinue treatment do so because of partner reluctance, perceived ineffectiveness of the drug, or lack of motivation. Up to one-third of men experience one or more adverse effects, but where effects do occur, they are mostly mild and transient (minutes to hours) (29,31). The frequencies of adverse effects vary from study to study and become more frequent where higher doses are used. Most common adverse effects are headaches (7–39%), facial flushing (7–35%), dyspepsia (7%), and rhinitis (4%) (22,29,32). These effects appear to be the result of a mild transient decrease in blood pressure because of the effect on peripheral vessel vasodilatation (31). Visual disturbances have also been reported by a small proportion of men, but these disturbances tend to be very transient, as a high plasma concentration is needed to affect PDE6 in the retina. Hypotension, orthostatic hypotension, and syncope have also been reported, but incidences were <2% and comparable to placebo (33). Very rarely, priapism (an erection lasting for >6 h) may occur and sildenafil should be used with caution in individuals who are predisposed to priapism (individuals with sickle cell anaemia, leukaemia, or multiple myeloma).

Sildenafil is effective for a large proportion of patients with psychogenic or organic causes for their ED. The highest proportion of positive responders is amongst men with a psychogenic etiology (84%) (34). Those with an organic etiology respond in 68% of cases, those with diabetes in 59%, and those with post-prostatectomy in 43%.

Prostate cancer: Whether prostate cancer is treated with the various surgical techniques available, radiotherapy or brachytherapy, up to 60% of all patients acquire ED within 18 months of treatment (35,36). Men with ED who have undergone a radical prostatectomy have an almost 100% occurrence of ED if the procedure was non-nerve-sparing. This is reduced to 40–70% if one or both nerve bundles are spared. Evidence from patients undergoing radical prostatectomy for cancer suggests that the neurovascular bundle must be intact on at least one side for sildenafil to have its effect (37,38). Nevertheless, Nehra and Goldstein (39) suggest that for post-prostatectomy patients, sildenafil should be the first line treatment regardless of the state of the neurovascular bundle. This is because there is evidence that with time, some function can return. If both nerve bundles are spared, then up to 80% of men respond to treatment, this figure is reduced to 15% if there is no sparing of the nerves during surgery. For the group of patients who receive radiotherapy as treatment for prostate cancer, studies show that the outcome of sildenafil use is dependent on the level of erectile function before treatment with sildenafil (40). Such patients should be started on a 50 mg dose and titrated up to 100 mg if required (36). Up to three-quarters of the radiotherapy group treated with sildenafil reported improvement.

Nightly dosing of sildenafil appears to increase the return of spontaneous nocturnal erections after nerve-sparing retropubic radical prostatectomy (NSRRP) (41).

Depressive disorder: Depression can be a complex problem to sort out but worth doing, since moderate to complete ED is 1.82 times more likely to occur in depressed men (8), and there is an increased incidence of depressive symptoms in men with ED (42). When associated with ED, it is important for the clinician to determine whether it is the causative factor of ED, a product of ED, or whether the two simply coexist. Treatment may then depend on what is considered to be the underlying causative factor. As an example, a man with limb loss may become depressed. He may then be treated with an antidepressant that results in a degree of ED [most classes of antidepressant cause some degree of ED (43), with the exception of bupropion and nefazodone (44)]. This further loss of sexual function then exacerbates the depression. This example illustrates one of the relationship models between depression and ED (i.e., ED due to antidepressant use). Note that many other medications are also responsible for ED, which affects treatment adherence. Other possibilities include depression secondary to ED or conversely ED as a symptom of depression. Depression resulting from another comorbidity which then manifests as ED is another possibility (45). It is therefore important to investigate for common risk factors such as diabetes (discussed subsequently). Assessment of nocturnal erections either by questioning or by investigation can occasionally lead to more discriminating questions about psychiatric state, since major depression can result in loss of nocturnal erections (46), which demonstrates an organic cause. One of the uses of sildenafil in cases of depression is to counteract the effect of antidepressants (47,48).

Diabetes mellitus: Diabetes is possibly the greatest risk factor for having ED (6). In a small-scale study using Rigiscan as an objective measure, it was found that sildenafil increases the period of penile rigidity in a dose dependent manner (25). In a much larger, double-blind, flexible dose-escalation study done over a 12 week period, diabetic men with ED were given sildenafil (49). Using the IIEF as a measure, 56% of diabetic men receiving sildenafil reported an improvement in their erections compared with only 10% in the placebo group. This figure was even higher when a diabetes type II group was studied independently (50). It was found that patients with fewer diabetic complications were more likely to benefit, probably because there is less neural and vascular damage. Many in the diabetes subgroup require the higher doses of sildenafil, and unsurprisingly, the proportion experiencing adverse effects tends to be greater than that seen in the general population (51). There appears to be little difference in the efficacy of sildenafil between type I and type II diabetes.

Hypertension: ED is commonly seen in patients with hypertension (6). In a retrospective analysis, Kloner et al. (52) examined the effect of antihypertensive medication on the efficacy of sildenafil. They found that sildenafil is effective in patients taking antihypertensives and is comparable to results seen in the general population of men taking sildenafil. There were no significant drug interactions between sildenafil and antihypertensive medications noted in the clinical trials that included men taking diuretics, beta-blockers, angiotensin converting enzyme inhibitors, calcium channel blockers, or nothing. There have been rare reports of spontaneous hypotensive events after the use of sildenafil in combination with alpha-blockers (30). However, generally it was found that regardless of whether the patient was taking a single antihypertensive drug, a combination of up to three different ones or none at all, about one-third experienced some adverse effects, mostly flushing and dizziness. Webb et al. (53) found that sildenafil can produce additive (but not synergistic) reductions in blood pressure when using amlodipine. Sildenafil does cause mild and transient decreases in blood pressure. The mean maximum fall in blood pressure observed with a 100 mg dose of sildenafil is a systolic decrease of 8.4 mmHg and a diastolic decrease of 5.5 mmHg (30). For this reason, it is inadvisable to give sildenafil to men with a blood pressure $\leq 90/50$ mmHg.

Cardiovascular disease: In patients with cardiovascular disease, it is important to determine whether any treatment for ED would be contraindicated (e.g., where sexual activity is inadvisable). Men with cardiovascular disease tend to have an increased number of risk factors such as smoking and diabetes. These men are also quite prone to depression, which compounds the problem (45). Nevertheless, those who have a low risk cardiovascular status that is stable and well controlled can be treated within the primary care setting (17). Those in the high risk category should be referred for specialist cardiac evaluation before treating ED. Specific contraindications in this group include hypotension, men with a recent history of stroke or myocardial infarction (within 6 months), and patients receiving nitric oxide donors (e.g., nicorandil and nebivolol) or organic nitrate therapy in any form including sprays and sublingual tablets. This is because organic nitrates increase available NO and PDE5 inhibitors increase the response to NO. A synergistic response occurs causing blood pressure to fall rapidly. If a nitrate is to be given after sildenafil administration, then a washout period of 25 h is a minimum requirement (i.e., five times the half-life of sildenafil). This period must be increased in patients who demonstrate decreased clearance of sildenafil as mentioned earlier.

Coronary heart disease: In a subanalysis of patients with coronary heart disease and ED, there was a 70% improvement in patient's erections (placebo 20%) (54). Much attention has been given by the media that sildenafil may increase the likelihood of a serious cardiovascular event such as a myocardial infarction or an ischaemic attack. This notion is not supported by evidence which concludes that the prevalence of such events in the treated and control group is similar (55,56). Recommendations from an independent expert panel agree that there is no evidence that there is any increase in risk to patients with or without diagnosed cardiovascular disease when using sildenafil (17).

Coronary artery disease: In patients with coronary artery disease, investigators found that there was no direct adverse effect on cardiovascular status in men with severe coronary artery disease. In addition, a small positive effect on coronary blood flow was seen (57). In a more recent study, the investigators concluded that sildenafil had no effect on rate of recovery from exercise, nor does it potentiate myocardial ischemia in patients with stable angina (who are not taking nitrates) (58). Data suggests that sildenafil is well tolerated and effective in heart transplantation patients who are fit for sexual activity (33,59).

Use in patients with a history of transient ischemic attacks (TIAs) has not been studied. Because some patients experience TIAs following a drop in blood pressure, sildenafil should be used with caution in these patients and should not be used in patients with a recent cerebral vascular accident.

Wagner and Mulhall (60) found that age does not seem to greatly influence therapeutic response to sildenafil. While ED is strongly associated with increasing age, it is not a direct consequence of it. In their study, Wagner and Mulhall found that 69% of elderly men with various comorbidities responded favorably to treatment. This compares well with the 74% of positive responders in the general population of men. The main point about elderly men is that there is often concurrent conditions that reduce response. Nevertheless, even in the most affected group (elderly men with diabetes), half of all those treated had some response. It should be remembered that elderly men have a reduced clearance to sildenafil, which results in increased efficacy and incidence of adverse events. With this in mind, the producers recommend that for men over the age of 65, a starting dose of 25 mg should be considered and only increased if the patient reports efficacy and tolerance (30).

Other conditions: Other conditions have been studied where sildenafil treatment has been used (29). In men with spina bifida, there is an 80% reported improvement in erections as well as a significant increase in sexual confidence. Men with SCI have shown improvement in their erections of between 75 and 94%, with up to 72% of SCI patients reporting successful attempts at intercourse (61). This shows that there is a high efficacy of sildenafil in SCI patients who have preserved reflexogenic erections. Men with multiple sclerosis show an 89% improvement after 12 weeks of treatment with sidenafil. In those patients who receive dialysis, 80% reported a 10-point increase in IIEF scores. One group in which caution should be exercised is men with Parkinson's disease. This is because those who have autonomic failure may suffer postural hypotension.

In men who were previously treated with intracavernous injections, 75% responded to sildenafil treatment, and of these, 64% were happy to continue oral therapy (29). Unfortunately, some remain resistant to first line oral therapy, and require second line intracavernous/intraurethral therapies.

It has been noted that sildenafil is available both on the internet and on the black market as a recreational drug. After more than 5 years on the market, it is now known that long term use is safe and that sildenafil remains effective over a period of years (32,62). Some men require an increased dose after some time of using the drug, but this is regarded as a consequence of underlying morbidity rather than a tachyphylaxis (62). As we have seen, use of other medications with sildenafil is safe in most cases. We have seen no studies done in men who use recreational drugs. Sildenafil treatment is not cheap; in the UK and most other countries, many men have to pay for their treatment because of government intervention. The economic validity of these restrictions is questionable when the impact of the psychological factors on individuals, their families, and their work are considered.

Sildenafil is not suitable for all patients. For those in whom it is not effective, they should move to another oral agent or to second and third line therapies or consider other salvage techniques (63).

Tadalafil (Cialis). The structure of tadalafil is shown in the Fig. 7.1 (64). This newer PDE5 inhibitor was introduced in the UK in 2003. The initial clinical trials have tested doses ranging from 2.5 to 25 mg (65,66). Investigators used IIEF scores, the Sex Encounter Profile (SEP), and Global Assessment Question (GAQ) to measure outcomes. The outcomes reported by men with various etiologies for their ED have indicated that the 10 and 20 mg doses are most effective, and these doses are now marketed. Tadalafil is rapidly absorbed and demonstrates a maximum response within 2 h. It has a half-life of 17.5 h. Brock et al. (65,66) team found that the longer half-life of the drug allowed 73% of their trial subjects to remain able to attempt intercourse over a period of 36 h when taking the 20 mg dose. The implication of this finding is that careful planning of the initiation of sexual activity is not necessary, and this is preferable to some patients.

As with the other PDE5 inhibitors, the liver p450 enzyme CYP3A4 metabolizes tadalafil, which neither inhibits nor induces the enzyme. Nevertheless, patients with diminished liver function should only be treated with caution. Another perceived advantage is that there is no pharmacodynamic interaction with alcohol, and so patients taking this oral therapy are not required to avoid alcohol (67). Food does not affect the rate and extent of absorption either.

Tadalafil appears to be well tolerated and has acceptable adverse effects as perceived by patients since in a series of five randomized, double-blind placebo-controlled trials (65) 89% of men completed the trial. The group receiving the maximum dose of 20 mg had the largest drop-out rate because of the associated increase in adverse effects. Nevertheless, where adverse effects do occur they are mild and transient and decrease in severity with continued treatment. The rarest effect was visual disturbance, with only one individual affected throughout the trials. The most common adverse effects were headache (14%) and dyspepsia (10%). Other less reported effects include back pain, nasal congestion, myalgia, and flushing. These last four effects were comparable to those reported by men taking placebo.

Further safety and efficacy trials have been conducted on volunteers with diabetes and cardiovascular disorders in whom ED can be a marker for cardiovascular disease.

Diabetes: In the diabetes group (68), 10 and 20 mg doses were tested on men with type I or type II diabetes mellitus with and without microvascular complications. Eight eight-percent of subjects completed the trial, 3% had recognized adverse events (although some were taking placebo), and 2% discontinued due to perceived lack of efficacy. Most success was reported in the 20 mg group, with two-thirds of men reporting significantly enhanced erections. The group receiving 10 mg had results that were comparable to men taking sildenafil at various doses.

Hypertension: Emmick et al. (69) worked with two groups of men who had stable angina and hypertension. Tadalafil had no clinically relevant effects on blood pressure in healthy subjects, but did have a mild vasodilator effect. When tested on patients with stable angina taking short-acting nitrates, there was a repeatable rapid decrease in the blood pressure of some men. With long-acting nitrates, the decrease was minimal and tolerance developed in some individuals by day 2. However, in a small subset of those tested, there was an appreciably large drop in blood pressure, and for this reason, men taking short- or long-acting nitrates should not be prescribed tadalafil. The group who had hypertension were monitored while they took tadalafil in combination with their antihypertensive medications. The study showed that there was no significant difference in blood pressure regardless of the number and classes of agents, although some men experienced flushing. This effect was also seen in men not taking concomitant therapy for hypertension. For all groups with stable angina or hypertension, there was no significant increase in cardiovascular adverse events. The number of events that did occur did not deviate from that expected after adjusting for differences in the population under investigation. More work involving larger numbers needs to be done with men taking antihypertensives. Studies should also be done to investigate the effect of tadalafil on men with other cardiovascular conditions. There is a great deal of safety and efficacy work yet to be done using tadalafil in patients with various conditions similar to what is outlined earlier about sildenafil.

Other areas of research outstanding for tadalafil include efficacy in men with depression, prostate cancer, ischemic heart disease, the elderly, those with SCI, and those who have undergone prostatectomy.

Vardenafil (Levitra).   The structure of vardenafil is shown in Fig. 7.1. This is another recently introduced PDE5 inhibitor. Various doses have been trialed and 5, 10, and 20 mg tablets are now available for prescription. Trials on vardenafil have also used the IIEF (EF Domain)2, SEP3, SEP, and GAQ questions to assess efficacy.

The pharmacokinetics of vardenafil are similar in many ways to those of sildenafil. Vardenafil is rapidly absorbed and reaches its peak plasma concentration around 1 h and 40 min after administration. Absorption is not compromised by a regular meal or by a moderate amount of alcohol, but this may be delayed when taken with a high-fat meal (>57% fat). Like the other PDE5 inhibitors, vardenafil is predominantly metabolized by the CYP34A isoform of cytochrome P450 with some contribution from CYP3A5 and CYP2C. The concomitant use of the potent CYP34A inhibitors ritonavir, indinavir, ketoconazole, and itraconazole (oral form) is contraindicated in men over the age of 75. When used with erythromycin, the dose should not exceed 5 mg. Use with alpha-receptor antagonists is not recommended as this may lead to a hypotensive episode. The half-life of vardenafil is ~5 h, slightly longer than that of sildenafil.

In clinical trials, tolerability has been demonstrated with adverse reactions similar to those seen with the other PDE5 inhibitors (70,71). Most common were headache (3–22%), flushing (0–10%), and nasal congestion (3–14%). Other effects with much less common occurrence include nausea, dyspepsia, dizziness, hypertension, photosensitivity reaction, visual disturbance, hypertonia, hypotension, syncope, and erectile disturbance (72). Adverse effects have a tendency to diminish with regular use of PDE5 inhibitors over a period of weeks. In the vardenafil trials, it was noted that for nasal congestion, the trend is fairly constant for doses >5 mg.

Although there is no significant effect on exercise induced ischemia in patients with coronary heart disease with vardenafil, it should not be given to those for whom sexual activity is not advised. Vardenafil does not significantly affect blood pressure and is safe to use for men taking one or more of the anti-hypertensive medications (73).

There is still a lot of research that must be done to test the safety and efficacy of vardenafil in certain groups of patients. Patients with severe renal or hepatic impairment, hypotension (with a blood pressure <90/50 mmHg), a recent history of stroke or myocardial infarction, unstable angina, and retinal disease have been excluded from trials done to date. Until these investigations are done, these conditions must be considered as contraindications.

Two "difficult to treat" groups of patients for whom vardenafil may be of benefit are those with diabetes and those who have undergone radical prostatectomy.

Post-radical prostatectomy: In a study by Brock et al. (65) it was found that post-radical prostatectomy patients were likely to suffer from ED in the "severe" category. Improved erections were reported in 71% of patients who had undergone a bilateral nerve-sparing procedure. Vardenafil treatment was able to move the majority into the moderate range for erectile function, and was also noted to have a positive effect on depressive symptoms in this group.

Diabetes mellitus: In another study conducted by Goldstein et al. (74) men who had diabetes and ED showed a significant improvement of their erections. Erectile function scores demonstrated that some of those treated moved from having moderate ED to mild ED and the change was appreciable by up to 72%. Two-thirds of diabetic men were able to penetrate their partner, and over half maintained the erection long enough to have successful intercourse. These results are comparable to those for sildenafil (75).

There is much more in depth research to be done on specific groups of men using vardenafil. Men with hypertension, depression, prostate cancer, ischemic heart disease, and SCI have yet to be studied, as have the elderly male population (though studies to date have included subgroups of patients aged >65).

Centrally Acting Oral Therapy

Apomorphine: Apomorphine is a drug used routinely in the treatment of patients with Parkinson's disease. Empirical evidence from a few Parkinson's patients treated with apomorphine has suggested that they experience increased sexual activity (76). Male patients with alcohol dependence treated with the same agent have also reported improved erectile function (77). Data from these two groups of patients suggest that apomorphine is able to induce erections.

While apomorphine is a derivative of morphine, it has greater structural and pharmacological similarities with dopamine, and acts as a dopamine agonist (78–80) (even in urine screening for opioids, apomorphine will rarely give a false positive). Dopamine and apomorphine act centrally on dopamine receptors (especially D1 and D2), and studies using rodents have demonstrated a role for dopamine in the control of sexual function in both sexes (76). This means that this drug works via a very different mechanism than most other pharmacological agents used in the treatment of ED. As we have already seen, many other agents act locally on smooth muscle to increase blood flow to the penis. While the exact mechanism of action of apomorphine is not fully understood, it appears to work on several areas of the brain to boost the neuronal signal involved in the erectile response (76). Recent large-scale trials have confirmed the connection between dopamine and sexual function in men because apomorphine is able to induce penile erections when they are sexually stimulated (81).

Apomorphine can be used to treat men with physical or psychological etiologies. It is important to note that like other oral treatments in use for ED, this drug requires the man to become sexually stimulated before an erection can be achieved. In this setting, apomorphine is self-administered sublingually (apo SL) as a 2 or 3 mg single dose, usually starting at 2 mg and only increasing to 3 mg if necessary (79,80). Good patient education is important to achieve optimum results. The tablet is placed under the tongue after a sip of water and allowed to dissolve slowly for up to 10 min without swallowing it. Best results are often not achieved until use of apo SL on the sixth occasion (82). By this point, over 90% (80) of correctly diagnosed users will achieve an erection and the majority of these will be within 20 min, making this a fast acting drug. This response is repeatable, so that by the sixth month of use there are still >90% of men able to achieve erections firm enough for intercourse [assessed using data from diary records from a double-blind placebo-controlled trial (81)].

Apo SL is rapidly absorbed and eliminated, and reaches a peak plasma concentration within 40–60 min, having a half-life of ~2–3 h (79). This means that apo SL can be taken every 8 h if required. Data suggests that no dose adjustment is required in elderly patients although this group is more prone to hypotensive episodes. There are few contraindications for use. Impaired hepatic function and renal insufficiency are not necessarily contraindicated but the dose should be limited to 2 mg. More work needs to be done in these areas, and until such time a careful assessment should be made to balance benefit against risk, especially in patients with hepatic insufficiency. There is also further work to be done to assess efficacy in patients with SCI and multiple sclerosis. The effect on patients who have had prostatectomy or pelvic surgery is also not known. Caution should be taken when treating patients with uncontrolled hypertension and patients with hypotension. Antihypertensives and nitrates (especially short-acting nitrates) do have the potential to cause an acute episode of hypotension. Caution also needs to be taken in patients who have penile deformity or other conditions that may predispose them to priapism. There are few absolute contraindications for use, but include combinations with other dopamine agonists or antagonists and patients with severe unstable heart conditions or other conditions where any sexual activity creates unacceptable risk. Excess alcohol should be avoided due to the increased risk of hypotension.

Because of the low doses involved in the therapeutic use of apo SL in the treatment of ED, there are few side effects (80). The most commonly seen are nausea (6.8%), headache (6.7%), and dizziness (4.4%). Nausea tends to diminish with subsequent dosing, so that by the eighth dose this is usually no longer a problem. Where nausea and emesis is a concern, it is safe to prescribe ondansetron hydrochloride, prochlorperazine maleate, or domperidone prophylactically (79). No other antiemetics have been tested for safety. Rhinitis and pharyngitis have been reported in a very small proportion on men, and in a very few cases (0.2%) syncope can occur.

There is more work to be done concerning the use of apo SL. But data published to date do indicate a good response (82,83). Responses from questionnaires such as the IIEF indicate that many patients and their partners report erectile function sufficient for penetration. The rapid onset of apo SL allows for a fair degree of spontaneity, and the response is predictable once satisfactory success has been achieved. This agent is available in the UK and Europe.

Yohimbine: Yohimbine (84) is an alpha2-selective antagonist currently unlicensed for use for men with ED. It is a naturally occurring alkaloid produced from the African yohimbe tree. It has been implicated as an aphrodisiac (85) but has not been properly considered as a therapeutic agent until recently. The proposed mechanism of action of yohimbine is to block presynaptic alpha2 receptors while sparing the postsynaptic alpha1 receptors. The effect of this is to enhance the release of norepinephrine in the central nervous system. It reaches a plasma concentration in just 10–15 min and has a very short half-life of just over 30 min. Previous research has shown that oral yohimbine can be used successfully to treat ED with a psychological basis. It has also been used to reverse antidepressant-induced sexual dysfunction.

Guay and Spark (84) suggest that previous studies using yohimbine have not been successful because their subjects included a large proportion of men who were smokers. They hypothesized that smoking reduces the effectiveness of yohimbine and so their study excluded this subgroup. In their small-scale study of 18 men aged between 34 and 69 years, they reported that use of low doses of yohimbine (5.4 or 10.8 mg) at home had resulted in nine of the men achieving successful penetration on 75% of occasions tried. They reported few side effects with the low doses used (mild anxiety in one subject and hot flashes in another). Also noted was a slight increase in serum cortisol. From their evidence, they suggested that yohimbine could be useful for a subset of men with mild disease or few risk factors, and recommended that yohimbine should be studied further. Random controlled trails would be useful to determine the safety and efficacy of this established pharmaceutical agent.

Second Line (Injectable and Intraurethral) Treatments

Injectable and intraurethral treatments for ED are now considered to be second line treatments after oral therapies have been tried or rejected. Also, these treatments are primarily for men with an organic cause for their ED. Patients need to be made aware of the potential for priapism. The initial doses of these agents are given under supervision as there is also a risk of a hypotensive episode needing medical attention. Patients must be taught how to inject safely and using a proper technique so as to avoid the problems of fibrosis which indicates that treatment must be discontinued.

Only alprostadil (prostaglandin E1) is licensed for use as an intracavernosal injection (ICI) in the UK and US. This drug utilizes cyclic adenosine monophosphate (cAMP) rather than cGMP (see Fig. 7.1). Prostaglandin E1 (PGE1) receptors are G-protein coupled receptors located at the surface of the smooth muscle cell. When stimulated, they activate adenylyl cyclase via the G-protein. This increases the concentration of intracellular cAMP, which acts as a second messenger in a cascade that ends with a decrease in intracellular calcium concentration and muscle relaxation. No sexual stimulation is required to elicit an erection using the ICI route of delivery. ICI alprostadil is marketed as 5, 10, 20, and 40 μg injections that have been proven to be effective and safe doses to give in the majority of cases (86). At the time of Linet and Ogrinc's studies, little else was available in the way of pharmacotherapies for ED. In the dose–response study of 296 men with various etiologies, they found that the erections would last longer the higher the dose injected. This pattern was repeated in their other placebo-controlled experiments with increasing numbers of subjects to determine optimum dose and to confirm efficacy and safety. In the largest of the trials with 683 men, 69% completed the 6 month study. There are adverse affects associated with ICI alprostadil use. The treatment was discontinued by 6% of men due to the main side effect, which is penile pain. This effect was actually experienced by half of the men participating, but not on all occasions. Most often, the men reported the pain as being mild. Five percent of the subjects experienced prolonged erections although most men continued the treatment. In the three studies, six individuals experienced priapism (an erection lasting >6 h). In the large study, 87% of men reported satisfactory sexual activity, and this was reflected in the partner's questionnaire. Other rare adverse effects occurred in 1% of the men and were thought to be related to hypotension. These included irregular pulse, lightheadedness, dizziness, diaphoresis, vasodilation, and vasovagal reaction. It is for this reason that the initial prescribed dose must be delivered in the clinical setting under medical supervision.

Alprostadil can also be delivered intraurethrally as MUSE (medicated urethral system for erection). This mode of delivery is recommended for a small subset of individuals who may have problems with injecting. PGE1 is delivered into the urethra immediately after urination (for lubrication and to help disperse the drug) using an applicator which the patient can be taught to use safely. Here, the drug is used at a much higher concentration at 125, 250, 500, or 1000 μg doses. Researchers have reported very different efficacies using MUSE in this way (87–89). Only Padma-Nathan et al., used a random controlled trial, and their subject recruitment was far greater than the other two groups (1511 vs. 100 and 103). Werthman and Rajfer (87) only reported making observations up to 10 min after administration of the drug whereas Padma-Nathan et al. (89) made observations up to 60 min after drug delivery. Also, Werthman and Rajfer's studies were conducted entirely in the clinical setting, which can inhibit the erections elicited by MUSE which often require sexual stimulation. Padma-Nathan et al., found that 65.9% of subjects had maximal penile responses (assessed on scale of 1–5) in the clinical setting. They increased the dose delivered to each individual up to a maximum of 1000 μg. The number of men achieving the maximum penile response rose linearly with increasing dose. Of this group, 35.7% of men experienced penile pain which was usually mild; 2.4% withdrew from the study because of the pain. Hypotension occured in 3.3% of the men, and syncope in 0.4% (for this reason, the initial prescribed dose must be delivered in the clinical setting under medical supervision). The study continued by giving further subjects MUSE to use in their own home. A 3 month trial of MUSE, was completed by 87.7% of these men with <2% discontinuing because of adverse effects. The success rate for intercourse for the home trial group was 64.9%, slightly lower than that indicated in the clinical setting. These men reported penile pain as the main adverse effect. The problems associated with ICI alprostadil, such as fibrosis, hematomas, and priapism, were not seen. Slight bleeding from the penis can occur, and this is probably due to minor trauma when inserting the MUSE applicator incorrectly (87).

Papaverine and phentolamine are not currently licensed in the UK for the treatment of ED, although they have been used for many years. Papaverine is closely related to morphine and originates from the opium poppy. However, its little understood pharmacology is very different from that of morphine. It is believed to inhibit phosphodiesterase in a similar fashion to sildenafil. The starting dose is dependent on local formulation but is usually ~20 mg in the alprostadil nonresponder, rising in increments to 50 mg. Phentolamine is a nonselective alpha adrenoceptor antagonist with a plasma half-life of 2 h and acts to relax smooth muscles (90). The starting dose is 0.5 mg which can be repeated after

20 min if there is no response. Typically, it may be necessary to combine two or more of the agents in the nonresponding patient (hence the tri-mix preparation). Injection into the cavernosal tissue is self administered after a clinic based trial of the drugs (often in combination with each other) under medical supervision. As with ICI alprostadil, complications can arise from repeated injections into the same site. These include nodule formation and indurations of the tunica albuginea resulting in a Peyronie's-like distortion of the penis. These affects should be checked for on follow-up visits. The nodules are painless and become more likely to occur as treatment continues over time (91). These complications alongside dislike of the technique by the man and his partner as well as "needle phobia" (increasing adrenergic outflow), all lead to a limited use of these effective agents.

Moxisylyte is an injectable alpha-blocking agent and is useful where there is considerable psychological etiology requiring evidence of an erection. Effective salvage therapy for intracavernosal injection nonresponse includes augmentation with sildenafil (92) or other combination therapies.

Third Line Therapies

Vacuum constriction devices and constriction rings for men with ED: A vacuum constriction device (VCD) (93) is simply a rigid tube that is placed over the penis. A vacuum is then created inside the tube either manually or by a battery-powered motor. The penis becomes erect when such a negative pressure surrounds it. This principle is not new, and was being used as a treatment for ED as far back as 1874. For some men, this vacuum is sufficient, but others need a "constriction ring" which when applied to the base of the erect penis, preventing venous leakage once the tube is removed for sexual activity to commence.

This device is useful as a treatment for men with ED who are unable to use oral therapies. It also avoids the use of ICI therapy, which some men find objectionable. It is fairly simple to use although it is somewhat obtrusive. One drawback of use with the constriction ring is that the erection pivots about the ring making it less natural. Its use has been studied in men with diabetes, SCI, explanted penile prosthesis, and requiring dialysis for various reasons. These studies have all reported high success rates of VCD use with approximately three-quarters of men. Partners too find the device an acceptable compromise.

As with all of the treatments, there are some contraindications to the use of VCDs. Sickle cell trait/disease, leukemia, and anticoagulation therapy are medical considerations that can be complicated by VCD use. In addition, men with poor manual dexterity may find the manual pump and the constriction ring difficult to use, although this need not be a problem for men with obliging partners!

For a few individuals who are able to achieve an erection but not maintain it, they can use the constriction ring without the vacuum tube. This will enhance the firmness and size of the penis. In all cases where a constriction ring is used, a time limit of 30 min must be strongly emphasized.

Some adverse affects are reported by some individuals using VCDs, but these tend to be painless and self-correcting. Ecchymoses is reported in 12%

of users, and 25% report petechiae. Other effects that can put some men off the idea include cold/numb penis, lack of ejaculation, pivoting of the penis and altered sensation at orgasm, which may be uncomfortable.

As with other treatments, VCD may be combined with other therapies to augment response such as with MUSE or psychosexual therapy (94).

Psychological Therapies for Men with ED

In the majority of cases of ED, psychological factors are involved in either the development of the disorder or the maintenance of the problem. While recognising that many men would not seek a psychological approach to resolving the condition, an outline of performance anxiety about continued erectile failure and the effect this has on their partner and their relationship, is often appreciated by the man. Difficulties with communication and the development of suspicion and mistrust between partners may need discussion, recognition, and specific intervention.

One group of men will experience ED almost entirely related to disease processes. These men are likely to have good interpersonal relationships which, if longstanding, will have been maintained with communication, respect, and intimacy. They are unlikely to need much in the way of sex counselling (if any).

A second group of patients will have ED as a consequence of a disease state but where there are also contributory psychological factors. Acknowledging with the patient that the ED may be having an adverse effect on his overall sex life may facilitate an interaction with the man (and often his partner) to find ways to re-establish the desired sexual relationship. Sometimes this will involve provision of basic educational information and guidance to enhance the sexual relationship. It may also be appropriate to consider a more integrative approach with the short-term prescription of an erectogenic agent to help restore sexual confidence and function.

The third group of men includes those with the presence of other psychological morbidity such as dysthymia or mild depression, substance misuse, relational problems, or other sexual problems such as loss of desire or ejaculatory disturbance. These may require a more proactive input from the psychosexual therapist, which may incorporate psychosexual therapy, relationship therapy, often integrated with management from one or more mental health professionals for any associated mental health disorders.

In each of these three situations, an integrative approach by the assessing clinician to ensure adequate assessment of both psychological and physical contributing factors may lead to more efficacious outcomes while recognising that the interventions themselves may be multiple, rather than relying on one treatment and progressing in a linear fashion to alternatives because of failure of "first line therapy." Helping the man to start to use his preferred treatment choice (such as sildenafil) and integrating this into his sexual repertoire with his partner can help the man and the couple to restart their sexual lives together and regain not only a good erection, but also good sex.

Psychosexual and Relationship Therapies for Men with ED

The clinician should try to encourage the man to be open and honest with his partner. This will allow the couple to identify together any anxieties or other issues that might be causing the problem. It is important to provide sufficient time for a psychosexual assessment and this is likely to be ~1 h. This will address predisposing, precipitating, and perpetuating factors.

Predisposing factors will include limited sexual education and childhood and pubertal sexual experiences including traumatic episodes of any kind and general life stressors. Environmental stressors may need addressing, such as financial, domestic, or children-related issues.

Common precipitating factors include deterioration in the general relationship; separation, divorce, or recent death of a partner; vocational failure; and onset of physical or psychiatric illness.

Sometimes there can be problems in their relationship. Couples therapy helps both partners to address the situation and this may be necessary before any specific psychosexual therapy. Issues may be limited to poor communication skills and ways of relating together but there may also be difficulties in other areas such as negotiating time apart (or together) or deciding the share of household duties. Systemic psychotherapy may be indicated.

There may be specific performance anxiety about recurrence of erectile disorder even after just one or two episodes (e.g., attempts at love making while intoxicated with alcohol), which maintains the problem. There may be fear of repeated failure with associated guilt and embarrassment. Once the problem has become established, a number of other maintaining factors may need addressing during therapy. Themes include loss of attraction to the partner, poor communication of likes and dislikes during foreplay and sex between the partners, limited sexual education and awareness, a fear of intimacy, and an impoverished self-image including concern about genital size (particularly penis size). There may be unrealistic expectations from sex as well as other lifestyle, cultural, and religious restrictions on sexual variety. Attraction towards others of the same sex may become evident.

Therapy is directed toward the relationship with agreed and realistic goals of therapy established fairly early in therapy. Specific techniques such as genital self-focus work and modified sensate focus may be helpful. Where therapy is successful, attention to relapse prevention work is recommended. A detailed description is provided elsewhere (95).

Comorbid sexual problems such as secondary early ejaculation or loss of desire as well as other psychological problems such as depression or social phobia and anxiety may be evident on assessment, which will require input from a sex therapist or mental health professional. Techniques including cognitive and behavioral therapy or psychoanalytical therapy may be indicated.

Integrated Therapies

Several workers have reported success from a combination of psychological and physical treatments for ED including sex therapy and ICI (96,97), psychotherapy and ICI (98,99), couple psychotherapy and VCD (94,100), sex therapy and sildenafil (101), short-term therapy and ICI (101), and ICI and counselling (102).

Other Unlicensed Treatment Therapies for Men with ED

Several new formulations are being developed, such as topical alprostadil and intra-nasal apomorphine. New agents are being developed, including selective PDE3/4/5 inhibitors: MS-223131 (Bristol-Myers Squibb), T-1032 (Tanabe Seiyaku), TA-1790 (Vivus), sildenafil nitrate (NCX-911) (NicOx); nonselective inhibitors of postsynaptic alpha-adrenoceptors within the corpus cavernosum: phentolamine (Vasomax; Schering Plough), melanocortin receptor agonists such as melatonan II (Palatin) (s.c. and intranasal)—increases erections and sexual drive/appetite (phase 2A)—and the 5HT1 agonist VML670 (Lily/Vernalis).

A recent review of herbal remedies has been scrutenized for potential benefit (103). Examples include L-arginine, yohimbine, and extracts of *Tribulus terrestris* L. (Protodioscin) that is metabolized to DHEA and which is reported to increase both erections and sexual drive.

Treatment for Priapism

For erections lasting over 4 h, apply cooling agents to the genitals and encourage moderate exercise to the legs to divert blood to the lower limbs. If the erection remains, aspirate 20–50 mL of blood from the corpus cavernosum using a 19–21 gage butterfly using a sterile technique. This may be followed by irrigation with heparinised saline. If necessary, repeat to the other side. If there is no response proceed to ICI alpha-adrenergic agents. Either phenylephereine [10 mg (1 mL) vial diluted to 10 mL with saline and 0.5 mg (0.5 mL) injected at a time to a maximum of 10 mg (10 mL)] or ephedrine [30 mg in 1 mL vial, using 15 mg (0.5 mL)] should be given, and repeated once if necessary. Monitor pulse and BP continuously. Proceed with extreme caution in patients with coronary heart disease, uncontrolled hypertension, or cerebral ischemia and in men taking MAOIs as hypertensive crises may occur. See also the latest AUA guidelines (104).

Surgical Interventions for Men with ED

Vascular Surgery

Penile arterial revascularization is only appropriate in young patients with demonstrable arteriogenic ED due to congenital vascular anomalies or traumatic injuries to the pudendal or penile arteries (e.g., after road traffic accidents).

Prostheses

There are three forms of penile prostheses available: semi-rigid, malleable, and inflatable. Typical candidates for a penile implant are patients with chronic disease states such as long-term diabetes and end-organ failure or severe arterio-genic impotence combined with severe veno-occlusive dysfunction and men with treatment unresponsive Peyronie's disease in combination with ED. Typical complications of prosthetic surgery are infections (1–5%) and mechanical failures (10–20%)

Special Situations Requiring Interventions for Men with ED

Depression and Serotonin Reuptake Inhibitors

Sexual dysfunction associated with the use of serotonin reuptake inhibitors has been reported in 30–70% of treated patients and is a significant contributor to discontinuation of these medications. A review of selective phosphodiesterase type-5 inhibitors for antidepressant-associated sexual dysfunction suggests treatmet of this side effect of antidepressant medication could improve depression disease management outcomes (105).

Testosterone Deficiency

Androgen replacement can improve libido, erection rigidity, and sexual satisfaction in men with demonstrable low serum levels of testosterone (106). In a large cohort of 1461 men presenting with ED, just over one-sixth (17.7%) at initial screening had biochemical evidence to suggest the possibility of hypogonadism. More rigorous estimation of serum testosterone, associated parameters, and the presence of clinical symptoms resulted in 3% of the population having a diagnosis of hypergonadotropic hypogonadism. Of these, one-fifth agreed to a trial of testosterone therapy but two-thirds of this eligible group also required another erectogenic agent to resolve the ED (107).

Treatment can be with daily 5 mg transdermal patches or gel or 250 mg intramuscular injection three times weekly. The dose may need adjustment depending on clinical and biochemical response. Monitoring of hematocrit, liver, prostate, and lipid parameters is mandatory.

CONCLUSION

ED is the most commonly presenting male sexual problem to clinicians. A thorough assessment of possible etiological factors and consideration of psychological, couple, and physical factors in the management of this disorder will allow sufferers of the condition an excellent opportunity for amelioration of the symptom. In many instances reassurance, educational advice, and the use of a PDE5 inhibitor will be sufficient as first line management of the condition.

APPENDIX

Management Recommendations for Men with ED and Cardiovascular Disease Based on Graded Cardiovascular Risk

Grading of risk	Cardiovascular status upon presentation	ED management recommendations for the primary care physician
Low risk	Asymptomatic, <3 major risk factors for CAD, excluding age and gender Controlled hypertension Mild, stable angina Post-successful coronary revascularization Mild valvular disease LVD/CHF (NYHA class I)	Manage within the primary care setting Review treatment options with patient and his partner (where possible)
Intermediate risk	Moderate, stable angina Recent MI or CVA (<6 weeks) LVD/CHF (NYHA class II) Murmur of unknown cause Asymptomatic but >3 risk factors for CAD, excluding gender and age	Specialized evaluation recommended (e.g., ETT for angina, Echo for murmur) Patient to be placed into high or low risk category, depending upon outcome of testing ED treatment can be initiated but exercise testing recommended to risk stratify
High risk	Unstable or refractory angina Uncontrolled hypertension (SBP > 180 mmHg) CHF (NYHA class III,IV) Recent MI or CVA (<2 weeks) High-risk arrhythmias Hypertrophic obstructive and other cardiomyopathies Moderate/severe valve disease	Refer for specialized cardiac evaluation and management Treatment for ED to be deferred until cardiac condition stabilized and/or specialist evaluation completed

Note: CAD, coronary artery disease; CHF, congestive heart failure; CVA, cerebral vascular accident; Echo, echocardiogram; ED, erectile dysfunction; ETT, exercise tolerance test; LVD, left ventricular dysfunction; NYHA, New York Heart Association; SBP, systolic blood pressure.
Source: Reproduced with permission from Jackson et al. (108).

REFERENCES

1. Morales A. Erectile dysfunction: an overview. Clin Geriatr Med 2003; 19(3):529–538.
2. Shabsigh R, Anastasiadis AG. Erectile dysfunction. Annu Rev Med 2003; 54:153–168.
3. Vroege JA, Gijs L, Hengeveld MW. Classification of sexual dysfunctions: towards DSM-V and ICD-11. Comp Psychiatry 1998; 39(6):333–337.

4. Melman A, Gingell JC. The epidemiology and pathophysiology of erectile dysfunction. J Urol 1999; 161:5–11.
5. NIH Consensus Conference. NIH consensus development panel on impotence. J Am Med Assoc 1993; 270:83.
6. Feldman HA, Goldstein I, Hatzichristou DG, Krane RJ, Mckinlay JB. Impotence and its medical and psychological correlates: results of the Massachusetts male aging study. J Urol 1994; 150:54–61.
7. Green JSA, Holden STR, Ingram P, Bose P, St. George DP, Bowsher WG. An investigation of erectile dysfunction in Gwent, Wales. BJU Int 2001; 88:551–553.
8. Araujo AB, Durante R, Feldman HA, Goldstein I, McKinley JB. The relationship between depressive symptoms and male erectile dysfunction: cross-sectional results from the Massachusetts Male Aging Study. Psychosom Med 1998; 60:458–465.
9. Kirby M, Jackson G, Betteridge J, Friedli K. Is erectile dysfunction a marker for cardiovascular disease? Int J Clin Prac 2001; 55(9):614–618.
10. Strand J, Wise TN, Fagan PJ, Schmidt CW Jr. Erectile dysfunction and depression: category or dimension? J Sex Marital Ther 2002; 28:175–181.
11. Kirby R, Carson C, Goldstein. Erectile dysfunction a clinical guide. Isis Medical Media 1999.
12. Guay AT, Perez JB, Heatley GJ. Cessation of smoking rapidly decreases erectile dysfunction. Endocr Pract 1998; 4:23–26.
13. Lue TF. Erectile dysfunction. N Engl J Med 2000; 342:1802–1813.
14. Andersson KE, Wagner G. Physiology of penile erection. Physiol Rev 1995; 75:191–236.
15. Lundberg PO, Ertekin A, Ghezzi A, Swash M, Vodusek D. Neurosexology. Guidelines for neurologists. Eur J Neurol 2001; 8(S3):2–24.
16. Heaton JP, Morales A. Endocrine causes of impotence (nondiabetes). Urol Clin North Am 2003; 30(1):73–81.
17. Jackson G, Betteridge J, Dean J, Eardley I, Hall R, Holdright D, Holmes S, Kirby M, Riley A, Sever P. A systematic approach to erectile dysfunction in the cardiovascular patient: a consensus statement—update 2002. Int J Clin Pract 2002; 56(9):669–671.
18. Rosen RC, Riley A, Wagner G, Osterloh IH, Kirkpatrick J, Mishra A. The international index of erectile function (IIEF): a multidimensional scale for assessment of erectile dysfunction. Urology 1997; 49(6):822–830.
19. Rosen RC, Cappelleri JC, Gendrano N III. The international index of erectile function (IIEF): a state-of-the-science review. Int J Impot Res 2002; 14:226–244.
20. Ogrinc FG, Linet OI. Evaluation of real-time Rigiscan monitoring in pharmacological erection. J Urol 1995; 154:1356–1359.
21. Lue TF, Basson R, Rosen R et al. Sexual Medicine 2004. Paris: Health Publications.
22. Goldstein I, Lue TF, Padma-Nathan H, Rosen RC, Steers WD, Wicker PA. Oral sildenafil in the treatment of erectile dysfunction. N Eng. J Med 1998; 338:1397–1404.
23. Ignarro LJ, Lippton H, Edwards JC, Baricos WH, Hyman AL, Kadowitz PJ, Gruetter CA. Mechanisms of vascular smooth muscle relaxation by organic nitrates, nitrites, nitroprusside and nitric oxide: evidence for the involvement of S-nitrosthiols as active intermediates. J Pharmacol Exp Ther 1981; 218:739–749.

24. Corbin JD, Sharron HF, Webb DJ. Phosphodiesterase type 5 as a pharmacologic target in erectile dysfunction. Urology 2002; 60(suppl 2B):4–11.
25. Boolell M, Allen MJ, Ballard SA, Gepi-Attee S, Muirhead GJ, Naylor AM, Osterloh IH, Gingell C. Sildenafil: an orally active type 5 cyclic GMP-specific phosphodiesterase inhibitor for the treatment of penile erectile dysfunction. Int J Impot Res 1996; 8:47–52.
26. McCullough AR, Barada JH, Fawzy A, Guay AT, Hatzichristou D. Achieving treatment optimization with sildenafil citrate (Viagra) in patients with erectile dysfunction. [Journal Article. Meta-Analysis] Urology 2002; 60(2 suppl 2):28–38.
27. Montorsi F, McDermott TED, Morgan R, Olsson A, Schultz A, Kirkeby HJ, Osterloh IH. Efficacy and safety of fixed-dose oral sildenafil in the treatment of erectile dysfunction of various etiologies. Urology 1999; 53:1011–1018.
28. Carson CC, Burnett AL, Levine LA, Nehra A. The efficacy of sildenafil citrate (Viagra) in clinical populations: an update. Urology 2002; 60(suppl 2B):12–27.
29. Hatzichristou DG. Sildenafil citrate: lessons learned from 3 years of clinical experience. Int J Impot Res 2002; 14(suppl 1):S43–S52.
30. Pfizer. Viagra—Summary of product characteristics.
31. Morales A, Gingell C, Collins M, Wicker PA, Osterloh IH. Clinical safety of oral sildenafil citrate (ViagraTM) in the treatment of erectile dysfunction. Int J Impot Res 1998; 10:69–74.
32. Padma-Nathan H, Eardley I, Kloner RA, Laties AM, Montorsi F. A 4-year update on the safety of sildenafil citrate (Viagra). Urology 2002; 60(suppl 2B): 67–90.
33. Wagoner LE, Giesting RM, Bell BJ, McGuire NC, Abraham WT. Is viagara (sildenafil) safe and effective in cardiac transplant recipients? Transplantation 1999; 67(7):S102.
34. Osterloh IH, Riley A. Clinical update on sildenafil citrate. Br J Clin Pharmacol 2002; 53:219–223.
35. Stanford JL, Feng Z, Hamilton AS, Gilliland FD, Stephenson RA, Eley JW, Albertson PC, Harlan LC, Potosky AL. Urinary and sexual function after radical prostatectomy for clinically localized prostate cancer. The prostate cancer outcomes study. J Am Med Assoc 2000; 283(3):354–360.
36. Zelefsky MJ, Mckee AB, Lee H, Leibel SA. Efficacy of oral sildenafil in patients with erectile dysfunction after radiotherapy for carcinoma of the prostate. Urology 1999; 53(4):775–778.
37. Zippe CD, Kedia AW, Kedia K, Nelson DR, Agarwal A. Treatment of erectile dysfunction after radical prostatectomy with sildenafil citrate (Viagra). Urology 1998; 52(6):963–966.
38. Zippe CD, Jhaveri FM, Klein EA, Kedia S, Pasqualotto FF, Kedia A, Agarwal A, Montague DK, Lakin MM. Role of viagra after radical prostatectomy. Urology 2000; 55(2):241–245.
39. Nehra A, Goldstein I. Sildenafil citrate (Viagra) after radical retropubic prostatectomy: Con. J Am Med Assoc 1999; 54(4):587–589.
40. Kedia S, Zippe CD, Agarwal A, Nelson DR, Lakin MM. Treatment of erectile dysfunction with sildenafil citrate (Viagra) after radiation therapy for prostate cancer. Urology 1999; 54(2):308–312.
41. Padma-Nathan H, McCullough A, Forest C. Erectile dysfunction secondary to nerve-sparing radical retropubic prostatectomy: comparative phosphodiesterase-5 inhibitor

efficacy for therapy and novel prevention strategies. Curr Urol Rep 2004; 5(6):467–471.

42. Shabsigh R, Klein LT, Seidman S, Kaplan SA, Lehrhoff BJ, Ritter JS. Increased incidence of depressive symptoms in men with erectile dysfunction. Urology 1998; 52:848–852.

43. Rosen RC, Lane RM, Menza M. Effects of SSRIs on sexual function: a critical review. J Clin Psychopharmacol 1999; 19(1):67–85.

44. Ferguson JM. The effects of antidepressants on sexual functioning in depressed patients: a review. J Clin Psychiatry 2001; 62(suppl 3):22–34.

45. Goldstein I. The mutually reinforcing triad of depressive symptoms, cardiovascular disease, and erectile dysfunction. Am J Cardiol 2000; 86(suppl):41F–45F.

46. Thase ME, Reynolds CF, Jennings JR, Frank E, Howell JR, Houck PR, Berman S, Kupfer DJ. Nocturnal penile tumescence is diminished in depressed men. Biol Psychiatry 1988; 24(1):33–46.

47. Nurnberg HG, Seidman SN, Gelenberg AJ, Fava M, Rosen R, Shabsigh R. Depression, antidepressant therapies, and erectile dysfunction: clinical trials of sildenafil citrate (Viagra) in treated and untreated patients with depression. Urology 2002; 60(suppl 2B):58–66.

48. Nurnberg HG, Gelenberg A, Hargreave TB, Harrison WM, Siegel RL, Smith MD. Efficacy of sildenafil citrate for the treatment of erectile dysfunction in men taking serotonin reuptake inhibitors. Am J Psychiatry 2001; 158(11):1926–1928.

49. Rendell M, Goldstein I, Collins O, Taylor T. Vardenafil significantly improved erectile function and quality of life in men with diabetes mellitus and erectile dysfunction. WCAM, 2002.

50. Boulton AJM, Salem J-L, Sweeney M, Ziegler D. Sildenafil citrate for the treatment of erectile dysfunction in men with Type II diabetes mellitus. Diabetologia 2001; 44:1296–1301.

51. Guay AT, Blonde L, Siegel R, Orazem J. Safety and tolerability of sildenafil citrate for treatment of erectile dysfunction in men with type 1 and type 2 diabetes mellitus. ADA, San Antonio, TX, 2000.

52. Kloner RA, Brown M, Prisant LM, Collins M. Effect of sildenafil in patients with erectile dysfunction taking antihypertensive therapy. Am J Hypertens 2001; 14:70–73.

53. Webb DJ, Freestone S, Allen MJ, Muirhead GJ. Sildenafil citrate and blood-pressure–lowering drugs: results of drug interaction studies with an organic nitrate and a calcium antagonist. Am J Cardiol 1999; 83:21C–28C.

54. Conti CR, Pepine CJ, Sweeney M. Efficacy and safety of sildenafil citrate in the treatment of erectile dysfunction in patients with ischaemic heart disease. Am J Cardiol 1999; 83:29C–34C.

55. Shakir SAW, Wilton LV, Boshier A, Layton D, Heeley E. Cardiovascular events in users of sildenafil: results from first phase of prescription event monitoring in England. Br Med J 2001; 322:651–652.

56. Zusman RM, Morales A, Glasser DB, Osterloh IH. Overall cardiovascular profile of sildenafil citrate. Am J Cardiol 1999; 83:35C–44C.

57. Herrmann HC, Chang G, Klugherz BD, Mahoney PD. Hemodynamic effects of sildenafil in men with severe coronary artery disease. N Engl J Med 2000; 342:1622–1626.

58. Arruda-Olsen AM, Mahoney DW, Nehra A, Leckel M, Pellikka PA. Cardio-vascular effects of sildenafil during exercise in men with known or probable coronary artery disease, a randomized crossover trial. J Am Med Assoc 2002; 287(6):719–725.

59. Chait J, Kobashigawa J, Chuang J, Moriguchi J, Kawata N, Laks H. Efficacy and safety of sildenafil citrate (Viagra) in male heart transplant patients. J Heart Lung Transplant 1999; 18(1):58.

60. Wagner G, Mulhall J. Pathophysiology and diagnosis of male erectile dysfunction. Br J Urol Int 2001; 88(suppl 3):3–10.

61. Derry F, Hultling C, Seftel AD, Sipski ML. Efficacy and safety of sildenafil citrate (Viagra) in men with erectile dysfunction and spinal cord injury: a review. Urology 2002; 60(suppl 2B):49–57.

62. Steers W, Guay AT, Leriche A, Gingell C, Hargreave TB, Wright PJ, Price DE, Feldman RA. Assessment of the efficacy and safety of Viagra (sildenafil citrate) in men with erectile dysfunction during long-term treatment. Int J Impot Res 2001; 13:261–267.

63. Kuan JK, Brock GB. Salvage of the sildenafil non-responder: the role of locally delivered therapies. Sexual Dysfunct Med 2001; 2:34–39.

64. Angulo J, Gadau M, Fernandez A, Gabancho S, Cuevas P, Martins T, Florio V, Ferguson K, Saenz de Tejada I. Tadalafil (IC351) enhances nitric oxide-mediated relaxation of human arterial and trabecular penile smooth muscle. 37th Annual Meeting of the European Association for the Study of Diabetes, 2001.

65. Brock GB, McMahon CG, Chen KK, Costigan T, Shen W, Watkins V, Anglin G, Whitaker S. Efficacy and safety of Tadalafil for the treatment of erectile dysfunction: Results of integrated analysis. J Urol 2002; 168:1332–1336.

66. Brock G, Iglesias J, Toulouse K, Ferguson KM, Pullman WE, Anglin G. Efficacy and safety of tadalafil (IC351) treatment for ED. 16th Congress of the European Association of Urology, 2001.

67. Patterson B, Bedding A, Jewell H, Payne C, Mitchell M. The effect of intrinsic and extrinsic factors on the pharmacokinetic properties of tadalafil (IC351) [abstract 16]. Int J Impot Res 2001; 13(suppl 5):S62.

68. Saenz de Tejada I, Anglin G, Knight JR, Emmick JT. Effects of tadalafil on erectile dysfunction in men with diabetes. Diabetes Care 2002; 25(12):2159–2164.

69. Emmick JT, Stuewe SR, Mitchell M. Overview of the cardiovascular effects of tadalafil. Eur Heart J 2002; 4(suppl H):H32–H47.

70. Sachse R, Rohde G. Safety, tolerability and pharmacokinetics of BAY 38-9456 in patients with erectile dysfunction. 95th AUA JTA, April 2000.

71. Porst H, Rosen R, Padma-Nathan H, Goldstein I, Giuliano F, Ulbrich E, Bandel T. The efficacy and safety of vardenafil, a new, oral, selective phosphodiesterase type 5 inhibitor, in patients with erectile dysfunction: the first at-home clinical trial. Int J Impot Res 2001; 13:192–199.

72. Hellstrom WJG, Gittelman GK, Segerson T, Thibonnier M, Taylor T, Padma-Nathan H. Vardenafil for treatment of men with erectile dysfunction: efficacy and safety in a randomized, double-blind, placebo-controlled trial. J Androl 2002; 23(6):763–772.

73. Padma-Nathan H et al. Efficacy and safety of vardenafil in men with ED on antihypertensive therapy. Am J Hypertension 2004; 15:48A (Am Soc Hypertens 2002).

74. Goldstein I, Fischer J, Taylor T, Thibonnier M. Influence of HbA1c on the efficacy and safety of vardenafil for the treatment of erectile dysfunction in men with diabetes. 61st ADA, June 2001.

75. Rendell MS, Rajfer J, Wicker PA, Smith MD. Sildenafil for treatment of erectile dysfunction in men with diabetes, a randomized controlled trial. J Am Med Assoc 1999; 281(5):421–426.

76. Giuliano F, Allard J. Dopamine and sexual function. Int J Impot Res 2001; 13(suppl 3):S18–S28.

77. Morales A. Apomorphine to Uprima: the development of a practical erectogenic drug: a personal perspective. Int J Impot Res 2001; 13(suppl 3):S29–S34.

78. Laurence DR, Bennett PN, Brown MJ. Clinical Pharmacology. 8th ed. Churchill: Livingstone, 1997.

79. Abbott Laboratories Ltd. *Uprima*. Summary of Product Characteristics 2001.

80. Bukofzer S, Livesey N. Safety and tolerability of apomorphine SL (Uprima). Int J Impot Res 2001; 13(suppl 3):S40–S44.

81. Dula E, Bukofzer S, Perdock R, George M, the apomorphine SL study group. Double-blind, crossover comparison of 3 mg apomorphine SL with placebo and with 4 mg apomorphine SL in male erectile dysfunction. Eur Urol 2001; 39:558–564.

82. Heaton JPW, Dean J, Sleep DJ. Rapid communication. Sequential administration enhances the effect of apomorphine SL in men with erectile dysfunction. Int J Impot Res 2002; 14:61–64.

83. Heaton JPW. Characterising the benefit of apomorphine SL (Uprima) amino as an optimized treatment for representative populations with erectile dysfunction. Int J Impot Res 2001; 13(suppl 3):S35–S39.

84. Guay AT, Spark RF, Jacobson J, Murray FT, Geisser ME. Yohimbine treatment of organic erectile dysfunction in a dose-escalation trial. Int J Impot Res 2002; 14:25–31.

85. Dahl R. My Uncle Oswald. Penguin Harmondsworth, 1980.

86. Linet OI, Ogrinc FG. Efficacy and safety of intracavernosal alprostadil in men with erectile dysfunction. N Engl J Med 1996; 334(14):873–877.

87. Werthman P, Rajfer J. MUSE therapy: preliminary clinical observations. Urology 1997; 50:809–811.

88. Porst H. Transurethral alprostadil with MUSE (medicated urethral system for erection) vs intracavernous alprostadil—a comparative study in 103 patients with erectile dysfunction. Int J Impot Res 1997; 9(4):187–192.

89. Padma-Nathan H, Hellstrom WJG, Kaiser FE, Labasky RF, Lue TF, Nolten WE, Norwood PC, Peterson CA, Shabsigh R, Tam PY, Place VA, Gesundheit N, Cowley C, Nemo KJ, Spivack AP, Stephens DE, Todd LK. Treatment of men with erectile dysfunction with transurethral alprostadil. N Engl J Med 1997; 336(1):1–7.

90. Rang HP, Dale MM, Ritter JM. Pharmacology. 3rd ed. Churchill: Livingstone, 1998.

91. Levine SB, Althof SE, Turner LA, Risen CB, Bodner DR, Kursh ED, Resnick MI. Side effects of self administration of intracavernous papaverine and phentolamine for the treatment of impotence. J Urol 1989; 141:54–57.

92. McMahon CG, Samali R, Johnson H. Treatment of intracorporeal injection nonresponse with sildenafil alone or in combination with triple agent intracorporeal injection therapy. J Urol 1999; 162(6):1992–1997.

93. von Buhler MAH. Vacuum and constriction devices for erectile disorder—an integrative view. Sexual Marital Ther 1998; 13(3):257–272.
94. Wylie KR, Jones RH, Walters S. The potential benefit of vacuum devices augmenting psychosexual therapy for erectile dysfunction: a randomized controlled trial. J Sex Marital Ther 2003; 29(3):227–236.
95. Rosen RC, Leiblum SR, Spector IP. Psychologically based treatment for male erectile disorder: a cognitive-interpersonal model. J Sex Marital Ther 1994; 20(2):67–85.
96. Kaplan HS. The combined use of sex therapy and intrapenile injections in the treatment of impotence. J Sex Marital Ther 1990; 16(4):195–207.
97. Hartmann U, Langer D. Combination of psychosexual therapy and intra penile injections in the treatment of erectile dysfunctions: Rationale and predictors of outcome. J Sex Educ Ther 1993; 19:1–12.
98. Colson MH. Intracavernous injections and overall treatment of erectile disorders: a retrospective study. Sexologies 1996; 5:11–24.
99. Lottman PE, Hendriks JC, Vruggink PA, Meuleman EJ. The impact of marital satisfaction and psychological counselling on the outcome of ICI treatment in men with ED. Int J Impot Res 1998; 10:83–87.
100. Segenreich E, Israilov SR, Shmueli J, Raz D, Servadio C. Psychotherapy combined with use of the vacuum constrictive device for erectile impotence. Harefuah. J Israel Med Assoc 1994; 126:633–636.
101. McCarthy BW. Integrating Viagra™ into cognitive behavioural couples sex therapy. J Sex Educ Ther 1998; 23:302–308.
102. van der Windt F, Dohle GR, van der Tak J, Slob AK. Intracavernosal injection therapy with and without sexological counselling in men with erectile dysfunction. BJU Int 2002; 89(9):901–904.
103. Rowland DL, Tai W. A review of plant-derived and herbal approaches to the treatment of sexual dysfunctions. J Sex Marital Ther 2003; 29(3):185–205.
104. Montague DK, Jarow J, Broderick GA, Dmochowski RR, Heaton JP, Lue TF, Nehra A, Sharlip ID. Members of the erectile dysfunction guideline update panel, Americal urological association. American urological association guideline on the management of priapism. J Urol 2003; 170:1318–1324.
105. Nurnberg HG, Hensley PL. Selective phosphodiesterase type-5 inhibitor treatment of serotonergic reuptake inhibitor antidepressant-associated sexual dysfunction: a review of diagnosis, treatment, and relevance. CNS Spectrosc 2003; 8:194–202.
106. Arver S, Dobs AS, Meikle AW, Allen RP, Sanders SW, Mazer NA. Improvement of sexual function in testosterone deficient men treated for 1 year with a permeation enhanced testosterone transdermal system. J Urol 1996; 155:1604–1608.
107. Wylie KR, Davies-South D. A study of treatment choices in men with erectile dysfunction and reduced androgen levels. J Sex Marital Ther 2004; 30:2.
108. Jackson G, Betteridge J, Dean J, Eardley I, Hall R, Holdright D, Holmes S, Kirby M, Riley A, Sever P. A systematic approach to erectile dysfunction in the cardiovascular patient: a consensus statement-update 2002. Int J Clin Practice 2002; 56:663–671.

8

Female Orgasm Dysfunction

Cindy M. Meston

University of Texas at Austin, Austin, Texas, USA

Roy J. Levin

University of Sheffield, Sheffield, UK

WHAT IS ORGASM?

Orgasm is a transient peak sensation of intense pleasure that is accompanied by a number of physiological body changes. In men, orgasm is normally accompanied by ejaculation, which makes the event easily identifiable. In women, however, the achievement of orgasm appears to be less facile than for males and recognizing that it has occurred is often difficult for some women. Objective indicators that orgasm has occurred have been sought for many years. Kinsey et al. (1) proposed "the abrupt cessation of the ofttimes strenuous movements and extreme tensions of the previous sexual activity and the peace of the resulting state" as the most obvious evidence that orgasm had occurred in women. Masters and Johnson (2) described the onset of orgasm as a "sensation of suspension or stoppage." In order to serve as a clear marker of orgasm, however, the indicator must involve a bodily change that is unique to orgasm. This necessarily rules out simple measures like peaks of blood pressure, heart and respiratory rates, or even a woman's own vocalizations because such events can occur during high levels of sexual arousal that fail to culminate in orgasm.

Remarkably, most of the so-called objective indicators of female orgasm rely on the original, nearly 40-year-old observations and descriptions of Masters and Johnson (2). They include physiological changes that indicate impending orgasm (prospective), occur during actual orgasm (current), and/or indicate that an orgasm has occurred (retrospective). With regard to prospective changes, during sexual arousal the labia become engorged with blood, increase in size, and undergo vivid color changes. The color changes (light pink to deep red) are presumably due to the changing hemodynamics of the tissue in relation to increased blood flow, tissue congestion, and tissue metabolism (oxygen consumption), indicating the balance between oxygenated (red/pink) and deoxygenated or reduced hemoglobin (blue). Following orgasm, the color of the labia rapidly changes (within 10–15 s) from deep red to light pink. There has been little detailed study of the minora labia apart from the suggested mechanism by which they become lubricated (3) and their increased temperature during sexual arousal has been used as an objective indicator of arousal (4) prior to and after orgasm (5).

Contractions of the vagina, uterus, and anal sphincter have been proposed as current indicators of orgasm. The resting vagina is a collapsed tube lined with a stratified squamous epithelium, approximating an elongated S-shape in longitudinal section and an H-shape in cross-section. It is anchored amid a bed of powerful, voluntary, striated muscles (pelvic diaphragm, consisting of the pubococcygeus and iliococcygeus muscle). According to Masters and Johnson [2, p. 118], contractions recorded in the vagina begin ~2–4 s after the subjective experience of the start of orgasm. They occur in many pre- and postmenopausal women and are due to the activation of the circumvaginal striated muscles which involuntarily contract in ~0.8 s repetitions. This squeezes the outer third of the vagina [designated the "orgasmic platform" by Masters and Johnson (2)] with a force that gradually becomes weaker as the interval between contractions increases. Vaginal rhythmic contractions vary greatly between women in their number and strength, and are dependent on the duration of the orgasm and the strength of the pelvic musculature. Masters and Johnson reported that the stronger the orgasm the greater the number of contractions and, thus indirectly, the longer the duration of orgasm (as each contraction was ~0.8 s apart). However, using physiological (pressure) recordings of the contractions, other researchers have failed to find a link between vaginal contractions and the perceived intensity or duration of the orgasm (6,7). Moreover, while Masters and Johnson proposed that vaginal contractions are a definitive sign of orgasm having occurred, other authors have noted that not all women who claim to experience orgasms show vaginal contractions (6–9). Uterine contractions have also been proposed as the terminative signal for sexual arousal in multiorgasmic women (10) but too few investigations have assessed orgasmic uterine contractions to make a definitive statement. While voluntary contractions of the anal sphincter can occur during sexual arousal and are sometimes used by women to facilitate or enhance arousal, involuntary contractions occur only during orgasm (2, p. 34). Such contractions are more frequently observed during masturbation than during coitus. As with uterine contractions, few studies on anal sphincter contractions during orgasm have been published (9).

A number of questionnaire studies have reported that orgasm through stimulation of the so-called G-spot (named after Ernst Grafenberg, who reportedly first described the phenomenon) causes a substantial number of women to expel fluid from their urethra (11). However, there has been no scientific evidence to support the assertion that women ejaculate a fluid distinguishable from urine at the time of orgasm. Moreover, there has not been consistent evidence for any anatomical structure or "spot" on the anterior vaginal wall apart from the known paraurethral glands and spongiosal tissue around the urethra, which could cause sexually pleasurable sensations when stimulated (12).

Physiological changes noted to occur after orgasm (retrospective) include areolae (the pigmented skin area around the nipple of the breasts) decongestion, enhanced vaginal pulse amplitude (measured by photoplethysmography), and raised prolactin levels. During sexual arousal, the primary areolae swell up, likely due to both vasocongestion and smooth muscle contraction. The volume expansion can become so marked that the swollen areolae hide a large part of the base of the erect nipples making it look as though they have lost their erection. At orgasm, the loss of volume is so rapid that the areolae become corrugated before becoming flatter. This provides a visual indicator that orgasm has occurred. In the absence of orgasm, the areolae detumescence is much slower and the corrugation does not develop. There has been minimal study of areolae changes during arousal and orgasm.

Changes in the blood supply to vaginal tissue before, during, and after orgasm were recorded by photoplethysmography in seven young women by Geer and Quartararo (13). Sexual arousal by masturbation caused an increase in the vaginal pulse amplitude signal compared to the basal values in all women. Immediately after the end of orgasm, however, vaginal pulse amplitude was actually significantly greater than before orgasm in five of the seven women (71%) and was not significantly less in the other two. The postorgasmic period of maximum amplitude lasts for $\sim 10-30$ s and then slowly returns to its resting level. Other recordings in the literature have shown similar changes.

Studies by Exton and colleagues (14) have reported that prolactin secretion (a peptide hormone secreted by the lactotrophic cells of the anterior pituitary gland) is not activated by sexual arousal *per se* but is specifically activated and doubled in plasma concentration with orgasm. This elevation occurs directly after orgasm and is maintained for ~ 60 min (14).

In summary, specific physiological indicators that orgasm has occurred include rapid color changes of the labia; contractions of the vagina, uterus, and anal sphincter; areolae decongestion; enhanced vaginal pulse amplitude; and raised prolactin levels.

What Causes Orgasm?

Orgasms can be induced via erotic stimulation of a variety of genital and nongenital sites. The clitoris and vagina (especially the anterior wall including Halban's fascia and urethra) are the most usual sites of stimulation, but stimulation of the periurethral glands (15), breast/nipple or mons (2, pp. 54, 67), mental-imagery or fantasy (2,16), or hypnosis (17) have also been reported to induce orgasm. Orgasms have been noted to occur during sleep (1,18,19), hence consciousness is not an absolute requirement. Cases of "spontaneous orgasm" have occasionally been described in the psychiatric literature where no obvious sexual stimulus can be ascertained (20). The precise mechanism that triggers orgasm has been a topic of debate for many years but, as of yet, no definitive mechanisms have been identified.

Only very recently have investigators examined the brain areas activated during orgasm in women (21). Compared to preorgasm levels of sexual arousal, the brain areas activated during orgasm in women included the paraventricular nucleus of the hypothalamus, the periaqueductal gray of the midbrain, the hippocampus, and the cerebellum. Other areas shown to be activated during sexual arousal include the amygdala, the anterior basal ganglia, and several regions of the cortex including the anterior cingulated, frontal, parietal, temporal, and insular cortices (22–24). Some of these areas may be more involved in the perception of sexual stimuli than with the actual triggering of orgasm. Further studies that compare brain imaging during sexual arousal without orgasm with brain imaging at orgasm are needed to determine whether there are any areas of the brain specifically involved in generating orgasm.

GENDER DIFFERENCES IN ORGASM

Although some therapists have suggested that different types of orgasm exist for men, it is generally believed that typologies of orgasm intriguingly exist only for women (25). Most of the research in this area is derived from self-reports of women who distinguish orgasmic sensations induced by clitoral stimulation (warm, ticklish, electrical, sharp) from those induced by vaginal stimulation (throbbing, deep, soothing, comfortable). Masters and Johnson (2) claimed that all orgasms in women were physiologically identical regardless of the source of stimulation. However, they did not have the instrumentation to obtain detailed muscular recordings for possible differences between clitoral- and vaginal-induced orgasms. There is now some limited physiological laboratory evidence to suggest that different patterns of uterine (smooth muscle) and striated pelvic muscular activity may occur with vaginal anterior wall stimulation as opposed to clitoral stimulation (15).

Several other physiological differences between male and female orgasms have been proposed. First, unlike men, women can have repeated (multiple) orgasms separated by very short intervals, and women can have extended orgasms that last for long periods of time (2). Secondly, men have a divided rhythmic pattern of muscular contractions that has not been noted in women (9). Thirdly, in men, once orgasm is initiated its further expression is automatic even if sexual stimulation is stopped. In contrast, if stimulation is stopped in the middle of either clitoral-induced or vaginal-induced orgasm, orgasm is halted in women (26).

In terms of gender differences in the psychological experience of orgasm, written descriptions of orgasms by men and women with any obvious gender clues removed could not be differentiated by sex, when read by other males and females (27). This suggests that men and women share common mental experiences during orgasm.

WHY DO WOMEN HAVE ORGASMS?

It is generally accepted that female orgasms are not essential for reproduction, and any benefit that they may have for female biology is, as yet, unclear. Early theorists believed that orgasm via intercourse activated ovulation and closed off the womb to air, thus facilitating conception (28). When it was later shown that the human female was a spontaneous ovulator at mid-cycle, and that this was unconnected to coitus, the discourse re-focused on the role of uterine suction created by orgasmic contractions in moving ejaculated spermatozoa through the cervix into the uterus and then fallopian tubes. However, there is now good evidence that the fastest transport of spermatozoa into the human uterus is actually in the sexually unstimulated condition (29).

An essential feature of sexual arousal of the female genitalia is to create the expansion of the vagina (vaginal tenting) and elevation of the uterocervix from the posterior vaginal wall. This reduces the possibility of the rapid entry of ejaculated spermatozoa into the uterus and gives time for the initiation of the decoagulation of semen and the capacitation of the spermatozoa to begin, decreasing the chance of incompetent sperm being transported too rapidly into the fallopian tubes (29). By dissipating arousal and initiating the resolution of the tenting, orgasm may allow the earlier entry of the spermatozoa into the cervical canal and their subsequent rapid transport to the fallopian tubes.

It has been suggested that women may use orgasm, initiated either from coitus or masturbation, as a way to manipulate the ejaculate in the vagina (30,31). This highly contentious concept is based on the amount of "flowback" (semen/fluid) lost from the vagina. The claim is that the amount of flowback containing spermatozoa varies with the precise timing of the woman's orgasm in relation to the time of deposition of the ejaculate into the vagina. Low sperm retention is thought to be associated with female orgasms that occur less than 1 min before vaginal deposition while maximum retention is thought to occur with orgasms occurring shortly after deposition. If orgasm occurs earlier than 1 min before the ejaculate, deposition sperm retention is the same as when there is no orgasm. According to Baker and Bellis (31) the effect of orgasm on sperm retention lasts only for the period of 1 min before semen deposition and up to 45 min later.

An additional function of women's orgasm, which may play a role in the reproductive process, is that if the woman attains orgasm during coitus, the associated contractions of the vagina can facilitate male ejaculation. This would allow the woman to capture the sperm of her chosen inseminator. In addition, as noted earlier, orgasm increases the secretion of prolactin. If prolactin in plasma is able to enter into the vaginal, cervical or uterine fluids, it may influence the entry of calcium into the sperm and this action could play a role in the activation of spermatozoa in the female tract (32).

There have been a number of other explanations offered for why women have orgasms. Some of those explanations are as follows. To the extent that orgasm is an intensely pleasurable sensation, it serves as a reward for the acceptance of the danger of coitus with its possibility of pregnancy and of possible death in childbirth. Orgasm serves as a means for resolving pelvic vasocongestion and vaginal tenting, and for inducing lassitude to keep the female horizontal and thereby reducing seminal "flowback." Through both psychological (loss of body boundaries and separateness) and physiological (oxytocin release) means, orgasm may enhance pair bonding. Lastly, by its activation of muscular contractions and the concomitant increased blood flow, orgasms maintain the functionality of the genital tract (33).

THE EFFECTS OF DRUGS ON WOMEN'S ORGASMIC ABILITY

A number of psychotherapeutic drugs have been noted to affect the ability of women to attain orgasm. The selective serotonin reuptake inhibitors (SSRIs) frequently affect orgasmic functioning, leading to delayed orgasm or anorgasmia. There is variability, however, in that some antidepressants have been associated with anorgasmia less frequently than others. For example, the antidepressant, nefazodone, has been reported to produce fewer sexual side effects in women (34) than many of the earlier-generation SSRIs. Nephazodone increases serotonin activity in general while simultaneously inhibiting serotonin activity at the serotonin$_2$ (5-HT$_2$) receptor. Stimulation of 5-HT$_2$ receptors has been reported to inhibit the release of both norepinephrine and dopamine from several brain areas (35). Because dopamine and norepinephrine have been reported to facilitate sexual behavior, the decrease in serotonergic activity at 5-HT$_2$ receptors (and consequent possible increase in dopamine and norepinephrine) could explain the decreased incidence of anorgasmia noted with nefazodone. Cyproheptadine is also a 5-HT$_2$ receptor antagonist and has been used with some success as an antidote to SSRI-induced orgasmic dysfunction.

Among the typical SSRIs, paroxetine has been reported to delay orgasm more frequently than fluvoxetine, fluoxetine, and sertraline (36) and more than nefazadone, fluoxetine and venlafaxine (37). One explanation for this greater impairment may be that paroxetine is a more potent inhibitor of the serotonin transporter than are fluoxetine and fluvoxetine, and does not inhibit the dopamine transporter, as does sertraline and, to a lesser degree, fluoxetine and fluvoxetine (38). As noted earlier, dopamine antagonists impair several aspects of sexual function. Women treated with fluoxetine, paroxetine, and sertraline for anxiety disorders reported delays in reaching orgasm and decreased quality of orgasm at 1 and 2 month follow-ups (39). However, the impairments in the fluoxetine group decreased by the end of the third month. In contrast to these findings of impaired orgasm with fluoxetine, one multicenter open-label study of fluoxetine reported an improvement in women's orgasmic ability associated with the amelioration of depression (40).

Several factors may explain the discrepancy between such studies. First, there may be individual differences in the numbers and anatomical distributions of receptor subtypes, and in the influence of the SSRI on subsequent dopamine and norepinephrine release. In addition, for some women, improvements in mood and interpersonal functioning, which result from the antidepressant properties of these drugs, may offset neurochemical changes that may adversely impact orgasmic ability.

Antipsychotic medications have also been reported to inhibit orgasm in women (41). This is likely attributable to the blockade of dopamine receptors in areas critical for sexual function (e.g., medial preoptic area, paraventricular nuclei), or indirectly from increased prolactin levels, extrapyramidal side effects, or sedation. A retrospective clinical study of women taking antiepilepsy drugs (primarily benzodiazepines) reported they found orgasm less satisfying than did the healthy, unmedicated controls (42). These effects were not attributable to alterations in free testosterone levels with antiepilepsy medication use.

Nitric oxide stimulates guanylate cyclase release, which triggers the conversion of guanosine triphosphate to cGMP. cGMP activity relaxes the smooth muscles of the penile tissue allowing vasocongestion and erection. Sildenafil (Viagra$^{®}$) potentiates the activity of cGMP by inhibiting phosphodiesterase type 5, the endogenous substance responsible for cGMP deactivation. This increases and prolongs cGMP activity, which increases and prolongs vasocongestion, and enables erection. There have been mixed reports of the effects of sildenafil on women's orgasmic function. Caruso et al. (43) found improved sexual arousal and orgasm with sildenafil. However, only a minority of women responded positively in several other studies (44,45). A number of case studies have reported a reversal of antidepressant-induced anorgasmia with sildenafil (46–49) but, to date, no placebo-controlled studies have been conducted.

Drugs that inhibit beta-adrenergic receptors do not seem to adversely impact women's orgasmic ability. In a retrospective questionnaire study of 1080 women, there were no reports of significant increases in difficulty achieving orgasm while taking hydralazine, beta-adrenergic antagonists, or methyldopa (50). In a prospective randomized double-blind study of 345 women over a period of 24 months (51), antihypertensive medications did not substantially impact orgasm ability. Similarly, atropine, a cholinergic acting agent, did not affect subjective sexual arousal or orgasm in women (52).

In an uncontrolled, open-label study, estrogen was reported to facilitate orgasmic function in 25% of 188 premenopausal women (53). However, a retrospective study of 66 women who had undergone hysterectomy and oophorectomy found no difference in orgasmic ability between the 33 who received conjugated estrogens and the 33 who did not (54). In a single blind study comparing estrogen plus progestin hormone replacement therapy (HRT) to tibolone, a drug which can be metabolized into estrogenic, androgenic, and progestogenic compounds, there was no effect of HRT or tibolone in 50 postmenopausal women (55). An open-label study of 48 women found a significant improvement after 3 months of tibolone treatment, but not HRT (56).

In a 3 month, prospective, open-label study of 44 women who had undergone hysterectomy and oophorectomy, monthly injections of estrogen and testosterone increased the rates of orgasm during the first 3 weeks following treatment, compared with the woman's own baseline and compared to estrogen alone or no treatment (57). Similar results were noted in a well-controlled study of 75 women who had undergone hysterectomy and oophorectomy (58). Conjugated estrogens were administered either alone or with testosterone (150 or 300 μg/day) in transdermal patches. The higher dose of testosterone improved orgasm pleasure. However, as was the case in the Sherwin and Gelfand study, the testosterone levels noted in this study were substantially greater than that regarded as being within the normal range for intact women. In an open-label, uncontrolled study, dehydroepiandrosterone (DHEA) (50 mg/day orally) was used to treat 113 women with low levels of testosterone and DHEA and complaints of orgasmic difficulty. After 3 months of treatment, the women reported a greater frequency of orgasm compared with pretreatment levels (59).

In summary, drugs that increase serotonergic activity (e.g., antidepressants), or decrease dopaminergic activity (e.g., antipsychotics) adversely impact female orgasm. The degree to which the former of these influences orgasm appears to be dependent upon which serotonin receptor subtype they activate/inhibit.

Beta-adrenergic drugs and estrogenic compounds do not seem to have a substantial impact on women's orgasm ability. High doses of testosterone seem to facilitate orgasmic ability but future controlled studies are needed to assess the impact of more moderate doses of testosterone on women's orgasmic ability.

PSYCHOSOCIAL FACTORS RELATED TO WOMEN'S ORGASM

Age, education, social class, religion, personality, and relationship issues are the psychosocial factors most commonly discussed in relation to female orgasmic ability. Laumann et al. (60) found only the youngest group of women (18–24 years) showed rates of orgasm lower than the older groups for both orgasm with a partner and orgasm during masturbation. This is likely to be attributable to age differences in sexual experience. There was no significant relation between education level and orgasmic ability with a partner, but substantial differences between education level and ability to attain orgasm during masturbation. Approximately 87% of women with an advanced degree reported "always" or "usually" attaining orgasm during masturbation compared with 42% of women with a high school education. The authors explained this finding as the better educated women having more liberal views on sexuality and being more likely to consider pleasure a major goal of sexual activity.

Research based on individuals presenting for sex therapy generally finds a negative relation between high religiosity and orgasmic ability in women. Sexual guilt is often used to explain this relation; the more religious a person, the more likely they are to experience guilt during sexual activity. Guilt could feasibly impair orgasm via a variety of cognitive mechanisms, in particular, distraction processes. A relation between improved orgasmic ability and decreased sexual guilt has also been reported (61). Laumann et al. (60) reported a substantially higher proportion (79%) of women with no religious affiliation reported being orgasmic during masturbation compared with religious groups (53–67%). Counterintuitive to these relations, Laumann et al. (60) found women without religious affiliation were much less likely to report always having an orgasm with their primary partner (22%) than were religious women (e.g., 33% for Type II Protestant women). The authors cautioned making assumptions based on these statistics given that there were substantial differences in education levels between religious categories.

In an extensive investigation of background and personality variables and women's orgasm, Fisher (25) found few significant associations, the most notable of which concerned the quality of the father/daughter relationship. Low orgasmic experience was consistently related to childhood loss or separation from the father, fathers who had been emotionally unavailable, or fathers with whom the women did not have a positive childhood relationship. Fisher explained this finding in terms of high arousal, presumably necessary for orgasm, creates a more vulnerable emotional state that is threatening to these women who are especially concerned with object loss. There has been no follow-up research on this finding. There have been no other personality or background variables consistently associated with orgasmic ability in women. A relation between childhood sexual abuse and various sexual difficulties has been reported, but reports of an association between early abuse and anorgasmia are inconsistent (62–64).

Relationship factors such as marital satisfaction, marital adjustment, happiness, and stability have been related to orgasm consistency, quality, and satisfaction in women [for review see Ref. (65)]. These findings are correlational in nature. Clearly, a satisfying marital relationship is not necessary for orgasm, particularly given rates of orgasm consistency in women are higher during masturbation than with a partner (60). A satisfying marital relationship most likely promotes orgasmic function via increased communication regarding sexually pleasurable activity, decreased anxiety, and enhancement of the subjective and emotional qualities of orgasm (65).

DEFINITION OF FEMALE ORGASMIC DISORDER

On the basis of findings from the National Social and Health Life Survey conducted in the early 1990s (60), orgasmic problems are the second most frequently reported sexual problems in US women. Results from this random sample of 1749 US women indicated 24% reported a lack of orgasm in the past year for at least several months or more. This percentage is comparable to the clinic-based data. Orgasmic problems were noted by 29% of 329 healthy women (ages 18–73) who attended an outpatient gynecological clinic (66) and by 23% of 104 women (18–65+) attending a UK general practice clinic (67). It is difficult to determine the precise incidence of orgasmic difficulties in women, however, because few well-controlled studies have been conducted and definitions of orgasmic disorder vary widely between studies depending on the diagnostic criteria used. The DSM-IV-TR (68) defines female orgasmic disorder (302.73) using the following diagnostic criteria:

1. Persistent or recurrent delay in, or absence of, orgasm following a normal sexual excitement phase. Women exhibit wide variability in the type or intensity of stimulation that triggers orgasm. The diagnosis of female orgasmic disorder should be based on the clinician's judgment that the woman's orgasmic capacity is less than would be reasonable for her age, sexual experience, and the adequacy of sexual stimulation she receives.
2. The disturbance causes marked distress or interpersonal difficulty.
3. The orgasmic dysfunction is not better accounted for by another Axis I disorder (except another sexual dysfunction) and is not due exclusively to the direct physiological effects of a substance (e.g., a drug of abuse, a medication) or a general medical condition. Female orgasmic disorder is further subtyped as lifelong vs. acquired, and generalized vs. situational.

Most studies examining orgasmic dysfunction in women refer to orgasm problems as either "primary orgasmic dysfunction" or "secondary orgasmic dysfunction." In general, the term primary orgasmic dysfunction is used to describe women who report never having experienced orgasm under any circumstances, including masturbation. According to the DSM-IV-TR, this would refer to those women who meet criteria for lifelong and generalized anorgasmia. Secondary orgasmic dysfunction relates to women who meet criteria for situational and/or acquired lack of orgasm. By definition, this encompasses a heterogeneous group of women with orgasm difficulties. It could, for example, include women who were once orgasmic but are now so only infrequently, women who are able to obtain orgasm only in certain contexts, with certain types of sexual activity, or with certain partners. Regarding women who can obtain orgasm during intercourse with manual stimulation but not intercourse alone, the clinical consensus is that she would not meet criteria for clinical diagnosis unless she is distressed by the frequency of her sexual response.

TREATMENT OF FEMALE ORGASMIC DISORDER

Female orgasmic disorder has been treated from psychoanalytic, cognitive-behavioral, pharmacological, and systems theory perspectives (69). Because substantial empirical outcome research is available only for cognitive-behavioral and, to a lesser degree, pharmacological approaches, only these two methods of treatment will be reviewed here.

Cognitive-Behavioral Approaches

Cognitive-behavioral therapy for female orgasmic disorder aims at promoting changes in attitudes and sexually relevant thoughts, decreasing anxiety, and increasing orgasmic ability and satisfaction. Traditionally, the behavioral exercises used to induce these changes include directed masturbation, sensate focus, and systematic desensitization. Sex education, communication skills training, and Kegel exercises are also often included in cognitive-behavioral treatment programs for anorgasmia.

Directed Masturbation

Masturbation exercises are believed to benefit women with orgasm difficulties for a number of reasons. To the extent that focusing on nonsexual cues can impede sexual performance (70), masturbation exercises can help the woman to direct her attention to sexually pleasurable physical sensations. Because masturbation can be performed alone, any anxiety that may be associated with partner evaluation is necessarily eliminated. Relatedly, the amount and intensity of sexual stimulation is directly under the woman's control and therefore the woman is not reliant upon her partner's knowledge or her ability to communicate her needs to her partner. Research that shows a relation between masturbation and orgasmic ability provides empirical support for this treatment approach. Kinsey et al. (1) reported that the average woman reached orgasm 95% of the time she engaged in masturbation compared with 73% during intercourse. More recently, in a random probability sample of 682 women, Laumann et al. (60) reported a strong relation between frequency of masturbation and orgasmic ability during masturbation. Sixty-seven percent of women who masturbated one to six times a year reported orgasm during masturbation compared with 81% of women who masturbated once a week or more.

LoPiccolo and Lobitz (71) were the first to outline a program of directed masturbation (DM). Since then, several other researchers have provided variations (72,73). The first step of DM involves having the woman visually examine her nude body with the help of a mirror and diagrams of female genital anatomy. During the next stage she is instructed to explore her genitals tactually as well as visually with an emphasis on locating sensitive areas that produce feelings of pleasure. Once pleasure-producing areas are located, the woman is instructed to concentrate on manual stimulation of these areas and to increase the intensity and duration until "something happens" or until discomfort arises. The use of topical lubricants, vibrators, and erotic videotapes are often incorporated into the exercises. Once the woman is able to attain orgasm alone, her partner is usually included in the sessions in order to desensitize her to displaying arousal and orgasm in his presence, and to educate the partner on how to provide her with effective stimulation.

DM has been used to effectively treat female orgasmic disorder in a variety of treatment modalities including group, individual, couples therapy, and bibliotherapy. A number of outcome studies and case series report DM is highly successful for treating primary anorgasmia. Heinrich (74) reported a 100% success rate for treating primary anorgasmia using therapist DM training at 2 month follow-up. The study was a controlled comparison of therapist-directed group masturbation training, self-directed masturbation training (bibliotherapy), and wait-list control. Forty-seven percent of the bibliotherapy subjects reported becoming orgasmic during masturbation compared with 21% of wait-list controls. In a randomized trial comparing written vs. videotaped masturbation assignments, the effects of self-directed masturbation training were further investigated (75). Sixty-five percent of women who used a text and 55% of women who used videotapes had experienced orgasm during masturbation and 50% and 30%, respectively, were orgasmic during intercourse after 6 weeks. None of the control women had attained orgasm. Few controlled studies have examined the exclusive effects of DM for treating secondary anorgasmia. Fichen et al. (76) compared minimal therapist contact bibliotherapy with a variety of techniques including DM and found no change in orgasmic ability. Hurlbert and Apt (77) recently compared the effectiveness of DM with coital alignment technique in 36 women with secondary anorgasmia. Coital alignment is a technique in which the woman assumes the supine position and the man positions himself up forward on the woman. After only four 30-min sessions, 37% of women receiving instructions on coital alignment technique vs. 18% of those receiving DM reported substantial improvements (>50% increase) in orgasmic ability during intercourse. The benefits of this technique are due to the fact that clitoral contact, and possibly paraurethral, stimulation are maximized.

In summary, DM has been shown to be an empirically valid, efficacious treatment for women diagnosed with primary anorgasmia. For women with secondary anorgasmia, who are averse to touching their genitals, DM may be beneficial. If, however, the woman is able to attain orgasm alone through masturbation but not with her partner, issues relating to communication, anxiety reduction, trust, and ensuring the woman is receiving adequate stimulation either via direct manual stimulation or engaging in intercourse using positions designed to maximize clitoral stimulation (i.e., coital alignment technique) may prove more beneficial.

Anxiety Reduction Techniques

Anxiety could feasibly impair orgasmic function in women via several cognitive processes. Anxiety can serve as a distraction that disrupts the processing of erotic cues by causing the woman to focus instead on performance related concerns, embarrassment, and/or guilt. It can lead the woman to engage in self-monitoring during sexual activity, an experience Masters and Johnson (78) referred to as "spectatoring". Physiologically, for many years it was assumed that the increased sympathetic activation that accompanies an anxiety state may impair sexual arousal necessary for orgasm via inhibition of parasympathetic nervous system activity. Meston and Gorzalka (79–81), however, have noted that activation of the sympathetic nervous system, induced via means such as 20 min of intense stationary cycling or running on a treadmill actually facilitates genital engorgement under conditions of erotic stimulation.

The most notable anxiety reduction techniques for treating female orgasmic disorder are systematic desensitization and sensate focus. Systematic desensitization for treating sexual anxiety was first described by Wolpe (82). The process involves training the woman to relax the muscles of her body through a sequence of exercises. Next, a hierarchy of anxiety-evoking stimuli or situations is composed and the woman is trained to imagine the situations while remaining relaxed. Once the woman is able to imagine all the items in the hierarchy without experiencing anxiety, she is instructed to engage in the activities in real life.

Sensate focus was originally conceived by Masters and Johnson (78). It involves a step-by-step sequence of body touching exercises, moving from nonsexual to increasingly sexual touching of one another's body. Components specific for treating anorgasmic women often include nondemand genital touching by the partner, female guidance of genital manual, and penile stimulation and coital positions designed to maximize pleasurable stimulation. Sensate focus is primarily a couple's skills learning approach designed to increase communication and awareness of sexually sensitive areas between partners. Conceptually, however, the removal of goal-focused orgasm, which can cause performance concerns, the hierarchical nature of the touching exercises, and the instruction not to advance to the next phase before feeling relaxed about the current one, suggest sensate focus is also largely an anxiety reduction technique and could be considered a modified form of *in vivo* desensitization.

The success of using anxiety reduction techniques for treating female orgasmic disorder is difficult to assess because most studies have used some combination of anxiety reduction, sexual techniques training, sex education, communication training, bibliotherapy, and Kegel exercises, and have not systematically evaluated the independent contributions to treatment outcome. Moreover, even within specific treatment modalities, considerable variation between studies exists. For example, systematic desensitization has been conducted both *in vivo* and imaginal, has used mainly progressive muscle relaxation but also drugs (83) and hypnotic techniques (84) to induce relaxation, and has varied somewhat in the hierarchical construction of events. Furthermore, the relative contribution of factors such as individual vs. group treatment, patient demographics (age, marital status, education, religion), precise diagnosis and severity of presenting sexual concerns, therapist characteristics (sex, theoretical orientation and training), treatment settings (private, hospital, university clinics), and length of treatment sessions and duration are often reported but systematic evaluation of many of these factors is missing from the literature. Finally, of the controlled studies that have included anxiety reduction techniques, few have differentiated between treatment outcomes for primary and secondary anorgasmic women. Across studies, women have reported decreases in sexual anxiety and, occasionally, increases in frequency of sexual intercourse and sexual satisfaction with systematic desensitization, but substantial improvements in orgasmic ability have not been noted. Similarly, of the few controlled studies that have included sensate focus as a treatment component, none have reported notable increases in orgasmic ability. These findings suggest that, in most cases, anxiety does not appear to play a causal role in female orgasmic disorder and anxiety reduction techniques are best suited for anorgasmic women only when sexual anxiety is coexistant.

Other Behavioral Techniques

As noted earlier, many treatment outcome studies for anorgasmia include a variety of treatment components, and the relevant individual contributions they make to treatment outcome success cannot be effectively evaluated. With this in mind, a number of additional treatment techniques warrant mention. Since Masters and Johnson's pioneering work (78), sex education has been a component of many sex therapy programs. Ignorance about female anatomy and/or techniques for maximizing pleasurable sensations can certainly contribute to orgasm difficulties. Jankovich and Miller (85) noted increases in orgasmic ability following an educational audiovisual presentation in seven of 17 women with primary anorgasmia. Kilmann et al. (86) compared the effectiveness of various sequences of sex education and communication skills vs. wait-list control on orgasmic ability in women with secondary anorgasmia. The authors found sex education to be beneficial for enhancing coital ability at posttest but not at 6 month follow-up. In a comparison study of the effectiveness of sex therapy vs. communication skills training for secondary anorgasmia, Everaerd and Dekker (87) found both treatments were equally effective in improving orgasmic ability. Kegel (88) proposed that conducting exercises that strengthen the pubo-coccygeous muscle could increase vascularity to the genitals and, in turn, facilitate orgasm. Treatment comparison studies have generally found no differences in orgasmic ability between women whose therapy included using Kegel exercises vs. those whose therapy did not. To the extent that Kegel exercise may enhance arousal and/or help the woman become more aware and comfortable with her genitals, these exercises may enhance orgasm ability (69). In summary, sex education, communication skills training, and Kegel exercises may serve as benefical adjuncts to therapy. Used alone, they do not appear highly effective for treating either primary or secondary anorgasmia.

Pharmacological Approaches

Of the few placebo-controlled studies examining the effectiveness of pharmacological agents for treating female orgasmic disorder, most examine the efficacy of agents for treating antidepressant-induced anorgasmia. Whether pharmacological agents would have the same treatment outcome effect on non-drug- vs. drug-induced anorgasmia is not known.

Modell et al. (89) reported no significant effect beyond placebo of either 150 or 300 mg/day bupropion-SR on orgasm in 20 women with delayed or inhibited orgasm. Ito et al. (90) conducted a double-blind, placebo-controlled study of ArginMax, a nutritional supplement comprising ginseng, *Ginkgo biloba*, Damiana leaf, and various vitamins, on sexual function in 77 women with unspecified sexual function. Approximately 47% of women treated with ArginMax reported an increase in the frequency of orgasm compared with ~30% of women treated with placebo—a marginally significant group difference. It cannot be determined from the report how many women would meet a clinical diagnosis for anorgasmia. To date, there have been no published placebo-controlled studies on sildenafil for female anorgasmia and findings from uncontrolled studies are equivocal. In an open-label trial, Kaplan et al. (44) reported a very modest 7.4% improvement in orgasm at 12 weeks with 50 mg sildenafil. Participants were 30 post-menopausal women with self-reported mixed sexual dysfunction.

As noted earlier, there is a high incidence of adverse sexual side effects noted with antidepressant treatment. A number of pharmacological agents have been prescribed along with the antidepressant medication in an effort to help counter these effects. Some such drugs include antiserotonergic agents such as cyproheptadine, buspirone, mirtazapine, and granisetron; dopaminergic agents such as amantadine, dextroamphetamine, bupropion, methylphenidate, and pemoline; adrenergic agents such as yohimbine and ephedrine; cholinergic agents such as bethanechol; and the selective cyclic-GMP catabolism inhibitor sildenafil. A number of case reports and open-label studies report success in alleviating SSRI-induced anorgasmia with some of these agents. Findings from the few placebo-controlled studies published are less optimistic. Michelson et al. (91) examined the comparative effects of 8 weeks of treatment with buspirone ($n = 19$), amantadine ($n = 18$), or placebo ($n = 20$) on fluoxetine-induced sexual dysfunction in premenopausal women reporting either impaired orgasm or sexual arousal. The authors reported all groups experienced an improvement in orgasm during treatment, but neither buspirone nor amantadine was more effective than placebo in restoring orgasmic function. It should be noted, however, that the doses of buspirone (20 mg/day) and amantadine (50 mg/day) administered were very low. At a higher dose level (mean daily dose $= 47$ mg), buspirone showed a marginally significant alleviation of sexual side effects in women taking either citalopram or paroxetine compared with placebo (92). The authors did not distinguish between orgasm and desire disorders in either the classification of patients or treatment outcome. In a randomized, double-blind, parallel, placebo-controlled study of mirtazapine (15 mg/day), yohimbine (5.4 mg/day), olanzapine (0.25 mg/day), or placebo for fluoxetine-induced sexual dysfunction, Michelson et al. (93) found no significant improvement in orgasmic ability beyond placebo in 107 women with either impaired orgasm or vaginal lubrication. Kang et al. (94) reported no significant effect of *Gingko biloba* beyond placebo in a small group of women with SSRI-induced sexual dysfunction. Meston (95) reported no significant effect of ephedrine (50 mg, 1 h prior to intercourse) beyond placebo on orgasmic function in 19 women with sexual side effects secondary to fluoxetine, sertraline, or paroxetine treatment. The study was conducted using a randomized, double-blind, placebo-controlled, cross-over design. In summary, to date there are no pharmacological agents proven to be beneficial beyond placebo in enhancing orgasmic function in women.

CONCLUSIONS

We conclude that DM is an empirically valid and efficacious treatment for lifelong female orgasmic disorder. To date, there are no empirically validated treatments for acquired female orgasmic disorder. Anxiety reduction techniques such as sensate focus and systematic desensitization have not been shown to be efficacious for treating either lifelong or acquired female orgasmic disorder. Anxiety reduction techniques may serve as beneficial adjuncts to therapy if the woman is experiencing a high level of anxiety. There is no direct empirical evidence to suggest that sex education, communication skills training, or Kegel exercises alone are effective for treating either lifelong or acquired female orgasmic disorder. Of the few studies examining the effects of pharmacological agents for female orgasmic disorder, none have been shown to be more effective than placebo. Placebo-controlled research is essential to examine the effectiveness of agents with demonstrated success in case series or open-label trials (i.e., sildenafil, testosterone) on orgasmic function in women.

REFERENCES

1. Kinsey AC, Pomeroy WD, Martin CE, Gebhard PH. Sexual Behaviour in the Human Female. Philadelphia: WB Saunders Company, 1953:628.
2. Masters WH, Johnson V. Human Sexual Response. Boston: Little, Brown & Co, 1966.
3. Levin RJ. Measuring the menopause genital changes: a critical account of laboratory procedures past and for the future. Menopause Rev 1999; 1V:49–57.
4. Henson DE, Rubin HB, Henson C, Williams JR. Temperature changes of the labia minora as an objective measure of female eroticism. J Behav Ther Exp Psychiatry 1977; 8:401–410.
5. Henson DE, Rubin HB, Henson C. Labial and vaginal blood volume responses to visual and tactile stimuli. Arch Sex Behav 1982; 11:23–31.
6. Bohlen GJ, Held JP, Sanderson MO. Response of the circumvaginal musculature during masturbation. In: Graber B, ed. Circumvaginal Musculature and Sexual Function. Basel: Kager, 1982:43–60.
7. Carmichael MS, Warburton VL, Dixen J, Davidson JM. Relationship among cardiovascular, muscular, and oxytocin responses during human sexual activity. Arch Sex Behav 1994; 23:59–79.
8. Levin RJ, Wagner G, Ottesen B. Simultaneous monitoring of human vaginal haemodynamics by three independent methods during sexual arousal. In: Hoch Z, Lief HI, eds. Sexology. Amsterdam: Elsevier Publishing Co, 1981:114–120.
9. Bohlen G, Held JP, Sanderson MO, Ahlgren A. The female orgasm: pelvic contractions. Arch Sex Behav 1982; 11:367–386.
10. Davidson JM. The psychobiology of sexual experience. In: Davidson JM, Davidson RJ, eds. The Psychobiology of Consciousness. New York: Plenum Press, 1980:271–332.
11. Ladas AK, Whipple B, Perry JD. The G-spot and Other Recent Discoveries About Human Sexuality. New York: Holt, Rinehart & Winston, 1982.
12. Hines TM. The G-spot: a modern gynecologic myth. Am J Obstet Gynecol 2001; 185:359–362.
13. Geer JH, Quartararo J. Vaginal blood volume responses during masturbation. Arch Sex Behav 1976; 5:403–413.
14. Kruger THC, Haake P, Hartman U, Schedlowski M, Exton MS. Orgasm-induced prolactin secretion: Feedback control of sexual drive? Neurosci Biobehav Rev 2002; 26:31–44.
15. Levin RJ. Sexual desire and the deconstruction and reconstruction of the human female sexual response model of Masters & Johnson. In: Everaerd W, Laan E, Both S, eds. Sexual Appetite, Desire and Motivation: Energetics of the Sexual System. Amsterdam: Royal Netherlands Academy of Arts and Sciences, 2001:63–93.
16. Whipple B, Ogden G, Komisaruk BR. Physiological correlates of imagery-induced orgasm in women. Arch Sex Behav 1992; 21:121–133.
17. Levin RJ. The mechanisms of human female sexual arousal. Annu Rev Sex Res 1992; 3:1–48.

18. Fisher C, Cohen HD, Schiavi RC, Davis D, Furman B, Ward K, Edwards A, Cunningham J. Patterns of female sexual arousal during sleep and waking: vaginal thermo-conductance studies. Arch Sex Behav 1983; 12:97–122.

19. Wells BL. Nocturnal orgasms: Females' perception of a "normal" sexual experience. J Sex Res 1983; 22:412–437.

20. Polatin P, Douglas DE. Spontaneous orgasm in a case of schizophrenia. Psychoanal Rev 1953; 40:17–26.

21. Whipple B, Komisaruk BR. Brain (PET) responses to vaginal-cervical self-stimulation in women with complete spinal cord injury: preliminary findings. J Sex Marital Ther 2002; 28:79–86.

22. Lane RD, Reiman EM, Ahern GL, Schwartz GE, Davidson RJ. Neuroanatomical correlates of happiness, sadness, and disgust. Am J Psychiatry 1997; 154:926–933.

23. Morris JS, Frith CD, Perrett DI, Rowland D, Young AW, Calder AJ, Dolan RJ. A differential neural response in the human amygdala to fearful and happy facial expressions. Nature 1996; 383:812–815.

24. Whalen PJ, Rauch SL, Etcoff NL, McInerney SC, Lee MB, Jenike MA. Masked presentations of emotional facial expressions modulate amygdala activity without explicit knowledge. J Neurosci 1998; 8:411–418.

25. Fisher S. The Female Orgasm. New York: Basic Books, 1973.

26. Sherfey MJ. The Nature and Evolution of Female Sexuality. New York: Vintage Books, Random House, 1972:121.

27. Vance EB, Wagner NN. Written descriptions of orgasm: a study of sex differences. Arch Sex Behav 1976; 5:87–98.

28. Laqueur T. Making Sex: Body and Gender from the Greeks to Freud. Cambridge, MA: Harvard University Press, 1990.

29. Levin RJ. The physiology of sexual arousal in the human female: a recreational and procreational synthesis. Arch Sex Behav 2002; 31:405–411.

30. Baker RR, Bellis MA. Human sperm competition: ejaculate manipulation by females and a function for the female orgasm. Anim Behav 1993; 6:887–909.

31. Baker RR, Bellis MA. Human Sperm Competition: Copulation, Masturbation and Infidelity. London: Chapman & Hall, 1995.

32. Reyes A, Para A, Chavarria ME, Goicoechea B, Rosado A. Effect of prolactin on the calcium binding and/or transport of ejaculated and epididymal human spermatozoa. Fertil Steril 1979; 31:669–672.

33. Levin RJ. Do women gain anything from coitus apart from pregnancy? Changes in the human female genital tract activated by coitus. J Sex Marital Ther 2003; 29(suppl):59–69.

34. Feiger A, Kiev A, Shrivastava RK, Wisselink PG, Wilcox CS. Nefazodone versus sertraline in outpatients with major depression: focus on efficacy, tolerability, and effects on sexual function and satisfaction. J Clin Psychiatry 1996; 57(suppl 2):53–62.

35. Alcantara AG. A possible dopaminergic mechanism in the serotonergic antidepressant-induced sexual dysfunctions. J Sex Marital Ther 1999; 25:125–129.

36. Montejo-Gonzalez AL, Llorca G, Izquierdo JA, Ledesma A, Bousono M, Calcedo A, Carrasco JL, Ciudad J, Daniel E, De la Gandara J, Derecho J, Franco M, Gomez MJ, Macias JA, Martin T, Perez V, Sanchez JM, Sanchez S, Vicens E. SSRI-induced sexual dysfunction: fluoxetine, paroxetine, sertraline, and fluvoxamine in a prospective, multicenter, and descriptive clinical study of 344 patients. J Sex Marital Ther 1997; 23:176–194.

37. Bobes J, Gonzalez MP, Bascaran MT, Clayton A, Garcia M, Rico-Villade Moros F, Banus S. Evaluating changes in sexual functioning in depressed patients: sensitivity to change of the CSFQ. J Sex Marital Ther 2002; 28:93–103.
38. Rosen RC, Lane RM, Menza M. Effects of SSRIs on sexual function: a critical review. J Clin Psychopharmacol 1999; 19:67–85.
39. Labbate LA, Grimes J, Hines A, Oleshansky MA, Arana GW. Sexual dysfunction induced by serotonin reuptake antidepressants. J Sex Marital Ther 1998; 24:3–12.
40. Michelson D, Schmidt M, Lee J, Tepner R. Changes in sexual function during acute and six-month fluoxetine therapy: a prospective assessment. J Sex Marital Ther 2001; 27:289–302.
41. Meston CM, Gorzalka BB. Psychoactive drugs and human sexual behavior: the role of serotonergic activity. J Psychoactive Drugs 1992; 24:1–42.
42. Duncan S, Blacklaw J, Beastall GH, Brodie MJ. Sexual function in women with epilepsy. Epilepsia 1997; 38:1074–1081.
43. Caruso S, Intelisano G, Lupo L, Agnello C. Premenopausal women affected by sexual arousal disorder treated with sildenafil: a double-blind, cross-over, placebo-controlled study. Int J Obstet Gynaecol 2001; 108:623–628.
44. Kaplan SA, Reis RB, Kohn IJ, Ikeguchi EF, Laor E, Te AE, Martins AC. Safety and efficacy of sildenafil in postmenopausal women with sexual dysfunction. Urology 1999; 53:481–486.
45. Berman JR, Berman LA, Lin H, Flaherty E, Lahey N, Goldstein I, Cantey-Kiser J. Effect of sildenafil on subjective and physiologic parameters of the female sexual response in women with sexual arousal disorder. J Sex Marital Ther 2001; 27: 411–420.
46. Ashton AK. Sildenafil treatment of paroxetine-induced anorgasmia in a woman [Letter]. Am J Psychiatry 1999; 156:800.
47. Nurnberg HG, Lauriello J, Hensley PL, Parker LM, Keith SJ. Sildenafil for iatrogenic serotonergic antidepressant medication-induced sexual dysfunction in 4 patients. J Clin Psychiatry 1999; 60:33–35.
48. Rosenberg KP. Sildenafil citrate for SSRI-induced sexual side effects [Letter]. Am J Psychiatry 1999; 156:157.
49. Shen WW, Urosevich Z, Clayton DO. Sildenafil in the treatment of female sexual dysfunction induced by selective serotonin reuptake inhibitors. J Reprod Med 1999; 44:535–542.
50. Bulpitt CJ, Beevers DG, Butler A, Coles EC, Hunt D, Munro-Faure AD, Newson RB, O'Riodan PW, Petrie JC, Rajagopalan B. The effects of anti-hypertensive drugs on sexual function in men and women: a report from the DHSS Hypertension Care Computing Project (DHCCP). J Hum Hypertens 1989; 3:53–56.
51. Grimm RH, Grandits GA, Prineas RJ, McDonald RH, Lewis CE, Flack JM, Yunis C, Svendsen K, Liebson PR, Elmer PJ. Long-term effects on sexual function of five antihypertensive drugs and nutritional hygienic treatment in hypertensive men and women. Treatment of Mild Hypertension Study (TOMHS). Hypertension 1997; 29:8–14.
52. Wagner G, Levin RJ. Effect of atropine and methylatropine on human vaginal blood flow, sexual arousal and climax. Acta Pharmacol Toxicol 1980; 46:321–325.
53. Eicher W, Muck AO. Treatment of estrogen deficiency-induced sex disorders. Gynakologisch-Geburtshilfliche Rundschau 1996; 36:83–89.

54. Nathorst-Boos J, von Schoultz B, Carlstrom K. Elective ovarian removal and estrogen replacement therapy: effects on sexual life, psychological well-being and androgen status. J Psychosom Obstet Gynecol 1993; 14:283–293.

55. Kokcu A, Cetinkaya MB, Yanik F, Alper T, Malatyalioglu E. The comparison of effects of tibolone and conjugated estrogen–medroxyprogesterone acetate therapy on sexual performance in postmenopausal women. Maturitas 2000; 36:75–80.

56. Wu MH, Pan HA, Wang ST, Hsu CC, Chang FM, Huang KE. Quality of life and sexuality changes in postmenopausal women receiving tibolone therapy. Climacteric 2001; 4:314–319.

57. Sherwin BB, Gelfand MM. The role of androgen in the maintenance of sexual functioning in oophorectomized women. Psychosom Med 1987; 49:397–409.

58. Shifren JL, Braunstein GD, Simon JA, Casson PR, Buster JE, Redmond GP, Burki RE, Ginsburg ES, Rosen RC, Leiblum SR, Caramelli KE, Mazer NA. Transdermal testosterone treatment in women with impaired sexual function after oophorectomy. N Engl J Med 2000; 343:682–688.

59. Munarriz R, Talakoub L, Flaherty E, Gioia M, Hoag L, Kim NN, Traish A, Goldstein I, Guay A, Spark R. Androgen replacement therapy with dehydroepiandrosterone for androgen insufficiency and female sexual dysfunction: androgen and questionnaire results. J Sex Marital Ther 2002; 28(suppl 1):165–173.

60. Laumann EO, Gagnon JH, Michael RT, Michaels S. The Social Organization of Sexuality: Sexual Practices in the United States. Chicago: University of Chicago Press, 1994.

61. Sholty MJ, Ephross PH, Plaut SM, Fischman SH, Charnas JF, Cody CA. Female orgasmic experience: a subjective study. Arch Sex Behav 1984; 13:155–164.

62. Bartoi MG, Kinder BN. Effects of child and adult sexual abuse on adult sexuality. J Sex Marital Ther 1998; 24:75–90.

63. Feinauer LL. Sexual dysfunction in women sexually abused as children. Contemp Fam Ther 1989; 11:299–309.

64. Meston CM, Heiman JR, Trapnell PD. The relation between early abuse and adult sexuality. J Sex Res 1999; 36:385–395.

65. Mah K, Binik YM. The nature of human orgasm: a critical review of major trends. Clin Psychol Rev 2001; 21:823–856.

66. Rosen RC, Taylor JF, Leiblum S, Bachman GA. Prevalence of sexual dysfunction in women: results of a survey study of 329 women in an outpatient gynecological clinic. J Sex Marital Ther 1993; 19:171–188.

67. Read S, King M, Watson J. Sexual dysfunction in primary medical care: prevalence, characteristics and detection by the general practitioner. J Public Health Med 1997; 19:387–391.

68. American Psychiatric Association. DSM-IV-TR: Diagnostic and Statistical Manual of Mental Disorders. 4th ed. Text revision. Washington, DC: American Psychiatric Association, 1994.

69. Heiman JR. Orgasmic disorders in women. In: Leiblum SR, Rosen RC, eds. Principles and Practice of Sex Therapy. 3rd ed. New York: Guilford Press, 2000.

70. Barlow DH. Causes of sexual dysfunction: the role of anxiety and cognitive interference. J Consult Clin Psychol 1986; 54:140–148.

71. LoPiccolo J, Lobitz WC. The role of masturbation in the treatment of orgasmic dysfunction. Arch Sex Behav 1972; 2:163–171.

72. Annon JS. The therapeutic use of masturbation in the treatment of sexual disorders. In: Rubin RD, Brady JP, Henderson JD, eds. Advances in Behavior Therapy. Vol. 4. New York: Academic Press, 1973.

73. Heiman JR, LoPiccolo L, LoPiccolo J. Becoming Orgasmic: A Sexual Growth Program for Women. Englewood Cliffs, NJ: Prentice-Hall, 1976.

74. Heinrich AG. The Effect of Group and Self-Directed Behavioral–Educational Treatment of Primary Orgasmic Dysfunction in Females Treated Without their Partners. Ph.D. dissertation, University of Colorado, Boulder, CO, 1976.

75. McMullen S, Rosen RC. Self-administered masturbation training in the treatment of primary orgasmic dysfunction. J Consult Clin Psychol 1979; 47:912–918.

76. Fichen CS, Libman E, Brender W. Methodological issues in the study of sex therapy: effective components in the treatment of secondary orgasmic dysfunction. J Sex Marital Ther 1983; 9:191–202.

77. Hurlbert DF, Apt C. Coital alignment technique and directed masturbation: a comparative study on female orgasm. J Sex Marital Ther 1995; 21:21–29.

78. Masters WH, Johnson VE. Human Sexual Inadequacy. London: Churchill, 1970.

79. Meston CM, Gorzalka BB. The effects of sympathetic activation following acute exercise on physiological and subjective sexual arousal in women. Behav Res Ther 1995; 33:651–664.

80. Meston CM, Gorzalka BB. The differential effects of sympathetic activation on sexual arousal in sexually functional and dysfunctional women. J Abnorm Psychol 1996a; 105:582–591.

81. Meston CM, Gorzalka BB. The effects of immediate, delayed, and residual sympathetic activation on physiological and subjective sexual arousal in women. Behav Res Ther 1996b; 34:143–148.

82. Wolpe J. Psychotherapy by Reciprocal Inhibition. Stanford: Stanford University Press, 1958.

83. Brady JP. Brevital-relaxation treatment of frigidity. Behav Res Ther 1966; 4:71–77.

84. Kraft T, Al-Issa I. Behavior therapy and the treatment of frigidity. Am J Psychol 1967; 21:116–120.

85. Jankovich R, Miller PR. Response of women with primary orgasmic dysfunction to audiovisual education. J Sex Marital Ther 1978; 4:16–19.

86. Kilmann PR, Mills KH, Caid C, Davidson E, Bella B, Milan R, Drose G, Boland J, Follingstad D, Montgomery B, Wanlass R. Treatment of secondary orgasmic dysfunction: an outcome study. Arch Sex Behav 1986; 15:211–229.

87. Everaerd W, Dekker J. Treatment of secondary orgasmic dysfunction: a comparison of systematic desensitization and sex therapy. Behav Res Ther 1982; 20:269–274.

88. Kegel AH. Sexual functions of the pubococcygeus muscle. West J Surg Obstet Gynecol 1952; 60:521–524.

89. Modell JG, May RS, Katholi CR. Effect of bupropion-SR on orgasmic dysfunction in nondepressed subjects: a pilot study. J Sex Marital Ther 2000; 26:231–240.

90. Ito TY, Trant AS, Polan ML. A double-blind placebo-controlled study of ArginMax, a nutritional supplement for enhancement of female sexual function. J Sex Marital Ther 2001; 27:541–549.

91. Michelson D, Bancroft J, Targum S, Kim Y, Tepner R. Female sexual dysfunction associated with antidepressant administration: a randomized, placebo-controlled study of pharmacologic intervention. Am J Psychiatry 2000; 157:239–243.

92. Landen M, Eriksson E, Agren H, Fahlen T. Effect of buspirone on sexual dysfunction in depressed patients treated with selective serotonin reuptake inhibitors. J Clin Psychopharmacol 1999; 19:268–271.

93. Michelson D, Kociban K, Tamura R, Morrison MF. Mirtazapine, yohimbine, or olanzapine augmentation therapy for serotonin reuptake-associated female sexual dysfunction: a randomized, placebo controlled trial. J Psychiatr Res 2002; 36:147–152.

94. Kang B, Lee S, Kim M, Cho M. A placebo-controlled, double-blind trial of ginkgo biloba for antidepressant-induced sexual dysfunction. Hum Psychopharmacol 2002; 17:279–284.

95. Meston CM. A randomized, placebo-controlled, crossover study of ephedrine for SSRI-induced female sexual dysfunction. J Sex Marital Ther 2004; 30:57–68.

9

Male Ejaculation and Orgasmic Disorders

Marcel D. Waldinger

Leyenburg Hospital, The Hague, The Netherlands

Utrecht Institute for Pharmaceutical Sciences and Rudolf Magnus Institute for Neurosciences, Utrecht University, Utrecht, The Netherlands

INTRODUCTION

Ejaculation and orgasm usually occur simultaneously in men even though ejaculation and orgasm are two separate phenomenona. Ejaculation occurs in the genital organs, whereas orgasmic sensations, being related to the genitals, are mainly a cerebral event which involves the whole body. In a few clinical syndromes, orgasm or ejaculation appears to exist independent of each other. For example, men with anesthetic ejaculation experience a normal ejaculation, but suffer from an absence of orgasmic sensation. On the other hand, men with premature ejaculation suffer from a disturbed speed of ejaculation, but do have intact orgasmic sensation.

It is very unfortunate that a clear distinction between orgasm and ejaculation has not been made in DSM-IV (American Psychiatric Association, 1994). In DSM-IV, ejaculation disorders are categorized under the heading of Orgasmic Disorders. Strangely, in DSM-IV retarded ejaculation has been called "male orgasmic disorder," analogous to "female orgasmic disorder," whereas premature ejaculation has not been called premature orgasm. Moreover, two rather rare syndromes, anesthetic ejaculation as well as partial ejaculatory incompetence, have not been mentioned at all in DSM-IV.

The synonymous terminology of ejaculation and orgasm in DSM-IV is not in line with current neurobiological thinking. In recent years, much has become known about the neurobiology and neuropharmacology of ejaculation. From a neurobiological perspective, it seems likely that orgasm and ejaculation are mediated by different neural circuits and various neurotransmitter systems.

In last century, ejaculatory disorders have been approached mainly from a psychological perspective. Although neuroscientists over the last 30 years have gained clear evidence of the important role of the central nervous system in ejaculation, it is only in the last decade that clinicians have begun to accept that ejaculatory disturbances are neurobiologically determined and can be treated by medication. However, in contrast with what is known about ejaculation, there is still limited information about the neurobiology of orgasm.

The history of ejaculatory and orgasm disturbances is colored with much speculations and particularly with a dramatic absence of evidence-based research. For example, many sexologists still believe in or favor one of the many psychological etiologies that have been put forward for the different ejaculatory disturbances. However, not one of these psychological hypotheses and associated treatments has been thoroughly investigated according to evidence-based medical principles. Most of these studies are characterized by very weak methodologies and designs.

I myself am convinced that evidence-based medical research is the only way to understand and investigate the efficacy of both drug- and psychological treatment of ejaculatory disturbances. Thus, I have written this chapter with a focus on methodology and design. Today, a clinical understanding of male ejaculatory and orgasm disturbances is no longer possible without a basic understanding of the neurophysiology, neuropharmacology, and neuroanatomy of serotonergic neurons in the brain. Therefore, I will start off by giving you a general explanation and overview of serotonergic neurotransmission, serotonergic receptors and how animal sexual behavior determines our understanding of sexual psychopharmacology. After this basic pharmacological introduction, I will describe the ejaculatory disturbances in rank order of frequency in the general population. As most research in recent years has been focused on premature ejaculation, it is inevitable that this disorder receives more attention than the other ejaculatory disorders.

NEUROPHYSIOLOGY

Ejaculation

The mechanism of ejaculation is conveniently divided into two phases, emission and expulsion.

Emission: During the emission phase, semen (e.g., sperm and seminal fluids) is deposited into the posterior urethra through contractions of the smooth muscles of the vasa deferentia, seminal vesicles, and prostate. At the same time, the internal sphincter of the urinary bladder is closed, thereby preventing retrograde passage of the semen into the bladder. The closure of the sphincter also prevents urine from mixing with the semen. Emission and bladder neck closure are mediated through the thoracolumbar sympathetic system. It is suggested that the sensation of ejaculatory inevitability parallels the emission phase.

Expulsion (or true ejaculation): Emission is immediately followed by expulsion. During expulsion, the semen is forcefully propelled along the urethra and out of the penis by clonic contractions of the striated bulbar muscles of the urethra and contractions of the striated muscles of the pelvic floor (mainly bulbospongiosus muscles).

Expulsion is mediated by the somatic nervous system. Orgasm is associated in timing with the expulsive phase.

Orgasm

There is limited knowledge about the physiological mechanisms and neurobiology underlying the sensation of orgasm. Orgasm is a complex response involving the whole body. During orgasm, there are changes in the genitalia, in skeletal muscle tone (characteristic spastic contractions of the feet), contractions of facial musculature, vocal reactions (moaning or sighing), semivoluntary movements, general cardiovascular (elevated systolic and diastolic blood pressure) and respiratory changes, somatic sensory experiences, and an altered consciousness.

The intense feelings of pleasure and desire accompanying orgasm are mediated by the brain.

NEUROBIOLOGY OF EJACULATION

Serotonin, 5-Hydroxytryptamine Neurotransmission and 5-HT Receptors

For a better understanding of the neurobiology of premature and delayed ejaculation and its treatments, it is a prerequisite to have some basic knowledge of what is happening in serotonergic neurons in the central nervous system (1,2).

Serotonergic neurons originate in the raphe nuclei and adjacent reticular formation in the brainstem. There is a clear dichotomy in the serotonergic (5-hydroxytryptamine, 5-HT) system neuronal cell groups (1). A rostral part with cell-bodies in the midbrain and rostral pons projecting to the forebrain and a caudal part with cell-bodies predominantly in the medulla oblongata with projections to the spinal cord. In the forebrain and spinal cord, the serotonergic neurons contact other serotonergic neurons. The location of connection is the synaps, in which the neurotransmitter serotonin provides information from one neuron to another. After its fabrication in the cell-body, serotonin runs through the serotonergic neuron to the presynaptic membrane, through which it is released into the synaps. In the synaps, serotonin proceeds to receptors at the opposite neuron (postsynaptic receptors) and after it has contacted these receptors serotonin runs back to the presynaptic membrane. Through the activity of serotonin transporters (5-HTT) in the presynaptic membrane, serotonin is brought back into the presynaptic neuron. The process of serotonin release and its action on postsynaptic receptors is called serotonergic neurotransmission.

There is normally a sort of equilibrium in the serotonergic neurotransmission system due to remarkable mechanisms. If too much serotonin is released from the presynaptic neuron into the synaps, the so-called 5-HT_{1B} autoreceptors, located in the presynaptic membrane, become activated. Their activation results in a diminished release of serotonin in the synaps. Consequently, the equilibrium is restored. This feedback mechanism of the cell, where the released 5-HT inhibits its own release, is a frequently occurring principle in neurotransmitter regulation and can allow the system with the possibility to prevent overstimulation of postsynaptic receptors (1).

However, serotonergic neurotransmission becomes seriously disturbed by the action of serotonergic antidepressants. Selective serotonin reuptake inhibitors (SSRIs) block the 5-HT transporters, both in the presynaptic membrane and around the cell-body. As a consequence, serotonin concentration increases outside the cell-body and in the synapses. Owing to the increased serotonin levels, 5-HT_{1A} autoreceptors at the surface of the cell-body and 5-HT_{1B} autoreceptors in the presynaptic membrane become activated. The activation of both the somatodendritic 5-HT_{1A} autoreceptors and the presynaptic 5-HT_{1B} autoreceptors results in an inhibition of 5-HT release into the synaptic cleft. Consequently, serotonin concentration in the synaps diminishes but remains slightly increased due to blockage of the 5-HT transporters leading to some stimulation of all postsynaptic 5-HT receptors. After some days, the 5-HT_{1A} and 5-HT_{1B} autoreceptors become desensitized resulting in a diminished inhibitory action of these receptors to 5-HT release. Consequently, serotonin again becomes released into the synaps. However, due to the SSRI-induced continuous blockade of the 5-HT transporters, serotonin cannot get back into the presynaptic neuron, and as a consequence serotonin levels in the synaps become higher. This increased serotoneric neurotransmission exerts a stronger effect on all postsynaptic receptors. It is the action of those postsynaptic receptors that determines the clinical effects of the SSRIs.

Male Rat Sexual Behavior

Male rat studies have demonstrated that serotonin (5-HT) and 5-HT receptors are involved in the ejaculatory process. As far as is currently known, 5-HT_{2C} and 5-HT_{1A} receptors determine the speed of ejaculation. For example, studies with D-lysergic acid diethylamide and quipazine, which are nonselective 5-HT_{2C} agonists, suggest that stimulating 5-HT_{2C} receptors delays ejaculation (3). However, 2,5-dimethoxy-4-iodophenyl-2-aminopropane, which equally stimulates 5-HT_{2A} and 5-HT_{2C} receptors, also increases ejaculation latency (4), whereas the selective 5-HT_{2A} receptor agonist 2,5-dimethoxy-4-methylamphetamine does not have this effect (3). On the other hand, activation of postsynaptic 5-HT_{1A} receptors by the selective 5-HT_{1A} receptor agonist 8-hydroxy-2-(di-*n*-propylaminotetralin) in male rats resulted in shorter ejaculation latency (3).

On the basis of these male rat studies, Waldinger (1,5) has hypothesized that premature ejaculation is related to a hypofunction of the 5-HT_{2C} receptor and/or a hyperfunction of the 5-HT_{1A} receptor. In contrast, delayed ejaculation is postulated to be related to a hyperfunction of the 5-HT_{2C} receptor and/or a hypofunction of the 5-HT_{1A} receptor.

Neuroanatomy

In recent years, much progress has been made in neuroanatomical research of ejaculatory processes. Most knowledge about the functional neuroanatomy of ejaculation is derived from male rat studies. With regard to male rat copulatory behavior, one has to distinguish among brain, brainstem, and spinal cord regions that become activated before and following ejaculation, when sensory information returns from the genitals (Fig. 9.1). The medial preoptic area (MPOA) in the rostral hypothalamus and the nucleus paragigantocellularis (nPGi) in the ventral medulla (6,7) are suggested as being important players in the process leading towards ejaculation. Electrical stimulation of the MPOA promotes ejaculation (8). It is hypothesized that ejaculation is tonically inhibited by serotonergic pathways descending from the nPGi to the lumbosacral motor nuclei. The present hypothesis is that the nPGi itself is inhibited by inhibitory stimuli from the MPOA. Disinhibition of the nPGi is supposed to lead to an ejaculation. The discovery of serotonergic neurons in the nPGi and the well-known ejaculation delay induced by serotonergic antidepressants suggests an action of the SSRIs on the nPGi. However, the precise location in the CNS on which SSRIs act to inhibit ejaculation has not yet been demonstrated.

On the other hand, brain areas activated as a result of the occurrence of one or more ejaculations have been observed in several mammals (9). Using expression of the immediate early gene, *c-fos*, as a marker for neural activity

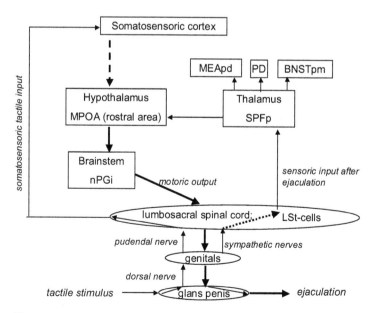

Figure 9.1 Cerebral areas and neuronal pathways mediating ejaculation according to animal research data.

in male rats, Coolen and co-workers (9–13) demonstrated the presence of distinct ejaculation-related neural activation in several brain regions following ejaculation: the *posteromedial* part of the bed nucleus of the stria terminalis (BNSTpm), a lateral subarea in the *posterodorsal* part of the medial amygdala (MEApd), the posterodorsal preoptic nucleus (PD), and the *medial* part of the parvicellular subparafascicular nucleus (SPFp) of the thalamus. These brain regions containing ejaculation-induced activation are extensively interconnected and reciprocally connected with the MPOA (12), forming an ejaculation-related subcircuit within the larger brain circuits underlying male sexual behavior (12). The functional significance of this ejaculation-subcircuit is still poorly understood but it might well be that these areas play a role in "satiety" and thus mediate the post-ejaculatory interval.

Truitt and Coolen (13) highlighted the role of the lumbar spinal cord in the processing of ejaculation. They identified a group of lumbar spinothalamic cells (LSt) that are specifically activated after ejaculation, and provide direct genital sensory inputs to the SPFp in the thalamus and the ejaculation-related subcircuit in the brain. The LSt cells also project to sympathetic and parasympathetic neurons related to the genitals. It is suggested that the LSt cells contribute to triggering the ejaculatory reflex and the sensation of ejaculation, that is, orgasm. These and other animal studies have clearly shown the existence of a neural circuitry for ejaculation in mammals.

Positron Emission Tomography-Scan Studies in Humans

Although male rat studies are of utmost importance for a better understanding of the neurobiology of ejaculation, brain imaging studies in humans are the tools which provide a better understanding of how the human brain mediates ejaculation and orgasm. Brain imaging studies will probably lead to a deeper insight into which parts of the brain mediate ejaculation and which parts are involved in the mechanism of orgasm, how these neural areas are linked to each other, and which parts are disturbed in the different ejaculatory and orgasm disturbances. The first Positron Emission Tomography (PET)-scan study during ejaculation has recently been conducted by Holstege et al. (14). Eleven healthy male volunteers were brought to ejaculation by manual stimulation of their female partner. The PET technique using radioactive water ($H_2^{15}O$) shows increases or decreases in blood flow in distinct parts of the brain, representing increases or decreases of activation of neurons in these areas. It was found that during ejaculation the strongest activation occurred in the so-called mesodiencephalic region, a brain area which comprises structures as the ventral tegmental area (VTA), also known as the "reward are" and the lateral central tegmental field. This area comprises dopaminergic neurons. The activation of the VTA shows that ejaculation leads to rewarding processes in the brain. Increased activation was also observed in the lateral putamen and adjoining parts of the claustrum and insula, and certain parts of the prefrontal, temporal, parietal, and insular cortexes. The meaning of all the activations of these various cortical areas is not yet clear. Further studies need to clarify whether associated sensations of orgasm are mediated by these cortical areas. Unexpectedly, a very strong activation was found in parts of the cerebellum, the meaning of it remaining unclear. Decreased blood flow, and thus less activity was found in the amygdala during sexual arousal, erection, and ejaculation. This may perhaps indicate that the brain looses a state of anxiety or fear during sexual activity. Hypothalamic involvement, as has been demonstrated in animal sexual behavior, has not been found in these male volunteers. Obviously, further PET-scan studies are needed to unravel this human and animal dichotomy.

PREMATURE EJACULATION

Premature ejaculation (ejaculatio praecox, rapid ejaculation, or early ejaculation) is the most frequent male ejaculatory disturbance. During the last century, premature ejaculation has been considered from both a medical and a psychological view, often resulting in contrasting psychotherapeutic and drug treatment approaches. For a better understanding of the current debate regarding its etiology and treatment, it is important to consider the history of how clinicians thought about and treated premature ejaculation.

History

Waldinger (5,15) distinguishes four periods in the approach to and treatment of premature ejaculation.

The First Period (1887–1917): Early Ejaculation

In 1887, Gross (16) described the first case of early ejaculation in medical literature. A second report of von Krafft-Ebing (17) followed in 1901. Although publications were rare, it is worth noting that during the first 30 years of its existence in the medical literature, early ejaculation was viewed as an abnormal phenomenon but not significantly as a psychological disturbance.

The Second Period (1917–1950): Neurosis and Psychosomatic Disorder

In 1917, Abraham (18) described early ejaculation as ejaculatio praecox and stated that it was a symptom of a neurosis caused by unconscious conflicts. Treatment should consist of classic psychoanalysis. On the other hand, some physicians stated that premature ejaculation was due to anatomical urological abnormalities, such as a too short foreskin frenulum or changes in the posterior urethra, which had to be treated with incision of the foreskin or electrocautery of the verumontanum. In 1943, Schapiro (19) argued that premature ejaculation was neither a pure psychological nor a pure somatic disorder, but a psychosomatic disturbance caused by a combination of a psychologically overanxious constitution and a weak ejaculatory system. Schapiro described two types of premature ejaculation, type B in which early ejaculation existed from the first intercourses and type A, which led to erectile dysfunction. Many years later, both types became distinguished as the primary (lifelong) and secondary (acquired) forms of premature ejaculation (20).

The Third Period (1950–1990): Learned Behavior

The biological component of premature ejaculation and therefore also drug treatment, advocated by Schapiro, was ignored by the majority of sexologists who advocated psychoanalytic treatment. This neglect became even more pronounced after Masters and Johnson (21) claimed the high success rates of behavioral therapy in the form of the squeeze technique, an adaptation of the stop–start technique published by Semans (22) in 1956. Masters and Johnson stated that men with premature ejaculation had learned this rapidity behavior as a result of their rushed initial experiences of sexual intercourse.

The Fourth Period (1990 to Present): Neurobiology and Genetics

Since the 1990s, there has been an increasing number of publications on the efficacy of SSRIs, clomipramine, and topical anesthetic creams in delaying ejaculation. At the same time, in 1998, Waldinger (1) postulated a new neurobiological view arguing that premature ejaculation is related to disturbance of serotonin (5-HT) receptors in specific areas of the central nervous system with a possible genetic vulnerability (5,23).

Prevalence

Premature ejaculation is often cited as being the most common male sexual dysfunction. The exact prevalence, however, is unknown as this appeared difficult to determine. Although it has been estimated that as many as 36% of all men in the general population experience premature ejaculation (24), other estimates have been lower. For example, Gebhard and Johnson (25), from a reanalysis of the Kinsey data, determined that 4% of the men interviewed reported ejaculating within 1 min of intromission. The large differences in prevalence numbers are mainly due to the use of various and often totally different definitions of premature ejaculation that have been used. Only by the general use of an empirically defined definition and identical tools to measure the ejaculation time, methodologically correct epidemiological studies can provide reliable prevalence data. Such studies have not been performed yet.

Evidence-Based Medicine

Evidence-based medicine means that the formulation of a seemingly attractive hypothesis of the cause of a disease is not enough for scientific acceptance. There needs to be empirical evidence, preferably replicated in various controlled studies.

For many decades, premature ejaculation was considered to be a psychological disorder that had to be treated with psychotherapy. However, psychological treatments and underlying theories mostly relied on case reports, series of case report studies, and opinions of some leading psychotherapists and sexologists. They were not based on controlled studies. I believe this to be a typical example of authority- or opinion-based medicine (15).

In contrast to authority-based medicine, evidence-based medicine (26) has been accepted today as the hallmark for clinical research and medical practice. Particularly in last decade, randomized clinical trials with clomipramine (27,28) and some SSRIs (29–33) have repeatedly demonstrated the efficacy of serotonergic antidepressants to delay ejaculation. In spite of these studies, the belief persists among those involved in sexology that premature ejaculation is a psychological disorder. In order to unravel this dichotomy, it is important to apply principles of evidence-based medicine to both the psychological and neurobiological approaches to premature ejaculation and its treatments.

Evidence-Based Research: Psychotherapy

The psychoanalytic idea of unconscious conflicts being the cause of premature ejaculation has never been investigated in a manner that allowed generalization, as only case reports on psychoanalytic therapy have been published.

But this is also true for behavioural therapy. Masters and Johnson (21) deliberately refuted a definition of premature ejaculation in terms of a man's ejaculation time duration. Instead, they insisted on defining premature ejaculation in terms of the female partner response, for example, as a male's inability to inhibit ejaculation long enough for the partner to reach orgasm in 50% of intercourses. It is obvious that their definition is inadequate because it implies that any male partner of females who have difficulty in reaching orgasm on 50% of intercourses suffers from premature ejaculation.

Masters and Johnson argued that premature ejaculation was conditioned by experiencing first sexual contacts in a rapid way (e.g., in the back seat of a car or with an impatient prostitute). However, Masters and Johnson, and sexologists who followed their ideas, have never provided any evidence-based data for this assumption. Regarding their proposed behavioral squeeze technique treatment, Masters and Johnson claimed a 97% success for delaying ejaculation. However, this very high percentage of success has never been replicated by others.

Usually, a lack of reproducible data leads to critical comments. This is one of the basic principles of evidence-based medicine. The effects of a treatment intervention should be reproducible by others. However, critical comments were not appreciated in the traditional sexological thinking of the late 20th century. This nonscientifically supported and uncritical belief in behavioral treatment still exists today, in spite of clear evidence-based medical research in favor of the neurobiological view. But the criticism is justified. The methodological insufficiencies of the report of Masters and Johnson are very serious. Their report on the efficacy of the squeeze method contains numerous biases.

First, there was a bias in selection and allocation of the subjects, the patients were not randomized to the new squeeze technique, or the older stop–start technique, or a nonsense behavioral technique. Second, the treatment design was open and not double-blinded. Further, the diagnosis of premature ejaculation was not quantified and therefore inaccurate, particularly since Masters and Johnson used an obscure definition of premature ejaculation. Baseline data were not reported, and inclusion and exclusion criteria were lacking. The assessment of success was subjectively reported without quantification or scoring scales. In addition, Masters and Johnson did not provide any information on their data processing. In spite of all these methodological flaws, their behavioral technique has received worldwide uncritical acceptance and been promoted as the best method of treatment. Even the very poor results of two studies (34,35) on behavioral therapy (also poorly designed) could not prevent sexologists from continuing to claim the squeeze technique as the best method of treatment. Not only the squeeze technique, but also all sorts of psychotherapy, including thought stopping, Gestalt therapy, transactional analysis, group therapy, and bibliotherapy, have been proposed as being effective (36–39). Also the efficacy of these psychotherapies has only been suggested in case reports and were never investigated in well-designed controlled studies.

In my opinion, the uncritical acceptance of the squeeze technique as first choice treatment is a clear example of the influence of opinion- or authority-based medicine, as in those years Masters and Johnson were famous for their new approaches in the treatment of sexual disorders (15). It did not seem to be an issue then that Masters and Johnson—these so highly esteemed sexologists—did not produce any evidence-based data for their claimed discovery.

Evidence-Based Research: Drug Treatment

In contrast with the easily accepted behavioral treatment by sexologists, drug treatment had to prove itself far more explicitly to avoid rejection by professionals in the field. Only a few physicians have tried to develop drug strategies to treat premature ejaculation. Currently, in spite of some residual ambiguous attitudes of many sexologists, drug treatment with serotonergic antidepressants are accepted as effective therapy. Despite of all circumstantial evidence, it should be emphasized that a scientific approach to investigating empirical evidence remains obligatory (40). To investigate how far differences in methodology may be of influence on clinical outcome of drug treatment studies, Waldinger and co-workers conducted an systematic review and meta-analysis of all drug treatment studies that were published between 1943 and 2003 (41).

In this study, several methodological evidence-based criteria were compared such as study design (single-blind and open-design vs. double-blind), tools for diagnostic testing (stopwatch vs. subjective reporting or questionnaire) and means of assessment (prospective vs. retrospective). The results revealed that from 79 publications on drug treatment, 35 studies involved serotonergic antidepressants. It was clearly demonstrated that both single-blind and open-design studies as well as studies using a questionnaire or subjective report on the ejaculation time led to a higher variability, that means exaggerated responses, in ejaculatory delay. Only eight studies (27,31,33,42–46) (18.5%) fulfilled all criteria of evidence-based medicine, for example, double-blind studies prospectively using real time stopwatch assessments at each intercourse both at baseline and during the drug trial. Regarding daily treatment, a similar efficacy for paroxetine, clomipramine, sertraline, and fluoxetine has been demonstrated, whereas the efficacy of paroxetine was found to be clearly stronger than all aforementioned drugs.

Operational Definition of Premature Ejaculation

For evidence-based research, it is of utmost importance to have a definition of premature ejaculation. However, because of conflicting ideas about the essence of premature ejaculation, sexologists have never reached an agreement on a definition.

DSM-IV (47) defines premature ejaculation as "persistent or recurrent ejaculation with minimal sexual stimulation before, upon, or shortly after penetration and before the person wishes it." Until recently, any scientific basis for the DSM-IV definition was lacking. For instance, the meaning of "persistent," "recurrent," "minimal," and "shortly after" is vague and certainly needs further qualification. In order to get an empirically operationalized definition, Waldinger and co-workers investigated 110 consecutively enrolled men with lifelong premature ejaculation (48). In this study, men and their female partners were instructed to use a stopwatch at home during each coitus for a period of 4 weeks (Fig. 9.2). It was found that 10% of these men ejaculated between 1 and 2 min but that the majority (90%) of them ejaculated within 1 min of intromission, and even 80% actually ejaculating within 30 s whereas 60% ejaculated within 15 s (48). The age of the men and duration of their relationship were not correlated with the ejaculation time. On the basis of this study, Waldinger and co-workers empirically defined lifelong premature ejaculation as an ejaculation that is <1 min in >90% of episodes of sexual intercourse, independent of age and duration of relationship (48). It has to be noted that this definition defines premature ejaculation as being an early ejaculation that is independent of psychological or relationship distress. Thus, assessment by stopwatch revealed that premature ejaculation is a matter of seconds and not of minutes. In this respect, the ICD-10 definition (e.g., ejaculation before or within 15 s) seems more appropriate than the DSM-IV definition, but both need to be adapted to these recent data.

The "Ejaculation Distribution Theory" of Premature Ejaculation

Waldinger (5,49) formulated a new theory on the etiology and genesis of lifelong premature ejaculation. He postulated that lifelong premature ejaculation is not an

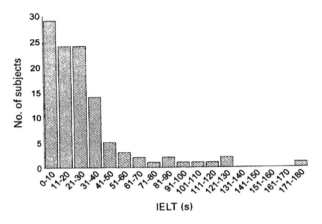

Figure 9.2 The IELT (29) measured by stopwatch in a sample of 110 Dutch males with lifelong premature ejaculation. Ninety percent ejaculates within 1 min and 80% ejaculates within 30 s (48).

acquired disorder due to habituation of initial hurried intercourses, as has been suggested by Masters and Johnson. Instead, Waldinger argues that early ejaculation is part of a normal biological variability of the intravaginal ejaculation latency time (IELT) in men, with a possible familial genetic vulnerability (5,23,49). In 1994, Waldinger et al., introduced and defined the IELT as a measure for pharmacological research (29). The IELT is the time between vaginal penetration and intravaginal ejaculation (29,31). According to Waldinger, early ejaculation is primarily a neurobiological phenomenon, which may or may not secondarily lead to psychological or psychosocial distress. Dependent on intra- and interpersonal and probably also cultural factors, early ejaculation may become perceived as premature ejaculation. Both animal and large-scale human epidemiological stopwatch studies are needed to demonstrate the existence of a biological continuum of the IELT.

On the basis of animal and human psychopharmacological studies, Waldinger and co-workers further postulated that lifelong premature ejaculation is related to decreased central serotonergic neurotransmission, and 5-HT_{2C} receptor hyposensitivity and/or 5-HT_{1A} receptor hypersensitivity (1,5,49,50a). Treatment should therefore consist of 5-HT_{2C} receptor stimulation and/or 5-HT_{1A} receptor inhibition.

Evidence for the role of the 5-HT_{2C} receptor has been found in four stopwatch studies in men with premature ejaculation (31,42–44). It was demonstrated that the 5-HT_{2C} receptor stimulating and the 5-HT_{2C} blocking antidepressants exerted an ejaculation delay and absence of ejaculation delay, respectively. In a double-blind placebo-controlled study with the $5\text{-HT}_{2C}/5\text{-HT}_{2A}$ receptor antagonist and 5-HT/noradrenaline reuptake inhibitor nefazodone, 400 mg nefazodone daily did not exert any ejaculation delay in contrast to a significant delay after 20 mg paroxetine daily and 50 mg sertraline daily (42). In a similar study, the $5\text{-}HT_{2C}/5\text{-}HT_3$ receptor antagonist, and noradrenergic and specific serotonergic antidepressant mirtazapine did not induce ejaculation delay compared with the significant delay resulting from 20 mg paroxetine daily (43). In both studies, nefazodone and mirtazapine did not delay ejaculation. Recent research suggests that $5\text{-}HT_{1A}$ receptors are likely to play a more important role than $5\text{-}HT_{2C}$ receptors in premature ejaculation and its treatment (50b). Further studies with selective $5\text{-}HT_{2C}$ and $5\text{-}HT_{1A}$ agonist and antagonists are encouraged to elucidate still undiscovered pharmacological mechanisms underlying the ejaculatory process.

Ejaculation Threshold Hypothesis

In order to understand the suggested biological variation of the IELT in relation to the serotonergic system, delaying effects of SSRIs and suggested genetics, Waldinger and co-workers have proposed the existence of a threshold of the IELT (5,49).

In the case of a low setpoint of the threshold, men can only sustain a small amount of sexual arousal prior to ejaculation. Whatever these men do or fantasize during intercourse, any control of ejaculation remains marginal and these men ejaculate easily even when they are not fully aroused. The low threshold is assumed to be associated with a low 5-HT neurotransmission and probably a hypofunction of the $5\text{-}HT_{2C}$ receptor and/or a hyperfunction of the $5\text{-}HT_{1A}$ receptor, as mentioned earlier.

In the case of a higher setpoint, men will experience more control over their ejaculation time. They can sustain more sexual arousal before ejaculating. In these men, 5-HT neurotransmission varies around a normal or averaged level and the $5\text{-}HT_{2C}$ receptor functions normally. The mean and range values of the setpoints that are considered to be normal or averaged are not known. These men have the neurobiological ability to voluntarily decide to get an ejaculation quickly or after a longer duration of intercourse.

In case of a high or very high setpoint, men may experience difficulty in ejaculating or cannot get an ejaculation even when fully sexually aroused. At a high setpoint, 5-HT neurotransmission is supposed to be increased, the $5\text{-}HT_{2C}$ receptor sensitivity is enhanced, and/or the $5\text{-}HT_{1A}$ receptor sensitivity is decreased.

According to this threshold hypothesis, it appears to be the level of $5\text{-}HT_{2C}$ and $5\text{-}HT_{1A}$ receptor activation that determines the setpoint and associated ejaculation latency time of an individual man. In case of men with premature ejaculation or any man using serotonergic antidepressants, the SSRIs and clomipramine activate the $5\text{-}HT_{2C}$ receptor and therefore switch the setpoint to a higher level leading to a delay in ejaculation. The effects of SSRIs on the setpoint appear to be individually determined; some men respond with extreme delay whereas others only experience a small delay at the same dose of the drug. Moreover, cessation of treatment results in a uniform reset of the setpoint within 3–5 days to the lower individually determined reference level, which is assumed genetically determined.

It is speculated that the threshold is mediated by serotonin neurotransmission and 5-HT receptors in the brainstem or spinal cord and may consist of serotonergic fibers that inhibit neurons that convey somatosensory information from the genitals. It is suggested that SSRIs enhance the inhibitory effects of these serotonergic neurons. However, also the cerebral cortex may mediate inhibitory impulses, but currently this has not been demonstrated. Apart from a suggested SSRI-induced increased inhibition of sensory input, the SSRIs might also delay ejaculation by interfering with spinal cord motoneurons of peripheral neurons that inhibit the internal genitals. Further studies are needed to unravel this important and intriguing question.

Course of Rapidity

It is generally believed that aging delays ejaculation. This assumption, might be true for men with a normal or average ejaculation time but has never been investigated in men with premature ejaculation. In a stopwatch study (48) of 110 consecutively enrolled men (aged 18–65 years) with lifelong premature ejaculation, 76% reported that throughout their lives, their speed of ejaculation had remained as rapid as at the first sexual contacts in puberty and adolescence, 23% reported that it had become even gradually faster with aging, and only 1% reported that it had become slower. From these data, it is questioned whether the fixed rapidity and even paradoxical shortening of the ejaculation latency time while getting older should be recognized as a part of the pathogenetic process of premature ejaculation. According to Waldinger, early ejaculation is thought of as a part of a normal biological variation of the IELT in men, but its paradoxical or fixed course through life is considered as being pathological. Chronic premature ejaculation appears to be the clinical syndrome of primary (lifelong) premature ejaculation. As yet, there is no real cure for lifelong premature ejaculation, though drugs may alleviate the symptoms, but only as long as they are being taken.

Premature Ejaculation and Genetics

In 1943, Schapiro noted that men with premature ejaculation seemed to have family members with similar complaints (19). Remarkably, this interesting observation has never been cited. To investigate the potential familial occurrence of premature ejaculation, I routinely asked 237 consecutively enrolled men with premature ejaculation about the family occurrence of similar complaints (23). Because of embarrassment only 14 men consented to ask male relatives about ejaculation latency. These 14 men reported a total of 11 first degree male relatives with information available for direct personal interview. In fact, 10 relatives fulfilled our strictly defined criterion of an ejaculation time of 1 min or less. In this small selected group of men, the calculated risk of having a first relative with premature ejaculation was 91% (CI 59–99). Therefore, the odds of family occurrence are much higher than the suggested population prevalence rate of 4–39%. Moreover, the high odds ratio indicates a familiar occurrence of the syndrome, far higher than by chance alone. On the basis of this preliminary observation, the influence of genetics gains substantial credibility (23).

Treatment

Drug Treatment for Premature Ejaculation

In 1943, Schapiro (19) described the use of topical anesthetic ointment to delay ejaculation. The use of anesthetics to diminish the sensitivity of the glans penis is probably the oldest form to treat premature ejaculation.

In 1973, the first report of successful ejaculation delay by clomipramine was published (51). However, in the 1970s and 1980s of the last century, drug treatment of premature ejaculation was not very popular. The introduction of the SSRIs meant a revolutionary change in the approach to and treatment of premature ejaculation. SSRIs encompass five compounds (citalopram, fluoxetine, fluvoxamine, paroxetine, and sertraline) with a similar pharmacological mechanism of action. In 1994, Waldinger and colleagues published the first double-blind study on the ejaculation delaying effect of paroxetine (29). In last decade, all other SSRIs and clomipramine have repeatedly been investigated in their propensity to delay ejaculation (27–33,42–46,52–62). There is some evidence that fluvoxamine and citalopram have less effect in delaying ejaculation than paroxetine, sertraline, and fluoxetine (31,44).

Although the methodology of the initial drug treatment studies was rather poor, later double-blind and placebo-controlled studies replicated the genuine effect of clomipramine and SSRIs to delay ejaculation.

In spite of a development towards more evidence-based drug treatment research, the majority of studies still lack adequate design and methodology (15,40,41,48,50a). For the interpretation of drug treatment studies, it is important to bear in mind that the outcome values of the ejaculation time are dependent on both gender (e.g., assessment by the male or his female partner) and method (e.g., assessment by subjective reporting, questionnaire, or stopwatch) (15,40,41,48,50a). Recently, Waldinger and colleagues conducted a systematic review and meta-analysis of all drug treatment studies (41), performed between 1943 and 2003, demonstrating that single-blind and open-design studies and studies using subjective reporting or questionnaires all showed a higher variability in ejaculation delay than double-blind studies in which the ejaculation delay was prospectively assessed with a stopwatch. Of all 79 studies, only 11 studies (14.4%) (27,31,33,42–46,63–65) have been performed in accordance with the established criteria of evidence-based medicine (41).

Nevertheless, in spite of the inaccurate assessment of delay in most drug treatment studies, three drug treatment strategies to treat premature ejaculation can be distinguished: (1) daily treatment with serotonergic antidepressants,

(2) as-needed treatment with antidepressants, and (3) as-needed treatment with anesthetic topical ointments.

Daily Treatment with Serotonergic Antidepressants

Daily treatment can be performed with paroxetine (20–40 mg), clomipramine (10–50 mg), sertraline (50–100 mg), and fluoxetine (20–40 mg). The recent meta-analysis of all drug treatment studies has demonstrated that paroxetine exerts the strongest ejaculation delay (41). Paroxetine, sertraline, and fluoxetine may give rise to side-effects like fatigue, yawning, mild nausea, loose stools, or perspiration. These side-effects often start in the first week after intake but gradually disappear within 2–3 weeks. Ejaculation delay with daily treatment usually manifests itself at the end of the first or second week. With the exception of fluoxetine, it is advised not to stop the SSRIs acutely but gradually within 3–4 weeks, in order to avoid withdrawal symptoms, like dizziness and tremors. Side-effects of clomipramine may consist of nausea, dry mouth, and fatigue. Sometimes clomipramine and the SSRIs may give rise to reversible feelings of diminished libido or moderate decreased rigidity of the penis. It is advised that patients are told about all aforementioned side-effects when starting the treatment.

The impressive ejaculation delay by daily treatment with paroxetine and the other SSRIs can be explained by the neuropharmacological processes that occur during chronic SSRI administration to serotonergic neurons. After chronic SSRI administration and through desensitization of the 5-HT_{1A} and 5-HT_{1B} autoreceptors, 5-HT levels in the synaps have increased highly. The higher levels of 5-HT consequently activate the postsynaptic 5-HT_{2C} and 5-HT_{1A} receptors (1,2). Not only in humans, but also in male rats it has been found that chronic administration of fluoxetine (66) and paroxetine (67) significantly delays ejaculation latency. Remarkably, chronic administration of fluvoxamine exerts only a mild change in male rat ejaculatory behavior (49,67).

As-Needed Treatment with Antidepressants

Since 1993, only eight studies (28,68–74) on as-needed (on-demand) treatment have been published. Owing to this limited number of studies and to inadequate designs, a meta-analysis was insufficiently powered to provide final conclusions with regard to difference in efficacy and dose relationships (41). In spite of these scientific limitations, it has been found that clomipramine (10–50 mg) taken minimally 4–6 h prior to intercourse may be efficacious in delaying ejaculation. However, in contrast with the positive results of a single-blind on-demand study by McMahon and Touma (61) with 20 mg paroxetine, Waldinger et al. (75) have found in a double-blind study that on-demand use of 20 mg paroxetine has no or just minimal ejaculation delaying effects after 5 h in men with a premature ejaculation of <1 min. It has to be noted that this lack of ejaculation delay after 5 h is in line with current knowledge of serotonin (5-HT) neurotransmission. After acute SSRI administration, there is no or only a mild increase of serotonergic neurotransmission in the synapse and no or only mild activation of postsynaptic 5-HT receptors. The lack of ejaculation delaying effects after acute paroxetine administration has also been found after acute treatment with SSRIs and clomipramine in male rats (76). Further well-controlled studies on acute SSRI treatment are needed to unravel the mean and range of the amount of ejaculation delay that can be accomplished with the on-demand strategy. However, it should be noted that due to pharmacodynamic limitations "on-demand" SSRI treatment, even with the new generation of SSRIs with a short half-life, will exert much less ejaculation delay than "daily" SSRI treatment (50b).

As-Needed Treatment with Anesthetic Topical Ointments

Only a few controlled studies have been performed with anesthetic ointments. In one study, the results of lidocaine–prilocaine cream 10 min before intercourse has been reported (77). In the Far East, there have been good results with SS cream according to evidence-based studies (41). SS cream is a locally produced cream consisting of various herbs, taken 1–2 h prior to intercourse (64,78–82).

Psychotherapy and Behavioral Therapy

Since the introduction of the SSRIs, the use of behavioral treatment has diminished as first choice of treatment for "lifelong" premature ejaculation. However, by many sexologists psychotherapy and behavioral treatment, including the stop–start strategy of Semans and squeeze-technique of Masters and Johnson, are still advocated as the first choice of treatment for "secondary" premature ejaculation. However, I would again like to emphasize that the use of behavioral treatment for "secondary" premature ejaculation is also not based on well-controlled studies.

I have previously stated that psychotherapy is only indicated in men or couples who cannot accept premature ejaculation (5,83). In contrast to the classic psychological view, I have suggested that the purpose of psychodynamic or cognitive psychotherapy is not to learn how to delay ejaculation, but has to be how to cope with premature ejaculation, for example, in cases where medication has no or insufficient effect. The latter purpose of psychotherapy requires much more effort and real knowledge of psychotherapy from a sexologist than just giving instructions to a man on how to make love and to have intercourse.

RETARDED EJACULATION

Many people believe that retarded ejaculation is not a real problem for a couple, as they argue that retarded ejaculation enables a man to go on enough time to enable his female partner to be satisfied with one or even multiple orgasms. The reality of this syndrome is different. Many men suffer from delayed ejaculation and their female partners are very frustrated by it. Quite a number of women think they are not attractive to their partner and that he will be able to ejaculate when making love with another woman. Obviously, if coitus goes on too long, it may become painful for her. The failure to conceive is often a reason to seek help.

Definition

In DSM-IV (American Psychiatric Association, 1994), retarded ejaculation is termed Male Orgasmic Disorder and defined as "a persistent or recurrent delay in, or absence of, orgasm in a male following a normal sexual excitement phase during sexual activity that the clinician, taking into account the person's age, judges to be adequate in focus, intensity, and duration." In more simple terms, retarded ejaculation means that a man finds it difficult or impossible to ejaculate, despite the presence of adequate sexual stimulation, erection, and conscious desire to achieve orgasm. Some of these men may struggle to ejaculate with such desperation that they may physically exhaust themselves, and sometimes even their partner, in the attempt. Delayed ejaculation may occur in coitus, masturbation (either by the patient or by the partner), as well as during anal or oral intercourse.

Throughout the years, a variety of terms have been used to refer to this ejaculatory disorder. Synonyms for delayed ejaculation are retarded ejaculation, inhibited ejaculation, difficult ejaculation, late ejaculation, and ejaculatio retarda or retardata. Other terms for failure of ejaculation are inability to ejaculate, no ejaculation, anejaculation, ejaculatory incompetence, impotentia ejaculandi or ejaculationis, ejaculatio deficiens or nulla, and lack (loss, failure, inability) of ejaculation.

It has to be noted that in DSM-IV there is no formal distinction between retarded ejaculation and failure of ejaculation. Both entities are erroneously termed male orgasmic disorder.

One distinguishes a lifelong (primary) and acquired (secondary) form. If the disorder has always been present, the disorder is termed as lifelong. In the acquired form, the disorder appears somewhere in life after previous normal ejaculatory functioning.

Symptoms

If ejaculation is delayed in all situations, in all sexual activities and with all partners, the disorder is "generalized." In contrast, the disorder is "situational" if the delayed ejaculation is limited to certain situations or with certain partners. Situational delayed ejaculation may therefore give rise to different clinical presentations: A man is unable to ejaculate intravaginally but can do so by masturbation, a man is able to ejaculate during sex with a man but not with a woman, a man is able to ejaculate with one woman but not another, a man is able to ejaculate with the same woman on one occasion but not the next, or a man can only ejaculate when the sexual act is accompanied by specific stimulation.

Prevalence

In contrast with premature ejaculation, lifelong delayed ejaculation is a relatively uncommon condition in clinical practice. In many studies on the distribution of diagnosis of sexual dysfunctions in males, delayed ejaculation is often among the least presented sexual disorders. The prevalence in the general population is also rather low. Regarding lifelong delayed ejaculation, Nathan (84) found a prevalence of 1.5 in 1000. Acquired delayed ejaculation has little higher prevalence of 3–4% in men below the age of 65.

Lifelong Delayed Ejaculation

Psychological Approach

According to the classical psychological view, lifelong delayed ejaculation is attributed to fear, anxiety, hostility, and relationship difficulties (85–87). Many different manifestations of anxiety and fear have been hypothesized, including fears of death and castration, fear of loss of self resulting from loss of semen, fear of castration by the female genitals, fear that ejaculation would hurt the female, fear of being hurt by the female, performance anxiety, unwillingness to give of oneself as an expression of love, fear of impregnating the female, and guilt secondary to a strict religious upbringing.

The psychological ideas and explanations may have face validity in some individual cases, but there are no well-controlled studies that support a generalization of any of the various psychological hypotheses. The psychological, cultural, and religious factors that may lead to lifelong delayed ejaculation clearly requires further investigations.

Neurobiological Approach

Waldinger (1,5) postulates that lifelong delayed ejaculation is part of the biological variability of the IELT in men. According to this view, there is a variability in the extent of delayed ejaculation, from mildly delayed to severely delayed and lastly a failure of ejaculation. I suggest that this biological variability is related to genetic factors. In case this is true, it means that men may be born with a biological vulnerability to develop delayed ejaculation. Whether environmental factors affect the neurobiological vulnerability remains to be understood.

From animal and human studies, it is known that in particular it is the serotonergic system which is involved in ejaculation. On the basis of animal studies, I suggest that lifelong delayed ejaculation is related to a hyperfunction of the 5-HT_{2C} receptor and/or a hypofunction of the 5-HT_{1A} receptor. Whether dopamine and oxytocine play a role in lifelong delayed ejaculation remains to be elucidated.

Unfortunately there is no drug treatment available for delayed ejaculation in men. In animals, the 5-HT_{1A} receptor agonist, 8-OH-DPAT, fastens the ejaculation latency, but such selective 5-HT_{1A} agonists are not yet available for safe human use. Another possibility is a selective blockade of the 5-HT_{2C} receptor. However, in a stopwatch controlled study in men with premature ejaculation, the 5-HT_{2C} receptor blocking antidepressants, nefazodone and mirtazapine, did not lead to either delayed ejaculation or a faster ejaculation time.

Treatment of Lifelong Delayed Ejaculation

With every man presenting with delayed ejaculation, it is essential to obtain a full sexual and medical history and clinical examination of the patient. It is important to find out the situations in which ejaculation is impaired (location, sexual activity, specific partner), the frequency with which ejaculation is inhibited, the degree of delay of orgasm, whether the complaint existed from the first sexual encounters (lifelong) or occurred later in life (acquired), and whether orgasm and ejaculation are both lacking.

Various treatments have been used to treat men with delayed ejaculation: Vibratory and electrical stimulation, a variety of sexual exercises, and a range of psychotherapeutic techniques (88–91). These treatments have been used separately or in combination with one or more others. Research on the effectiveness of these treatments is limited to uncontrolled studies on individual patients or short series of patients (92). Controlled studies are not available.

By vibratory stimulation (93) of the penis an ejaculation can be induced. The percentage of success to cure lifelong delayed ejaculation, however, is unknown. Electrical stimulation (94) of the internal ejaculatory organs by a transrectal electrical probe (electro-ejaculation) is mainly used to obtain semen in paraplegic men. This intervention is extremely painful in men with normal sensation and is not an option to treat lifelong delayed ejaculation. Masturbation exercises have been extensively used in the treatment of delayed ejaculation. Kaplan (85) describes a method in which a period of undemanding sensate focus exercises is followed by a period in which a man masturbates, initially alone and subsequently in circumstances in which he becomes gradually closer to his female partner. Once the patient has had an orgasm in the presence of his partner, he masturbates in a number of steps in which the penis is closer to the vagina during masturbation. Finally, he enters the vagina and combined coital and manual stimulation is then used to induce ejaculation. Apart from masturbation exercises, individual psychodynamic psychotherapy, marital therapy, rational emotive therapy, and social skills training have been used to treat delayed ejaculation. Because controlled studies are not available, it is very difficult to evaluate the results. The overall impression of these different approaches is that some patients are actually cured after treatment although most patients are only somewhat improved or unchanged. In the absence of comparative studies, it is not possible to compare the effectiveness of different treatments. A major methodological impairment is that in most studies, outcome is assessed by means of a single statement ("improved," "cured," or "unchanged"), more specific information on ejaculation is lacking, and that treatment has not been standardized in most studies. Because of these methodological deficiencies, no firm conclusion or recommendation on the optimal treatment approach can be given (92). Currently, the best way to treat men with lifelong delayed ejaculation is to inform patients beforehand that success of psychotherapy cannot be guaranteed, but that it may be worth trying, as effective drug treatment is not yet available. At present, a combination of masturbation exercises and general therapeutic interventions may have a chance for success.

In spite of the above-mentioned treatment options, it is generally believed that lifelong retarded ejaculation is difficult to treat. In my opinion, continuous psychological, cultural of religious factors prohibiting sexual feelings may perhaps lead to a release of stress hormones that might disturb the full development of or even damage cerebral areas and neuronal pathways that are important for the ejaculation process. This might be one of the reasons that although psychological factors may heavily contribute to retarded ejaculation, psychotherapy alone is often hardly effective. Further research of lifelong retarded ejaculation is of utmost importance to unravel the neurobiology and interaction with psychological factors of this distressing ejaculatory disorder.

Acquired Delayed Ejaculation

Psychological Factors

The only way to determine the cause(s) of delayed ejaculation is the clinical interview. There are no specific characteristics of psychologically induced acquired delayed ejaculation. Obviously, the ejaculation disturbance has not existed previously. In addition, the onset may be sudden, the delay may be situational and also intermittent. Some factors may be related to the development of acquired delayed ejaculation, such as a psychological trauma (for example, the discovery of the partner's infidelity), or lack of sexual and psychological stimulation (inadequate technique or lack of attention on sexual cues).

Organic Factors

The onset of ejaculation delay may be sudden or gradual and deteriorates progressively to global unremitting ejaculatory inhibition. A rather normal delay of ejaculation occurs during aging. Androgen deficiency or hypogonadism may be accompanied by loss of sexual desire and delay of ejaculation. Any neurological disease, injury, or surgical procedure that traumatizes the lumbar sympathetic ganglia and the connecting nerves (multiple sclerosis, diabetic neuropathy, abdominoperineal resection, lumbar sympathectomy) may lead to a delay or failure of ejaculation. A wide range of drugs (SSRIs, tricyclic antidepressants, antipsychotics, alpha-sympathicolytics) can impair the ejaculatory process through central and peripheral mechanisms. Alcohol can delay or abolish ejaculation by a direct effect after acute abuse and indirectly by neurological or hormonal disturbances during chronic abuse.

Treatment of Acquired Delayed Ejaculation

In order to exclude pharmacological causes of delayed ejaculation, one has to carefully review the patients concomitant drugs that are likely to inhibit ejaculation. In those cases, an alternative drug should be tried, or in case of antidepressants, reduction of dose or antidote may be required (95). Neuropathic inhibition of ejaculation is usually irreversible and the patient should be counseled to optimize his and his partner's enjoyment from the residual sexual functioning. Androgen deficiency requires appropriate testosterone replacement therapy. In the case of inadequate stimulation, pelvic floor exercises may be helpful. Most patients require general advice on reducing precipitating factors, reduction in alcohol use, finding more time for sexual activity when not fatigued.

Research and Methodology

Research on lifelong delayed ejaculation is scarce. Most of the literature consists of hypotheses that have not been investigated according to methodological well-designed studies. Several factors may have contributed to this state of affairs. Delayed ejaculation is a relatively rare condition. Both in the general population and in the clinical practice, the prevalence of delayed ejaculation is rather low (84). Furthermore, delayed ejaculation is known as a disorder that is relatively difficult to treat (92). Although controlled studies do not exist, clinical experience suggests that the outcome is rather poor (92). A major problem in the research of lifelong delayed ejaculation is the absence of an empirically derived operational definition of delayed ejaculation.

The DSM-IV criteria are arbitrary and not based on quantified research. For example, consider the sentence "orgasm in a male following a normal sexual excitement phase during sexual activity that the clinician, taking into account the person's age, judges to be adequate in focus, intensity, and duration," what one wonders is meant by "normal" and how may a clinician judge that the excitement phase has been adequate in focus, intensity, and duration. There are no well-controlled studies regarding average or "normal" time of stimulation and therefore it is difficult to determine what is a delayed time of stimulation.

In the absence of objective standards on orgasmic latency, the clinician must rely on the subjective judgment of the patient. Generally, if the patient feels that it takes too long to reach orgasm, the diagnosis of delayed orgasm will be considered.

RETROGRADE EJACULATION

Definition

Retrograde ejaculation (ejaculation sicca, dry orgasm) is the propulsion of semen from the posterior urethra into the bladder instead of being ejected externally from the urethra (96).

Symptoms

Men with retrograde ejaculation do experience emission and expulsion and do feel the subjective feeling of orgasm, but semen is not propelled from the penis. Some men may be able to urinate during erection.

A definite diagnosis is made when examination of the urine following orgasm shows the presence of fructose and spermatozoa. The sperm, however, may be absent in cases of genital duct obstruction.

Etiology

Owing to a congenital or acquired anatomical and/or functional failure of closure of the internal sphincter of the bladder ("bladderneck") during the ejaculatory process, sperm passes into the bladder. Most frequently the cause is a transurethral prostatectomy, a surgical treatment of benign prostatic hypertrophy. But any traumatic, neurogenic or drug-induced interference with the thoracolumbar sympathetic nervous system may lead to retrograde ejaculation. Spinal cord injury through trauma, birth defect, neoplasm, or surgery and abdominopelvic surgery, retroperitoneal lymph node dissection or total lymphadenectomy, and diabetes may also result in retrograde flow of semen.

The medications that may give rise to retrograde ejaculation include alpha-adrenergic blockers (e.g., prazosin, tamsulosin), peripheral sympatholytics (e.g., guanethidine), and antipsychotics (e.g., thioridazine).

Treatment

Treatments for retrograde ejaculation focus on closing the bladder neck using surgical bladder reconstruction or pharmacotherapy with sympathicomimetic agents (e.g., ephedrine) or anticholinergics (e.g., imipramine). If sperm is needed for procreation and retrograde ejaculation cannot be corrected pharmacologically, vibratory stimulation of the penile shaft and glans penis (93) can be used. For those men who fail vibrator therapy, transrectal stimulation (94) may be used to obtain sperm.

ANESTHETIC EJACULATION (EJACULATORY ANHEDONIA)

Definition

Men with anesthetic ejaculation have a normal propulsive ejaculation, but the accompanying sensation of orgasm is absent. The mechanism of the emission and expulsion phase of ejaculation are intact (97).

Symptoms

Both at masturbation and at intercourse, ejaculation occurs without sense of pleasure or orgasmic sensation. The lack of enjoyable ejaculation may lead to a rather indifferent attitude of some of these men to have intercourse.

Etiology

Anesthetic ejaculation is probably a rare syndrome. Only 4 publications, describing a total of 13 cases, have been published. In 1923, Stekel (98) described one case. In 1975, Dormont (99), using the term ejaculatory anhedonia, described four cases and suggested that the problem was distinctly psychological in nature but concluded that the condition is very difficult to treat. Williams (97) described seven case vignettes. He could not find any organic causative factors or common psychological dynamics. Treatment of these patients with various sex therapy procedures was ineffective. In contrast, Garippa (100) published a successful sextherapy of a man with anesthetic ejaculation.

In my opinion, it may well be possible that anesthetic ejaculation is due to a disturbance in the neural circuitry that mediates the sensation of orgasm, leaving the circuitry of ejaculation intact. One of the ways to elucidate the neurobiological cause of this syndrome is to perform a PET-scan study in these men during orgasm.

Treatment

There are no controlled studies supporting a psychological cause and success of psychotherapy for this disorder. The most ethical way is to inform the patient that the syndrome is rare, the cause is unknown, that psychotherapy has no guarantee for success and that drug treatment is as yet not available.

PARTIAL EJACULATORY INCOMPETENCE

Definition

Men with partial ejaculatory incompetence lack a forceful propulsive ejaculation, by which semen seeps out of the penis. The associated orgasmic experience may be weak or absent (85).

Symptoms

Semen seeps out of the penis instead of being propelled. The associated orgasmic experience is weak or absent.

Etiology

In partial ejaculatory incompetence, there is a normal emission of ejaculate, but the expulsion phase of ejaculate is impaired. The patient experiences the sensations of ejaculatory inevitability but fails to experience true orgasmic ejaculatory sensation.

Treatment

Although hardly any study has been published, case reports suggest that psychotherapy and drug treatment may be beneficial. According to Kaplan (85), partial ejaculatory incompetence is frequently psychogenic and responds favorably to psychotherapeutic intervention. Riley and Riley (101) mentioned 11 cases of partial ejaculatory incompetence; 2 men responded to behavioral therapy, 3 men were lost to follow up. The remaining 6 men did not respond to psychotherapy, antidepressant therapy or ephedrine taken before intercourse. A placebo-controlled study with the selective alpha-adrenoceptor agonist midodrine in 6 patients was effective.

PAINFUL EJACULATION

Definition

In painful ejaculation, there is a sharp painful sensation in the penis during or shortly after ejaculation.

Symptoms

During or immediately following ejaculation, there is a sharp or burning pain in the urethra.

Etiology

Pain during ejaculation can be due to strictures of the urethra and if there is infection in the bladder, seminal vesicles, prostate or urethra, intense burning immediately following ejaculation may occur. With gonococcal infection, this pain can be severe. In rare cases, painful ejaculation may also be a side-effect of tricyclic antidepressant drugs (102).

Treatment

Following bacteriological investigation, appropriate antibiotical treatment needs to be prescribed. Painful ejaculation induced by tricyclic antidepressants seems to be dose-dependent. Treatment should therefore consist of discontinuing or reducing the dosage of the antidepressant.

POSTORGASMIC ILLNESS SYNDROME

Definition

In postorgasmic illness syndrome (103), the patient feels extremely fatigue and develops a flu-like state immediately or 20–30 min after the occurrence of ejaculation and/or orgasm. There are no disturbances in the sexual performance itself.

This peculiar syndrome has been discovered and described for the first time by Waldinger and Schweitzer in 2002.

Symptoms

Immediately or 20–30 min after the occurrence of ejaculation and/or orgasm, the patient feels extremely tired, and may develop symptoms of a flu-like rhinitis, sneezing, painful muscles, iching eyes. It is often associated with irritability and a depressed mood and may last 3–7 days after which the symptoms gradually disappear. These patients very characteristically plan their intercourses in order not the get in trouble with their work in the days after.

Etiology

The etiology is unknown. The syndrome is probably very rare.

Treatment

No treatment is available yet.

CONCLUSIONS

In this chapter, I omitted all sorts of methodologically weak publications in the field of psychotherapy that have been published during the last 30 years. Unfortunately, in last decade hardly any or even no progress has been made in the development of evidence-based research into the psychology and psychotherapy of ejaculatory disturbances. Instead, I have tried to provide you with up-to-date knowledge about the neurobiology and pharmacological treatment of ejaculatory disorders. Most of it, however, pertains to premature ejaculation. I hope and am also convinced that in the near future, with the development of new animal models of ejaculatory disturbances, the use of brain-imaging techniques in humans, and interest of pharmaceutical companies, also the other ejaculatory and orgasm disturbances, will become amenable for effective drug treatment. Nevertheless, one should always "talk" with patients, inform them about the most recent knowledge of their ejaculatory problem, and most of all "listen" to their complaints.

REFERENCES

1. Waldinger MD, Berendsen HHG, Blok BFM, Olivier B, Holstege G. Premature ejaculation and SSRI-induced delayed ejaculation: the involvement of the serotonergic system. Behav Brain Res 1998; 92:111–118.
2. Olivier B, van Oorschot R, Waldinger MD. Serotonin, serotonergic receptors, selective serotonin reuptake inhibitors and sexual behavior. Int Clin Psychopharmacol 1998: 13(suppl 6):S9–S14.

3. Ahlenius S, Larsson K, Svensson L, Hjorth S, Carlsson A, Linberg P et al. Effects of a new type of 5-HT receptor agonist on male rat sexual behavior. Pharmacol Biochem Behav 1981; 15:785–792.
4. Foreman MM, Hall JL, Love RL. The role of the 5-HT2 receptor in the regulation of sexual performance of male rats. Life Sci 1989; 45:1263–1270.
5. Waldinger MD. The neurobiological approach to premature ejaculation (review). J Urol 2002; 168:2359–2367.
6. Marson L, McKenna KE. The identification of a brainstem site controlling spinal sexual reflexes in male rats. Brain Res 1990; 515:303–308.
7. Yells DP, Prendergast MA, Hendricks SE, Nakamura M. Fluoxetine-induced inhibition of male rat copulatory behavior: modification by lesions of the nucleus paragigantocellularis. Pharmacol Biochem Behav 1994; 49:121–127.
8. MacLean PD. Brain mechanisms of primal sexual functions and related behavior. In: Sandler M, Gessa GL, eds. Sexual Behavior: Pharmacology and Biochemistry. New York: Raven Press, 1975.
9. Veening JG, Coolen LM. Neural activation following sexual behavior in the male and female rat brain. Behav Brain Res 1998; 92:181–193.
10. Coolen LM, Peters HJ, Veening JG. Fos immunoreactivity in the rat brain following consummatory elements of sexual behavior. Brain Res 1996; 738:67–82.
11. Coolen LM, Olivier B, Peters HJ, Veening JG. Demonstration of ejaculation-induced neural activity in the male rat brain using 5-HT1A agonist 8-OH-DPAT. Physiol Behav 1997; 62:881–891.
12. Coolen LM, Peters HJ, Veening JG. Anatomical interrelationships of the medial preoptic area and other brain regions activated following male sexual behavior: a combined fos and tract-tracing study. J Comp Neurol 1998; 397:421–435.
13. Truitt WA, Coolen LM. Identification of a potential ejaculation generator in the spinal cord. Science 2002; 297:1566–1569.
14. Holstege G, Georgiadis JR, Paans AMJ, Meiners LC, van der Graaf FHCE, Reinders AATS. Brain activation during human male ejaculation. J Neurosci 2003; 23:9185–9193.
15. Waldinger MD. Lifelong premature ejaculation: from authority-based to evidence-based medicine. BJU Int 2004; 93:201–207.
16. Gross S. Practical Treatise on Impotence and Sterility. Edinburgh: YJ Pentland, 1887.
17. von Krafft-Ebing RF. Psychopathia Sexualis. 11th ed. Germany: Publishing Hause Enke in Stuttgart, 1901.
18. Abraham K. Ueber Ejaculatio Praecox. Zeitschrift fur Aerztliche Psychoanalyse 1917; 4:171.
19. Schapiro B. Premature ejaculation: a review of 1130 cases. J Urol 1943; 50:374–379.
20. Godpodinoff ML. Premature ejaculation: clinical subgroups and etiology. J Sex Marital Ther 1989; 15:130–134.
21. Masters WH, Johnson VE. Premature ejaculation. In: Masters WH, Johnson VE, eds. Human Sexual Inadequacy. Boston, MA: Little, Brown and Co, 1970:92–115
22. Semans JH. Premature ejaculation: a new approach. South Med J 1956; 49:353–357.
23. Waldinger MD, Rietschel M, Nothen MM, Hengeveld MW, Olivier B. Familial occurrence of primary premature ejaculation. Psychiatric Genet 1998; 8:37–40.
24. Frank E, Anderson C, Rubinstein D. Frequency of sexual dysfunction in "normal" couples. N Engl J Med 1978; 299:111–115.

25. Gebhard PH, Johnson AB. The Kinsey Data: Marginal Tabulations of the 1938–1963 Interviews Conducted by the Institute for Sex Research. Philadelphia: W.B. Saunders, 1979.

26. Sackett DL, Rosenberg WMC, Muir Gray JA, Haynes RB, Richardson WS. Evidence based medicine: what it is and what it isn't. BMJ 1996; 312:71–72.

27. Althof SE, Levine SB, Corty EW, Risen CB, Stern EB. A double-blind crossover trial of clomipramine for rapid ejaculation in 15 couples. J Clin Psychiatry 1995; 56:402–407.

28. Segraves RT, Saran A, Segraves K, Maguire E. Clomipramine vs placebo in the treatment of premature ejaculation: a pilot study. J Sex Marital Ther 1993; 19:198–200.

29. Waldinger MD, Hengeveld MW, Zwinderman AH. Paroxetine treatment of premature ejaculation: a double-blind, randomised, placebo-controlled study. Am J Psychiatry 1994; 151:1377–1379.

30. Waldinger MD, Hengeveld MW, Zwinderman AH. Ejaculation retarding properties of paroxetine in patients with primary premature ejaculation: a double-blind, randomised, dose-response study. Br J Urol 1997; 79:592–595.

31. Waldinger MD, Hengeveld MW, Zwinderman AH, Olivier B. Effect of SSRI antidepressants on ejaculation: a double-blind, randomized, placebo-controlled study with fluoxetine, fluvoxamine, paroxetine and sertraline. J Clin Psychopharmacol 1998; 18:274–281.

32. Mendels J, Camera A, Sikes C. Sertraline treatment for premature ejaculation. J Clin Psychopharmacol 1995; 15:341–346.

33. Kara H, Aydin S, Agargun Y, Odabas O, Yilmiz Y. The efficacy of fluoxetine in the treatment of premature ejaculation: a double-blind, placebo controlled study. J Urol 1996; 156:1631–1632.

34. DeAmicis LA, Goldberg DC, LoPiccolo J, Friedman J, Davies L. Clinical follow-up of couples treated for sexual dysfunction. Arch Sex Behav 1985; 14:467–490.

35. Hawton K, Catalan J, Martin P, Fagg J. Prognostic factors in sex therapy. Behav Res Ther 1988; 24:377–385.

36. Trudel G, Proulx S. Treatment of premature ejaculation by bibliotherapy: an experimental study. Sex Marital Ther 1987; 2:163.

37. Mosher DL. Awareness in Gestalt sex therapy. J Sex Marital Ther 1979; 5:41–56.

38. Zeiss RA, Christensen A, Levine AG. Treatment for premature ejaculation through male-only groups. J Sex Marital Ther 1978; 4:139–143.

39. Lowe CJ, Mikulas WL. Use of written material in learning self control of premature ejaculation. Psychol Rep 1975; 37:295–298.

40. Waldinger MD. Towards evidence-based drug treatment research on premature ejaculation: a critical evaluation of methodology. Int J Impot Res 2003; 15:309–313.

41. Waldinger MD, Zwinderman AH, Schweitzer DH, Olivier B. Relevance of methodological design for the interpretation of efficacy of drug treatment of premature ejaculation: a systematic review and meta-analysis. Int J Impot Res 2004; 16:369–381.

42. Waldinger MD, Zwinderman AH, Olivier B. Antidepressants and ejaculation: a double-blind, randomized, placebo-controlled, fixed-dose study with paroxetine, sertraline, and nefazodone. J Clin Psychopharmacol 2001; 21:293–297.

43. Waldinger MD, Zwinderman AH, Olivier B. Antidepressants and ejaculation: a double-blind, randomized, fixed-dose study with mirtazapine and paroxetine. J Clin Psychopharmacol 2003; 23:467–470.

44. Waldinger MD, Zwinderman AH, Olivier B. SSRIs and ejaculation: a double-blind, randomised, fixed-dose study with paroxetine and citalopram. J Clin Psychopharmacol 2001; 21:556–560.

45. Novaretti JPT, Pompeo ACL, Arap S. Selective serotonin uptake inhibitor in the treatment of premature ejaculation. Braz J Urol 2002; 28:116–122.

46. Atmaca M, Kuloglu M, Tezcan E, Semercioz A. The efficacy of citalopram in the treatment of premature ejaculation: a placebo-controlled study. Int J Impot Res 2002; 14:502–505.

47. American Psychiatric Association. Diagnostic and statistical manual of mental disorders. 4th ed. Washington, DC: American Psychiatric Association, 1994.

48. Waldinger MD, Hengeveld MW, Zwinderman AH, Olivier B. An empirical operationalization study of DSM-IV diagnostic criteria for premature ejaculation. Int J Psychiatry Clin Pract 1998; 2:287–293.

49. Waldinger MD, Olivier B. Selective serotonin reuptake inhibitors (SSRIs) and sexual side effects: differences in delaying ejaculation. In: Sacchetti E, Spano P, eds. Advances in Preclinical and Clinical Psychiatry, Vol I: Fluvoxamine: Established and Emerging roles in Psychiatric Disorders. Milan, Italy: Excerpta Medica, 2000:117–130.

50a. Waldinger MD, Olivier B. Selective serotonin reuptake inhibitor-induced sexual dysfunction: clinical and research considerations. Int Clin Psychopharmacol 1998; 13(suppl 6):S27–S33.

50b. Waldinger MD, Schweitzer DH, Olivier B. On-demand SSRI treatment of premature ejaculation: pharmacodynamic limitations for relevant ejaculation delay and consequent solutions. J Sex Medicine 2005; 2:120–130.

51. Eaton H. Clomipramine in the treatment of premature ejaculation. J Int Med Res 1973; 1:432–434.

52. Goodman RE. An assessment of clomipramine (Anafranil) in the treatment of premature ejaculation. J Int Med Res 1980; 3:53–59.

53. Porto R. Essai en double aveugle de la clomipramine dans l'éjaculation premature (French). Med Hyg 1981; 39:1249–1253.

54. Girgis SM, El-Haggen S, El-Hermouzy S. A double-blind trial of clomipramine in premature ejaculation. Andrologia 1982; 14:364–368.

55. Assalian P. Clomipramine in the treatment of premature ejaculation. J Sex Res 1988; 24:213–215.

56. Haensel SM, Klem TMAL, Hop WCJ, Slob AK. Fluoxetine and premature ejaculation: a double-blind, crossover, placebo-controlled study. J Clin Psychopharmacol 1998; 18:72–77.

57. Biri H, Isen K, Sinik Z, Onaran M, Kupeli B, Bozkirli I. Sertraline in the treatment of premature ejaculation: a double-blind placebo controlled study. Int Urol Nephrol 1998; 30:611–615.

58. McMahon CG. Treatment of premature ejaculation with sertraline hydrochloride. Int J Impot Res 1998; 10:181–184.

59. Kim SC, Seo KK. Efficacy and safety of fluoxetine, sertraline and clomipramine in patients with premature ejaculation: a double-blind, placebo controlled study. J Urol 1998; 159:425.

60. Ugur Y, Tatlisen A, Turan H, Arman F, Ekmekcioglu O. The effects of fluoxetine on several neurophysiological variables in patients with premature ejaculation. J Urol 1999; 161:107–111.

61. McMahon CG, Touma K. Treatment of premature ejaculation with paroxetine hydrochloride. Int J Impot Res 1999; 11:241–246.
62. Rowland DL, De Gouveia Brazao CA, Slob AK. Effective daily treatment with clomipramine in men with premature ejaculation when 25 mg (as required) is ineffective. BJU Int 2001; 87:357–360.
63. Cooper AJ, Magnus RV. A clinical trial of the beta blocker propranolol in premature ejaculation. J Psychosom Res 1984; 28:331–336.
64. Choi HK, Jung GW, Moon KH, Xin ZC, Choi YD, Lee WH et al. Clinical study of SS-cream in patients with lifelong premature ejaculation. Urology 2000; 55:257–261.
65. Greco E, Polonia-Balbi P, Speranza JC. Levosulpiride: a new solution for premature ejaculation. Int J Impot Res 2002; 14:308–309.
66. Matuszcyk JV, Larsson K, Eriksson E. The selective serotonin reuptake inhibitor fluoxetine reduces sexual motivation in male rats. Pharmacol Biochem Behav 1998; 60:527–532.
67. Waldinger MD, Plas A vd, Pattij T, Oorschot RV, Coolen LM, Veening JG, Olivier B. The SSRIs fluvoxamine and paroxetine differ in sexual inhibitory effects after chronic treatment. Psychopharmacology 2001; 160:283–289.
68. Haensel SM, Rowland DL, Kallan KTHK, Slob AK. Clomipramine and sexual function in men with premature ejaculation and controls. J Urol 1996; 156:1310–1315.
69. Strassberg DS, de Gouveia Brazao CA, Rowland DL, Tan P, Slob AK. Clomipramine in the treatment of rapid (premature) ejaculation. J Sex Marital Ther 1999; 25:89–101.
70. Kim SW, Paick J-S. Short-term analysis of the effects of as needed use of sertraline at 5 PM for the treatment of premature ejaculation. Urology 1999; 54:544–547.
71. McMahon CG, Touma K. Treatment of premature ejaculation with paroxetine hydrochloride as needed: 2 single-blind, placebo-controlled, crossover studies. J Urol 1999; 161:1826–1830.
72. Abdel-Hamid IA, El Naggar EA, El Gilany AH. Assessment of as needed use of pharmacotherapy and the pause-squeeze technique in premature ejaculation. Int J Impot Res 2001; 13:41–45.
73. Chia SJ. Management of premature ejaculation—a comparison of treatment outcome in patients with and without erectile dysfunction. Int J Androl 2002; 25:301–305.
74. Salonia A, Maga T, Colombo R, Scattoni V, Briganti A, Cestari A et al. A prospective study comparing paroxetine alone versus paroxetine plus sildenafil in patients with premature ejaculation. J Urol 2002; 168:2486–2489.
75. Waldinger MD, Zwinderman AH, Olivier B. On-demand treatment of premature ejaculation with clomipramine and paroxetine: a randomized, double-blind fixed-dose study with stopwatch assessment. Europ Urol 2004; 46:510–516.
76. Mos J, Mollet I, Tolboom JT, Waldinger MD, Olivier B. A comparison of the effects of different serotonin reuptake blockers on sexual behavior of the male rat. Eur Neuropsychopharmacol 1999; 9:123–135.
77. Berkovitch M, Keresteci AG, Koren G. Efficacy of prilocaine–lidocaine cream in the treatment of premature ejaculation. J Urol 1995; 154:1360–1361.
78. Xin ZC, Choi YD, Lee SH, Choi HK. Efficacy of a topical agent SS-cream in the treatment of premature ejaculation: preliminary clinical studies. Yonsei Med J 1997; 38:91–95.

79. Choi HK, Xin ZC, Choi YD, Lee WH, Mah SY, Kim DK. Safety and efficacy study with various doses of SS-cream in patients with premature ejaculation in a double-blind, randomised, placebo controlled clinical study. Int J Impot Res 1999; 11:261–264.

80. Choi HK, Xin ZC, Cho IR. The local therapeutic effect of SS-cream on premature ejaculation. Korean J Androl Soc 1993; 11:99–106.

81. Xin ZC, Seong DH, Minn YG, Choi HK. A double blind study of SS-cream on premature ejaculation. Korean J Urol 1994; 35:533–537.

82. Xin ZC, Choi YJ, Choi YD, Ryu JK, Seong DH, Choi HK. Local anesthetic effects of SS-cream in patients with premature ejaculation. J Korean Androl Soc 1995; 13:57–62.

83. Waldinger MD. Klaar is Kees: Een Nieuwe Visie op Vroegtijdige Zaadlozing. Amsterdam: Uitgeverij de Arbeiderspers, 1999.

84. Nathan SG. The epidemiology of the DSM-III psychosexual dysfunctions. J Sex Marital Ther 1986; 12:267–281.

85. Kaplan HS. Retarded ejaculation (chapter 17). In: Kaplan HS, ed. The New Sex Therapy. New York: Brunner/Mazel, 1974:316–338.

86. Munjack DJ, Kanno PH. Retarded ejaculation: a review. Arch Sex Behav 1979; 8:139–150.

87. Shull GR, Sprenkle DH. Retarded ejaculation reconceptualization and implications for treatment. J Sex Marital Ther 1980; 60:234–246.

88. Delmonte MM. Case reports on the use of meditative relaxation as an intervention strategy with retarded ejaculation. Biofeedback and self-regulation 1984; 9:209–214.

89. Delmonte M, Braidwood M. Treatment of retarded ejaculation with psychotherapy and meditative relaxation: a case report. Psychol Rep 1980; 47:8–10.

90. Gagliardi FA. Ejaculatio retardata; conventional psychotherapy and sex therapy in a severe obsessive-compulsive disorder. Am J Psychother 1976; 30:85–94.

91. Apfelbaum B. Retarded ejaculation: a much-misunderstood syndrome. In: Leiblum R, Rosen RC, eds. Principles and Practice of Sex Therapy. Update for the 1990s. 2nd ed. New York/London: The Guilford Press, 1989:168–206.

92. Dekker J. Inhibited male orgasm (Chapter 10). In: O'Donohue W, Geer JH, eds. Handbook of Sexual Dysfunctions. Massachusetts: Simon and Schuster, Inc., 1993:279–301.

93. Beckerman H, Becher J, Lankhorst GJ. The effectiveness of vibratory stimulation in an ejaculatory man with spinal cord injury. Paraplegia 1993; 31:689–699.

94. Brindley GS. Reflex ejaculation: its technique, neurological implications and uses. J Neurol Neurosurg Psychiatry 1981; 44:9–18.

95. Waldinger MD. Use of psychoactive agents in the treatment of sexual dysfunction. CNS Drugs 1996; 6:204–216.

96. Sandler B. Idiopathic retrograde ejaculation. Fertil Steril 1979; 32:474–475.

97. Williams W. Anesthetic ejaculation. J Sex Marital Ther 1985; 11:19–29.

98. Stekel W. Die Storungen des Orgasmus beim Manne. In: Die Impotenz des Mannes. Wien, Austria: Verlag der Psychotherapeutischen Praxis, 1923:347–391.

99. Dormont P. Ejaculatory anhedonia. Medical Aspects of Human Sexuality 1975; 9:32–48.

100. Garippa PA. Case report: anesthetic ejaculation resolved in integrative sex therapy. J Sex Marital Ther 1994; 20:56–60.

101. Riley AJ, Riley EJ. Partial ejaculatory incompetence: the therapeutic effect of Midodrine, an orally active selective alpha-adrenoceptor agonist. Eur Urol 1982; 8:155–160.

102. Aizenberg D, Zemishlany Z, Hermesh H, Karp L, Weizman A. Painful ejaculation associated with antidepressants in four patients. J Clin Psychiatry 1991; 52:461–463.

103. Waldinger MD, Schweitzer DH. Postorgasmic illness syndrome: two cases. J Sex Marital Ther 2002; 28:251–255.

10

Dyspareunia

Caroline F. Pukall

*Queen's University, Kingston, Ontario, Canada and
McGill University, Montreal, Quebec, Canada*

Kimberley A. Payne and Alina Kao

McGill University, Montreal, Quebec, Canada

Samir Khalifé

*McGill University and Sir Mortimer B. Davis
Jewish General Hospital, Montreal, Quebec, Canada*

Yitzchak M. Binik

*McGill University and McGill University Health Center
(Royal Victoria Hospital), Montreal, Quebec, Canada*

INTRODUCTION

What Does the Term "Dyspareunia" Mean?

In 1874, Barnes (1) coined the term dyspareunia. He felt that it would be a convenient way of summarizing the different conditions underlying painful intercourse: " . . . just as 'dyspepsia' is used to signify difficult or painful digestion, we want a word to express the condition of difficult or painful performance of the sexual function" (p. 68). Although the usefulness of the term dyspepsia is a matter of some controversy (2), the diagnosis of dyspareunia has not been seriously challenged and is still used by all major classificatory systems, such as the DSM-IV-TR (3) and the ICD-10 (4). The lack of specificity of the word dyspareunia is evidenced by the growing number of overlapping terms (e.g., vulvodynia, vulvar vestibulitis syndrome, dysesthetic vulvodynia, vestibulodynia) denoting presumed "disease entities." The majority of these terms originate from a recent renewed interest in painful vulvar conditions. Even prior to this increased interest, the term dyspareunia was often used interchangeably with the terms vaginismus or chronic pelvic pain. This unrestricted creation of diagnostic labels plagues many mental health and medical domains and often results in much confusion. In our view, the term dyspareunia has outlived its utility as a nosological entity. Although this suggestion might be considered radical, we believe that it is justifiable both on the basis of logical/theoretical considerations as well as on empirical data.

In this chapter, we will standardize our use of the terminology as follows: The term dyspareunia denotes any form of recurrent or chronic urogenital pain that interferes with sexual and nonsexual activities in women of any age, and which may be experienced in a variety of different locations (e.g., at the vaginal opening or deep inside the pelvic area) with various qualities and patterns (e.g., as an acute stabbing sensation on contact, or a chronic throbbing pain that waxes and wanes throughout the day). It is important to note that dyspareunia also occurs in men (5), but is relatively rare compared with its frequency in women. Why there is such a gender disparity remains unclear and is worthy of study; however, this chapter will focus on dyspareunia in women. Following the criteria outlined by Friedrich (6), vulvar vestibulitis syndrome refers to severe pain experienced in the vulvar vestibule upon contact. Unlike vestibulitis, vulvodynia denotes chronic vulvar pain or discomfort that can occur in the absence of overt stimulation.

Why Is it Important to Study and Treat Dyspareunia?

Recent epidemiological surveys indicate that dyspareunia affects between 15% and 21% of women between the ages of 18 and 59 (7–9). Although dyspareunia is a common problem, many sufferers do not pursue treatment because of the embarrassment associated with talking about genital pain and sexuality. Of those who do consult, many do not receive adequate care; it is reported that 40% of dyspareunic women who sought treatment did not receive any diagnosis even after multiple consultations (8). These women may also be told, after several potentially invasive and painful evaluations, that all is well physically, implying either that their pain is "not real" or that they suffer from psychological problems.

In addition to problems encountered in the health care system, women with dyspareunia suffer negative impacts in both sexual and nonsexual areas of their lives. In terms of sexuality, women with dyspareunia report lower frequencies of intercourse, lower levels of sexual desire, arousal, and pleasure, and less orgasmic success than non-affected women (10–12). It is therefore not surprising that women with dyspareunia also report difficulties with relationship adjustment and psychological distress, including depression and anxiety (10). Outside of sexuality and intimate relationships, activities such as gynecological examinations, bicycle riding, or sitting for long periods of time may also be affected (10,11,13,14). Given the significant negative impact dyspareunia can have on multiple aspects of life, it is crucial to provide women suffering from this condition with information, validation of their pain, and appropriate treatment. However, the classification of dyspareunia has precluded this in many cases by focusing on the sexual aspects of dyspareunia, to the exclusion of focusing on the pain and the complexity of factors (e.g., emotional, interpersonal) that are involved.

CLASSIFICATION

Barnes derived the term dyspareunia from the Greek term meaning "difficult or painful mating" (1). This definition, based on interference with sexual intercourse, is understandable given that it is this interference that brings many women to clinical attention. Unfortunately, the focus on "difficult mating" has resulted in the classification of dyspareunia as a sexual dysfunction (3), and has deflected attention away from the major clinical symptom of pain. The nosological questions concerning dyspareunia are further complicated by a more general theoretical issue: the distinction between organic and psychogenic. For example, both the DSM-IV-TR (3) and the ICD-10 (4) differentiate between organic (i.e., due to a medical condition) and idiopathic (i.e., no known physical cause, usually attributed to psychogenic origin) dyspareunia. The apparent presumption in the case of psychogenic dyspareunia is that it is a distinct category, though there is little specification of its underlying determinants. In contrast, organic dyspareunia is seen as the result of many underlying types of gynecological pathologies, as well as a symptom of inadequate lubrication or of naturally occurring menopausal vulvovaginal atrophy.

The reality of the situation is that there are no empirically or theoretically valid guidelines to distinguish psychogenic vs. organic dyspareunia. The notion that these terms reflect easily diagnosable qualitative categories is questionable both on empirical and theoretical grounds. The typical presumption made by many health professionals and the general public is that there must be an underlying physical cause for the pain. In clinical practice, this typically results in numerous physical investigations ranging from standard gynecological examinations and tests for infections, to invasive procedures such as colposcopy and laparoscopy. If such investigations yield negative findings, the default is to assume a psychogenic causation ("it is all in your head") and refer the patient to a mental health professional. Depending on the orientation of the mental health professional, dyspareunia may be attributed to factors ranging from inadequate arousal to childhood sexual abuse. Because most women with dyspareunia present without an identifiable physical explanation for their pain, rarely is there a primary focus on the pain or on direct pain control in the case of dyspareunia. However, other idiopathic pain conditions are afforded this approach. For example, 85% of back pain patients present without identifiable pathology (15), yet they are still provided with treatment alternatives, such as analgesic medication and/or physical therapy.

As in the case of back pain, we recommend a similar multidimensional pain approach to the understanding and treatment of dyspareunia (16). This approach is consistent with current biopsychosocial pain perspectives that evolved from the

Gate Control Theory of Pain, which states that the experience of pain includes sensory and emotional components and that psychological factors play a role in pain control (17). This theory has helped explain the powerful influence of cognitive processes on pain perception via descending modulation from the brain, and scientists have since learned that the complex experience of pain cannot be simply equated with tissue damage (18). The Classification of Chronic Pain manual published by the International Association for the Study of Pain (IASP) (19) has also inspired a new multidimensional approach for dyspareunia treatment and research (16). According to the IASP classification system, pain is defined as "an unpleasant sensory and emotional experience associated with actual or potential tissue damage, *or described in terms of such damage*" (italics added; page 210). The italicized portion of this definition is reserved for pain patients without identifiable physical pathology, as in most cases of dyspareunia and other chronic pain conditions. Within this framework, the study of underlying physiology is ascribed great importance, but is not sufficient in order to characterize the whole pain experience. Therefore, pain classification is further organized according to five axes assessing the region affected, system involved, temporal characteristics, intensity, and duration.

ASSESSMENT AND DIAGNOSIS

Once treatable causes for the pain of dyspareunia (e.g., infections, dermatological conditions, sexually transmitted diseases) are ruled out, the pain needs to be carefully characterized. Questions about the location, quality, and temporal characteristics (e.g., When did the pain start? When does the pain occur? How long does it last?) of the pain are crucial to obtain a solid understanding of the pain experienced and may also help in diagnosis. In terms of pain history, many women link the pain onset to their first intercourse experience, but it may actually have long preceded this. Similarly, women with vulvar vestibulitis have been found to describe their pain in a consistent manner (14). Some patients, however, may have limited knowledge of their pelvic/genital anatomy, in which case a diagram is often helpful. It is also important for the physician to try and locate the affected region by attempting to replicate the pain through palpation and/or pelvic examination. This, however, can be a very painful and upsetting experience for the patient, therefore, it is vital to adequately prepare the patient and inquire about the intensity of the pain prior to the examination. If upon examination, pain is experienced, the physician should then determine whether this is the same pain experienced during intercourse. This can be assessed by inquiring about pain location, quality, and intensity during both intercourse and examination. In the case that the gynecologist fails to replicate the pain, it is important to clarify to the patient that the gynecological examination is not the same scenario as the bedroom and that there are many factors that could produce variability in the pain experienced. For example, emotional reactions to the pain may vary; some women may react very strongly by vocalizing and moving away from the painful stimulation, whereas others may "grin and bear it." It is therefore necessary to distinguish between the intensity of the pain and the unpleasantness associated with it, as these two components form separate dimensions of the pain experience. A further assessment of these factors includes inquiring about activities that produce the pain (e.g., different sexual positions, certain kinds of exercise) and assessing the temporal characteristics of the pain (e.g., does the pain vary with menstrual cycle) to name a few. To this end, keeping a pain diary can be extremely informative for both the physician and the patient.

Asking questions about the pain not only provides useful diagnostic information, but is also of therapeutic benefit to the patient by validating her experience, since many times, the pain is the last thing that medical professionals may inquire about, if at all. Asking about past treatments, previous diagnoses, and remedies that helped/worsened the pain are also key in obtaining a complete picture of the problem. Furthermore, careful questioning about how the pain has affected the patient's relationships, sexuality, psychological well-being, and overall quality of life will provide a more thorough understanding of the pain and clarify potential treatment options (e.g., physical therapy, psychological treatment for the pain and/or couple problems).

Vulvar Vestibulitis Syndrome

Case Study

Following numerous yeast infections after using a new oral contraceptive pill 2 years ago, Sandra, a 25-year old primary school teacher, started experiencing an intense burning pain at the entrance of her vagina during sexual intercourse. The pain started with initial penetration, lasted throughout intercourse, and was present for ~30 min afterwards. Thinking that it was caused by yet another yeast infection, Sandra purchased her usual treatment from the pharmacy: over-the-counter antifungal vaginal suppositories. However, this only increased her pain to the point that, 6 months later, she had become apprehensive about sexual activity with her long-term partner. She also noticed a "tensing up" of her pelvic floor muscles while engaging in foreplay and a marked decrease in her sexual desire and arousal levels, which further contributed to her pain. Sandra began avoiding all sexual activities, even nonpenetrative ones. She sought treatment from several medical professionals, underwent several painful examinations, and tried various topical creams and lubricants without any improvement in her pain or answers as to what her pain was. She began doubting her love for her partner, thinking that the pain was indicative of relationship problems. Finally, through one of her friends at work, Sandra obtained the phone number of a gynecologist who diagnosed her with vulvar vestibulitis syndrome and recommended physical therapy and pain relief therapy.

Diagnosis

Friedrich (6) proposed the following diagnostic criteria for vulvar vestibulitis: (1) severe pain upon vestibular touch or attempted vaginal entry, (2) tenderness to pressure localized within the vulvar vestibule, and (3) physical findings limited to vestibular erythema of various degrees. Although the third criterion has not received much support in terms of its validity and reliability, the first two have (14). Typically, vestibulitis patients present with provoked pain at the entrance of the vagina, their main complaint usually being painful intercourse. The cotton-swab test, a standard gynecological tool for diagnosing vestibulitis, consists of the application of a swab to various areas of the genital region. If the woman reports pain when pressure is applied to the vestibule during this test, then the diagnosis of vestibulitis is made. The cotton-swab test is usually performed in a clockwise manner around the vestibule; however, research has shown that pain ratings increase with each successive palpation. Therefore, we recommend a randomized order of cotton-swab application with adequate pauses after each palpation to avoid sensitization of the vulvar vestibule and unnecessary pain to the patient (16,20).

Although the cotton-swab test for the diagnosis of vulvar vestibulitis syndrome is considered the clinical method of choice since it is fast and easy to perform, it is not necessarily the standard tool for research purposes. First, the amount of pressure applied during the cotton-swab test is not standardized either between or within gynecologists (16,20,21). Indeed, it has been shown that different gynecologists apply different pressures and can elicit significantly different pain ratings in the same women (16,20). Second, the amount of pressure applied using this method are above pain threshold level, that is, the point at which women report the first sign of pain, making the cotton-swab test highly painful and distressing for patients. In order to overcome these problems, Pukall et al. (20) have developed a device called a vulvalgesiometer, which holds much promise in terms of standardized genital pain measurement by allowing for the application of known pressures using a spring-based device. The vulvalgesiometer replicates the quality of pain that women with vulvar vestibulitis report experiencing during intercourse, and is currently being used in numerous studies.

Vulvodynia

Case Study

Joanne, a 39-year-old lawyer, reported a constant tingling and burning sensation over her entire vulvar area, including her labia, perineum, vestibule, and clitoris, for the past 3 years. The sensations started progressively, initially with short periods of discomfort, but gradually became more frequent and intense to the point that she always felt some degree of pain during a 24-h period. The pain increased sharply with both sexual and nonsexual activities (e.g., walking or sitting for long periods of time), but she sometimes experienced these increases without provocation. She, like Sandra, underwent many invasive examinations and received numerous treatments, none of which helped. Joanne found that all aspects of her life were negatively affected; she had difficulties working, sleeping, and engaging in sexual activities. The pain was always on her mind, and although she obtained some relief from applying ice packs wrapped in towels to her vulva, this solution was only temporary and limited to her home environment. She lost interest in sex and began reducing her sexual activities, as they would exacerbate her pain. Desperate, she waited 1 year on a waiting list at a chronic pain service and was finally diagnosed with vulvodynia. She was prescribed a low dose of Elavil to help her sleep and to decrease the amount of pain she was experiencing, and was given a recommendation to join a vulvodynia support group to learn more about her condition and to meet others who experienced difficulties similar to hers.

Diagnosis

The diagnosis of vulvodynia is a diagnosis of exclusion, meaning that other causes for the pain (e.g., infections, inflammation, postherpetic neuralgia) must be ruled out, as in the case of vulvar vestibulitis syndrome. It is based on the description, quality, and location of the pain. Vulvodynia sufferers report chronic vulvar discomfort characterized by a burning sensation that is not contact-dependent. The pain is diffuse, often covering the vulvar area and including the perineum and may or may not lead to dyspareunia. Some vulvodynia sufferers also meet the diagnostic criteria for vulvar vestibulitis syndrome. It is crucial to rule out pruritus vulvae, which affects the same region as vulvodynia but is characterized by an itching sensation, and is often associated with skin changes, including excoriation and erythema (13,22). In addition, pudendal neuralgia must also be ruled out. In this condition, pain radiates from the vulva to the rest of the perineum, groin, and/or thighs and hyperesthesia is present in a saddle distribution. McKay (13) recommends the following evaluation for vulvodynia: examination of the skin for dermatoses and a careful search for infectious agents likely to cause inflammation. This is followed by nerve assessment, and by a careful anatomic distribution of involved areas, as locations and patterns of discomfort have been shown to be important in differential diagnosis (13).

Postmenopausal Dyspareunia

Case Study

Brenda (age 55) and Alexander (age 57) had been married for 30 years when they were referred to a sex and couple therapy clinic for dyspareunia by her gynecologist. A comprehensive pain assessment revealed that Brenda experienced a "rubbing, cutting, and sometimes burning" pain upon penetration and a deeper "dull, pulling pain" during intercourse. She reported that the pain started 4 years ago, at a time when she began to experience hot flashes and irregular periods, with an increase in intensity of the superficial pain over the last year. Attempts to lessen the pain through the use of water-based lubricants and topical estradiol cream had not been successful, and she did not wish to try systemic hormone replacement therapy for fear of developing breast cancer. A detailed sexual history revealed that Brenda had suffered from intermittent pain during intercourse for at least 15 years but had never complained about it, and that Alexander had always had difficulties with ejaculatory control. Over the past 4 years, Brenda reported difficulty getting sexually aroused, diminished lubrication, postcoital bleeding, and less interest in sex. Their current sexual frequency was less than once every 3 months, a frustrating situation for Alexander, who had hoped that their youngest child leaving home in the previous year would result in more frequent sexual activity. In the previous 5 years, the couple had also experienced significant life stressors including the sudden death of Brenda's mother and major financial problems. The couple was seen in therapy to help overcome their sexual difficulties, to manage the pain, and to receive support and advice concerning their stressful life situation.

Diagnosis

As women approach middle-age and menopause, physiological aging, psychosocial factors, and declining levels of endogenously produced sex hormones caused by ovarian senescence can exert significant effects on their sexual response cycle. As such, comprehensive enquiry of dyspareunic pain characteristics and history, climacteric symptoms, as well as changes in sexual functioning, urogenital anatomy, marital/partner relations that have occurred are essential in the assessment of postmenopausal dyspareunia. The many anatomical changes, within but not limited to the urogenital region, experienced by aging women (e.g., reduced vaginal and/or clitoral size, loss of fat and subcutaneous tissue from the mons pubis, arteriosclerosis) can result in decreased sexual arousal, vaginal dryness, and dyspareunia (23). Dyspareunia may also result from iatrogenic efforts, including pelvic or cervical surgery and radiotherapy, and pharmacotherapy (24). Moreover, it is considered a secondary symptom of atrophic vaginitis, often accompanied with postcoital bleeding (25). Physical examination following reliable criteria such as the Vaginal Atrophy Index (26), hormonal assays, and cytological evaluation (i.e., pap smear) are essential in the diagnosis of vulvovaginal atrophy.

Psychosocial difficulties that commonly affect postmenopausal women may impinge on sexual functioning and affect pain perception. Intrapersonal issues, such as negative perceptions of menopause, body image, and postreproductive sexuality, often function as self-fulfilling prophecies and foster sexual dysfunction in the menopause (27). Interpersonal factors such as marital/relationship difficulties, partner's sexual dysfunction (e.g., erectile dysfunction, decreased desire), and loss of social support may also be implicated (28). Clinicians should carefully assess for possible non-biomedical factors that may play a role in maintaining postmenopausal dyspareunia before making a diagnosis or prescribing treatment.

ETIOLOGY

Vulvar Vestibulitis Syndrome

Vulvar vestibulitis syndrome is believed to be the most common form of painful intercourse in premenopausal women (10), affecting an estimated 12% in the general population (8). Women with vulvar vestibulitis typically experience a severe sharp, burning pain localized at the entrance of the vagina (i.e., the vulvar vestibule) (14). This pain occurs upon contact, through both sexual and nonsexual stimulation (10,14). Approximately half of the women with vulvar vestibulitis syndrome have "primary" vestibulitis, that is, they have experienced the pain from their first intercourse attempt, whereas the other half of the sufferers develop the pain after a period of pain-free intercourse, termed "secondary" vestibulitis (29,30).

Characteristics of the Vulvar Vestibule in Affected and Non-affected Women

To answer the question of what causes vulvar vestibulitis, it is necessary to start with where the vulvar vestibule is located and its normal tissue characteristics. The vulvar vestibule (Fig. 10.1) is a part of the external genitalia (i.e., the vulva). It extends from the inner aspects of the labia minora to the hymen, is bordered anteriorly by the clitoral frenulum and posteriorly by the fourchette, and includes the vaginal and urethral openings (31). The vestibule is innervated by the pudendal nerve (32) and contains free nerve endings, the majority of which are believed to be C-fibers, otherwise known as pain fibers (33). Although the vulvar vestibule is composed of visceral tissue, it has a nonvisceral innervation

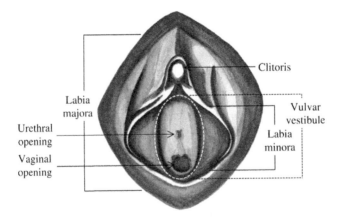

Figure 10.1 The vulva. Parts of the vulva are shown, including the vulvar vestibule (indicated by dotted lines), clitoris, urethral and vaginal openings, and the labia majora and minora. The vulvar vestibule extends laterally from the base of the labia minora, and is bordered anteriorly by the clitoral frenulum and posteriorly by the fourchette. [Image courtesy of Katherine Muldoon.]

(34). Therefore, sensations of touch, temperature, and pain are similar to those evoked in the skin.

The suffix "-itis" refers to conditions of inflammatory origin and, in the case of vulvar vestibulitis, implies that the pain is due to an inflammation of vestibular tissue. However, studies examining indices of inflammation in this tissue suggest that inflammatory infiltrates are common in the vestibule, and thus, not necessarily related to the pain (35,36). Other controlled investigations of vestibular tissue suggest that altered pain processing plays a role in the development and/or maintenance of vulvar vestibulitis. Evidence for this includes the following: a heightened innervation of intraepithelial nerve fibers (33,37), an increase in blood flow and erythema (38), nociceptor sensitization (39), the presence of calcitonin gene-related peptide (i.e., a peptide that exists in pain nerves) (40), and lower pain thresholds (41). These tissue properties would lead to an increase in sensation in response to vestibular pressure, consistent with the clinical picture of provoked pain in women with vestibulitis. Taking a cotton-swab, for example, and touching different areas of the vestibule in a non-affected woman is perceivable but not painful, but this same stimulation in the vestibule of a vestibulitis sufferer is perceived as excruciatingly painful.

Etiological Theories: Physical Explanations for the Pain

Yeast infections: Many etiological theories exist regarding what initiates the increase in sensitivity of the vulvar vestibule in sufferers (42,43). One of the most consistently reported findings associated with the onset of vulvar vestibulitis is a history of repeated yeast infections (44). However, it is not clear whether the culprit is the yeast itself or treatments undertaken which can sensitize the vestibular tissue or an underlying sensitivity already present in the tissue (29,45,46). Many women, like Sandra, when they feel the irritation during intercourse do not go to the doctor's office to have a culture taken before they treat what they think is a yeast infection with over-the-counter remedies from the local drugstore. At the same time, some gynecologists may not perform the culture themselves, and on the basis of symptomatic description alone, suggest to the woman that she has a yeast infection (47). It is vital that both the woman and her health care professional ensure that treatment is not being undertaken without reason, as this can aggravate the problem.

Hormonal factors: Hormonal factors have also been found to be associated with vestibulitis in controlled studies. Bazin et al. (30) and Bouchard et al. (48) found that women who used oral contraceptives had an increased risk of developing vestibulitis later in life, with those starting before the age of 16 being especially at risk. Early menarche (i.e., before the age of 11) and painful menstruation were also associated with an increased risk of vestibulitis (8,30). These findings suggest that hormonal factors may play a role in the increase in sensitivity of the vulvar vestibule, but the question of how hormones are involved remains to be elucidated.

Genetic factors: In one controlled study, Jeremias et al. (49) found that affected women have a high incidence of a genetic allele that is involved in the regulation of inflammation and is associated with chronic inflammatory conditions (e.g., ulcerative colitis, inflammatory bowel disease) (50,51). It is possible that women with this allele are genetically susceptible to the development of vestibulitis, but may only develop it after some injury to the vulvar vestibule, whether through repeated infections, local treatments, hormonal factors, early age at first intercourse, early age at first tampon use, and/or difficulty with or pain during first tampon use (8,9,30). Although these findings need to be replicated, they lead to several possible explanations for the development of vulvar vestibulitis. For example, women with this particular gene profile may have an abnormality in the regulation of inflammation, which has recently been shown in vestibulitis sufferers (52–54). This would allow vulvar vestibulitis to be one of many expressions of this gene; others would include colitis and inflammatory bowel disease. In addition, it would imply that women with vulvar vestibulitis might have associated pain problems and/or sensory abnormalities. Although just beginning to be examined, controlled studies support this implication. Women with vulvar vestibulitis have a higher sensitivity to vestibular touch (41), a higher sensitivity to nonvestibular touch, painful pressure, and heat pain (41,55), in addition to more somatic pain-related complaints (41,56) when compared with non-affected women.

Other factors: Many other physically based etiological theories of vulvar vestibulitis exist; however, they are based on uncontrolled studies and should be interpreted with caution. These include human papillomavirus infection (57), faulty immune system functioning/allergies (6,58), urethral conditions (e.g., interstitial cystitis) (59), vaginismus (46), sexual abuse (44,60), and psychological factors (e.g., somatization disorder) (46). It is important to note that controlled studies of sexual abuse (10,12) show no difference between affected and non-affected women, although a history of depression and physical abuse has been linked to vulvar vestibulitis (8). Furthermore, an increase in pelvic floor muscle tension (61,62) has also been associated with vulvar vestibulitis. Although the tensing of pelvic floor musculature may represent a protective reaction against, or a conditioned response to vulvar pain, this increase in tension is likely to only exacerbate the pain.

Etiological Theories: Psychosocial Explanations for the Pain

Psychological and cognitive factors: In accordance with current chronic pain models, there is much more to the experience of dyspareunia than the pain and its possible physiological underpinnings. This point is illustrated by a recent functional magnetic resonance imaging study of women with vulvar vestibulitis (63), demonstrating that both sensory and affective brain areas are activated in response to painful genital stimulation. These findings are consistent with results from other pain imaging studies (64–67) and support the multidimensional conceptualization of dyspareunia proposed in this chapter.

Factors such as psychological distress, anxiety, depression, low sexual self-esteem, harm avoidance, somatization, shyness, and pain catastrophization (41,55,56,60,68,69) have been found in women with vulvar vestibulitis. Whether they precede or develop subsequent to the pain remains to be elucidated; however, it is crucial to investigate the role of these factors in the maintenance of dyspareunia as negative affect has been shown to modulate pain intensity (70). Negative affect is also associated with an increase in attention towards pain stimuli, otherwise known as hypervigilance (71), which in turn can increase perceived pain intensity (72). In a recent study (73), hypervigilance for pain stimuli was examined in women with vestibulitis and matched control women. Results indicated that women with vulvar vestibulitis syndrome reported hypervigilance to coital pain and exhibited a selective attentional bias towards pain stimuli, an effect mediated by anxiety and fear of pain. These results suggest that anxiety and fear-mediated hypervigilance represent important factors for pain perception in vulvar vestibulitis. Furthermore, hypervigilance to pain stimuli could exacerbate sexual impairment in women suffering from dyspareunia by distracting attentional resources away from erotic cues, a cognitive bias that has been associated with impaired sexual arousal (74–76). The role of sexual arousal in vulvar sensation has not yet been established; however, many theoretical models posit arousal as a key factor in preparing the female reproductive system for the "trauma" of coitus. Therefore, hypervigilance to pain stimuli in women with VVS may result in both a heightened awareness of pain and a distraction away from sexual stimuli, resulting in impaired sexual arousal which may further aggravate the pain experience.

Relationship factors: The examination of relationship factors has been quite limited despite the tremendous impact dyspareunia has on intimate relationships. Seventy-four percent of vestibulitis sufferers report that the pain impacts their relationships (77), although they do not typically report significant levels of dyadic distress. In addition, high dyadic adjustment is related to decreased pain severity in women with dyspareunia (78), whereas psychosocial attributions for the pain are associated with dyadic distress, suggesting an interaction between pain coping style and relationship adjustment (79). Further research is currently underway to clarify the complex relationship among pain severity, relationship adjustment, and coping styles in this population of women.

Vulvodynia

Wesselmann and colleagues (5,80) classify vulvodynia as a "dynia," a group of well described but poorly understood chronic pain syndromes. Vulvodynia is defined as noncyclic, chronic vulvar discomfort extending to the urethral and rectal areas, characterized by the patient's complaint of burning, stinging, irritation, or rawness (81). Light touch of the vulvar area often exacerbates the ongoing pain. A recent epidemiological study estimated that vulvodynia affects 6–7% of women in the general population, with a higher prevalence in women over the age of 30 (8). The onset of vulvodynia is usually acute, without a precipitating event. When such an event is recalled, it is often linked to episodes of local treatments, such as vulvar cream application or laser surgery (80). Little is known about the etiology of vulvodynia. McKay (82) proposed that the pain results from altered cutaneous perception, such as in neuropathic pain syndromes.

Postmenopausal Dyspareunia

Recurrent pain during intercourse occurring for the first time within or subsequent to the menopausal transition is typically attributed to vulvovaginal and urogenital atrophy (also referred to as atrophic vaginitis) (83). These conditions are manifestations of tissue aging, cytological changes, and chemical transformations within the vagina, urethra, and bladder, which result from declining levels of endogenously produced estrogens at menopause (84,85). Both the DSM-IV-TR (3) and the ICD-10 (4) specifically mention this problem but do not classify it as dyspareunia. In the DSM-IV-TR, it would be termed a "sexual dysfunction due to a general medical condition," whereas in the ICD-10, it is classified as "postmenopausal atrophic vaginitis." These classifications and descriptions appear to be based on clinical experience since there is, in fact, very little systematic research evidence to support a strong link between declining estrogen levels, vulvovaginal atrophy, and recurrent pain during intercourse (86–88).

Comment

Regardless of etiology, many areas of these women's lives must be addressed simultaneously in order to achieve therapeutic success. Once the pain is consistently present, a vicious cycle is put into motion (Fig. 10.2), involving physical, muscular, psychological, sexual, and relationship factors.

CURRENT TREATMENT STRATEGIES

As with classification and diagnostic approaches to dyspareunia, treatment approaches have historically adopted a similar dualistic approach by attempting to alleviate the pain via a variety of medical interventions, failing which, psychotherapy is recommended. Typical medical treatment is characterized by a focus on the vestibule to the exclusion of other systems that may be involved (e.g., pelvic floor musculature). In addition, current medical interventions have not incorporated empirically based treatments for dyspareunia, which have recently been published.

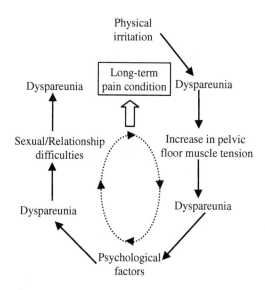

Figure 10.2 The vicious cycle of pain. Once the experience of pain is initiated (shown here as starting from a physical irritation) and continues without appropriate treatment, it begins to encompass many different factors, including physical, muscular, psychological, sexual, and sexual/relationship. The involvement of these different systems usually leads to increases in the amount of pain and distress experienced, and can explain pain maintenance in the absence of physical findings, as in most cases of dyspareunia and back pain. Although this figure indicates that the initiating symptom can evolve into a complex cycle, theoretically, the cycle can start at any point or at multiple points simultaneously.

Vulvar Vestibulitis Syndrome

Medical Interventions

Treatment for vestibulitis is typically guided by the medical model. This model follows a traditional strategy of starting with conservative, non-invasive treatments and progressing to more invasive ones (89). Palliative interventions (e.g., sitz baths) to reduce the pain are the first-line treatment choice for dyspareunia. If these are not effective, treatment progresses to topical interventions (e.g., lidocaine, corticosteriods), systemic medications (e.g., oral corticosteriods, antifungals), followed by injectable medical treatments (e.g., interferon), "neurophysiological" treatments (e.g., biofeedback, pharmacotherapy), and ending with surgical intervention (e.g., vestibulectomy). However, there is little evidence to support the use of topical, systemic, or injectable treatments. Although one placebo-controlled study of the effectiveness of cromolyn cream (90) and one randomized trial of fluconazole (91) found these treatments to be ineffective for relieving the symptoms of vulvar vestibulitis, one study found that long-term lidocaine ointment application decreased pain scores and re-established sexual activity in a group of vestibulitis sufferers (92). Follow-up data and a randomized clinical trial are needed in order to fully assess the effects of this kind of treatment, as local and systemic medications, such as creams, antibiotics, and injectable medical treatments may cause more harm than benefit (5). In addition, there is no empirical evidence for the success of any medication, such as antidepressants, for the pain of vestibulitis.

Cognitive-Behavioral Interventions

Cognitive-behavioral interventions for vulvar vestibulitis syndrome include cognitive-behavioral pain management, sex therapy, and pelvic floor biofeedback to target both pain reduction and sexual functioning. Success rates ranging from 43% to 86% have been reported in two uncontrolled studies in which sex therapy and pain management were combined (93,94). In 1996, Weijmar Schultz et al. (95) published a prospective and partially randomized treatment outcome study investigating the effectiveness of behavioral intervention with or without surgery. Results from this study indicated that women in both groups benefited in terms of pain reduction, with no significant differences between women who had undergone the behavioral intervention alone vs. those who underwent the combined treatment of behavioral intervention and surgery. The authors suggest that the behavioral approach should be the first line of treatment for vestibulitis sufferers, with the surgery acting as an additional form of treatment for refractory cases.

Biofeedback training has been used in an effort to reduce hypertonicity of the pelvic floor muscles (61). With the aid of a vaginal sensor, the patient is provided with direct visual feedback regarding their level of muscle tension, facilitating muscle training with respect to contraction, relaxation, and the acquisition of voluntary control. After $\sim$4 months of training, subjective pain reports decreased an average of 83%, with 52% of the women reporting pain-free intercourse, and 79% of women who were abstaining from intercourse resuming activity posttreatment. However, this study contained a mixed group of women with vulvar pain and likely contained a high proportion of vaginismic women, considering that many participants were not engaging in intercourse at the beginning of the study. The effectiveness of physical therapy, which includes a pelvic floor biofeedback component in addition to soft tissue mobilization and other techniques specific to this treatment, has recently been evaluated in a retrospective study of vestibulitis sufferers (96). Results indicated that after an average of 16 months of treatment, physical therapy yielded a moderate to great improvement in over 70% of participants. Treatment resulted in significant pain reduction during intercourse and gynecological examinations, and increases in intercourse frequency and levels of sexual desire and arousal. These findings indicate that physical therapy is indeed a promising treatment modality for women who suffer from vulvar vestibulitis syndrome, although prospective studies are needed.

Surgical Intervention

Vestibulectomy has been the most investigated treatment for vulvar vestibulitis to date with over 20 published outcome studies, yielding success rates ranging from 43% to 100% (42). This minor surgical procedure, preformed as day surgery under general anesthesia, consists of the excision of the hymen and sensitive areas of the vestibule to a depth of $\sim$2 mm, with some procedures involving the mobilization of the vaginal mucosa to cover the excised area. Following this procedure, women are generally instructed to abstain from all forms of vaginal penetration for 6–8 weeks.

Our research group conducted a randomized treatment outcome study of vulvar vestibulitis comparing vestibulectomy, group cognitive-behavior therapy, and pelvic floor biofeedback (97). At posttreatment and 6-month follow-up, there was significant pain reduction for all three treatment groups. However, vestibulectomy resulted in approximately twice the pain reduction (47–70% depending on the pain measure) of the two other treatments (19–38%); it was characterized by a high success rate and by elevated percentages of pain reduction. In addition, there were significant improvements in overall sexual functioning and self-reported frequency of intercourse at the 6-month follow-up, with no treatment differences. However, means for intercourse frequency for all three groups remained below the mean frequency of intercourse for healthy women of similar age. In a 2.5-year follow-up of this study (98), members of all three treatment groups continued to improve over time. Vestibulectomy remained superior to the other two treatments with respect to pain ratings on the cotton-swab test, whereas women in the group therapy condition reported equal improvements in terms of self-report measures of painful intercourse. Changes in overall sexual functioning and intercourse frequency were maintained, with no group differences. These results suggest that although the benefits of group therapy may take longer to appear, it can be just as effective as surgery in reducing the pain experienced during intercourse.

Alternative Treatments

Alternative treatments for vulvar vestibulitis syndrome include acupuncture and hypnotherapy. Although few studies currently exist, there are promising data regarding the effect of acupuncture on pain reduction and overall quality of life (99). In addition, a recently published case study indicated that hypnosis reduced pain and helped re-establish sexual pleasure (100). Randomized controlled trials are needed in order to truly establish the effectiveness of these treatments. Alternative treatments seem promising, yet to date, only cognitive-behavioral therapy, biofeedback, and vestibulectomy have been empirically validated. It is also likely that concurrent treatment with multiple non-invasive methods may be even superior to single treatments, though this has yet to be investigated.

Vulvodynia

Little information exists with respect to validated treatments for vulvodynia. McKay (13) recommends low-dose amitriptyline for symptom control in vulvodynia. This treatment is effective for neuropathic pain syndromes (101), which have a similar pain presentation to vulvodynia. Glazer (102) reported that pelvic floor muscle rehabilitation reduced pain and improved sexual functioning in vulvodynia sufferers. However, no randomized controlled trials have been conducted with respect to any treatment for vulvodynia. Despite the lack of knowledge concerning valid treatments for this condition, there is much agreement that it should be multidisciplinary (5,80,81).

Postmenopausal Dyspareunia

Postmenopausal dyspareunia is considered a major indicator for hormonal treatment (103). If nonhormonal vaginal lubricants, such as Replens, are not adequate, then estrogen-based creams or estradiol inserts in ring or tablet format are often recommended. In principle, systemic estrogen-based hormone replacement therapy may also be prescribed. Significant reduction of urogenital atrophy can be obtained through estrogen supplementation, which may, in turn, provide the context for improvements in sexual functioning (104). Presently, evidence from randomized controlled trials is tenuous regarding the benefit of hormone replacement for dyspareunic pain (105). Beyond alleviating symptoms of urogenital atrophy that may subsequently lead to sexual impairment, hormonal supplementation has not been found to substantially contribute to postmenopausal sexual functioning (104–106).

FUTURE DIRECTIONS

Major confusion exists in the literature with respect to the nomenclature and classification of dyspareunia. The DSM-IV-TR classifies idiopathic dyspareunia as a sexual dysfunction (3), whereas the ICD-10 (4) distinguishes between organic and psychogenic dyspareunia, neither of which are explicitly defined. In addition, the current nomenclature with respect to dyspareunia subtypes is confusing and fails to clearly differentiate among the various conditions (16). We suggest that a careful characterization of the pain associated with these conditions will clarify this diagnostic labeling confusion and help to unify the field. Throughout this chapter, we have established the complexity of dyspareunia and how this class of disorders can affect a woman's life on multiple physiological, emotional, cognitive, and interpersonal levels. Given the large prevalence of women suffering from dyspareunia, it is essential for primary health care providers to become familiar with these conditions and to establish collaborations with other health professionals in order to provide their patients with multidisciplinary treatment options.

Given the physiological, cognitive, affective, and interpersonal complexity of dyspareunia, it is likely that no one "cure" for dyspareunia or for other chronic pain conditions will be found. Thus, we propose a multimodal treatment approach for all types of urogenital pain discussed in this chapter, tailored to each patient, and including careful assessment of the different aspects of the pain experience. Clinicians should also educate their patients as to the multidimensional nature of chronic pain so that the treatment of so-called psychological or relationship factors is not experienced as invalidating. Although pain reduction is an important goal, sexual functioning should also be worked on simultaneously through individual or couple therapy, as it has been shown that pain reduction does not necessarily restore sexual functioning (97).

Further research is needed to further examine the pain component of dyspareunia using standardized tools in an effort to more fully understand the mechanisms involved in the development and maintenance of this painful and disruptive condition. Currently, we are investigating the effects of sexual arousal on genital and nongenital sensation, baseline measures of vestibular blood flow through thermal and laser Doppler imaging techniques, and sensitivity to body-wide pressure in women with vulvar vestibulitis syndrome. We hope to extend these research avenues to include the examination of women suffering from vulvodynia and postmenopausal dyspareunia in the near future. In addition, our research group is presently conducting a randomized treatment outcome study of women with vestibulitis, examining the effects of pain relief therapy compared with typical medical treatment. Future treatment outcome studies will include the investigation of the effects of physical therapy, as well as combined treatments, in an effort to develop and implement effective treatment strategies for the numerous women suffering from dyspareunia.

REFERENCES

1. Barnes R. A Clinical History of the Medical and Surgical Diseases of Women. Philadelphia: Henry C. Lea, 1874.
2. Heading RC. Definitions of dyspepsia. Scand J Gastroenterol 1991; 182(Suppl):1–6.
3. American Psychiatric Association. Diagnostic and Statistical Manual of Mental Disorders. 4th ed. Text Revision. Washington, DC: Author, 2000.
4. World Health Organization. Manual of the International Statistical Classification of Diseases, Injuries, and Causes of Death. 10th ed. Geneva: Author, 1992.
5. Wesselmann U, Reich SG. The dynias. Semin Neurol 1996; 16:63–74.
6. Friedrich EG Jr. Vulvar vestibulitis syndrome. J Reprod Med 1987; 32:110–114.
7. Laumann EO, Paik A, Rosen RC. Sexual dysfunction in the United States. J Am Med Assoc 1999; 281:537–544.
8. Harlow BL, Wise LA, Stewart EG. Prevalence and predictors of chronic lower genital tract discomfort. Am J Obstet Gynecol 2001; 185:545–550.
9. Harlow BL, Stewart EG. A population-based assessment of chronic unexplained vulvar pain: have we underestimated the prevalence of vulvodynia? J Am Med Womens Assoc 2003; 58:82–88.

10. Meana M, Binik YM, Khalifé S, Cohen D. Biopsychosocial profile of women with dyspareunia. Obstet Gynecol 1997; 90:583–589.
11. Reed BD, Advincula AP, Fonde KR, Gorenflo DW, Haefner HK. Sexual activities and attitudes of women with vulvar dysesthesia. Obstet Gynecol 2003; 102:325–331.
12. Reissing ED, Binik YM, Khalifé S, Cohen D, Amsel R. Etiological correlates of vaginismus: sexual and physical abuse, sexual knowledge, sexual self-schema, and relationship adjustment. J Sex Marital Ther 2003; 29:47–59.
13. McKay M. Vulvodynia: diagnostic patterns. Dermatol Clin 1992; 10:423–433.
14. Bergeron S, Binik YM, Khalifé S, Pagidas K, Glazer HI. Reliability and validity of the diagnosis of vulvar vestibulitis syndrome. Obstet Gynecol 2001; 98:45–51.
15. Deyo RA. The early diagnostic evaluation of patients with low back pain. J Gen Intern Med 1986; 1:328.
16. Pukall CF, Payne KA, Binik YM, Khalifé S. Pain measurement in vulvodynia. J Sex Marital Ther 2003; 29(s):111–120.
17. Melzack R, Casey KL. Sensory, motivational, and central control determinants of pain: a new conceptual model. In: Kenshalo D, ed. The Skin Senses. Illinois: Thomas, 1968:423–443.
18. Coderre TJ, Mogil JS, Bushnell MC. The biological psychology of pain. In: Gallagher M, Nelson RJ, eds. Handbook of Psychology. Vol. 3. Biological Psychology. New York: John Wiley & Sons, Inc., 2003:237–268.
19. Merskey H, Bogduk N. Classification of Chronic Pain. 2nd ed. Washington, DC: IASP Press, 1994.
20. Pukall CF, Binik YM, Khalifé S. A new instrument for pain assessment in vulvar vestibulitis syndrome. J Sex Marital Ther 2004; 30:69–78.
21. Eva LJ, Reid WM, MacLean AB, Morrison GD. Assessment of response to treatment in vulvar vestibulitis syndrome by means of the vulvar algesiometer. Am J Obstet Gynecol 1999; 181:99–102.
22. McKay M. Vulvodynia versus pruritus vulvae. Clin Obstet Gynecol 1985; 28:123–133.
23. Baram DA. Sexuality, sexual dysfunction, and sexual assault. In: Berek JS, ed. Novack's Gynecology. 13th ed. Philadelphia: Lippincott Williams & Wilkins, 2002:295–321.
24. Graziottin A. Etiology and diagnosis of coital pain. J Endocrinol Invest 2003; 26:115–121.
25. Soper DA. Genitourinary infections and sexually transmitted diseases. In: Berek JS, ed. Novack's Gynecology. 13th ed. Philadelphia: Lippincott Williams & Wilkins, 2002:453–470.
26. Leiblum S, Bachmann G, Kemmann E, Colburn D, Swartzman L. Vaginal atrophy in the postmenopausal woman: the importance of sexual activity and hormones. J Am Med Assoc 1983; 249:2195–2198.
27. Bachmann GA, Burd ID, Ebert GA. Menopausal sexuality. In: Lobo RA, Kelsey J, Marcus R, eds. Menopause: Biology and Pathobiology. San Diego: Academic Press, 2002:383–393.
28. Lamont JA. Sexuality. In: Stewart DE, Robinson GE, eds. A Clinician's Guide to Menopause. Washington: American Psychiatric Press Inc., 1997:63–75.
29. Goetsch MF. Vulvar vestibulitis: prevalence and historic features in a general gynecologic practice population. Am J Obstet Gynecol 1991; 164:1609–1616.

30. Bazin S, Bouchard C, Brisson J, Morin C, Meisels A, Fortier M. Vulvar vestibulitis syndrome: an exploratory case–control study. Obstet Gynecol 1994; 83:47–50.
31. Friedrich EG Jr. The vulvar vestibule. J Reprod Med 1983; 28:773–777.
32. Krantz KE. Innervation of the human vulva and vagina: a microscopic study. Obstet Gynecol 1958; 12:382–396.
33. Bohm-Starke N, Hilliges M, Falconer C, Rylander E. Increased intraepithelial innervation in women with vulvar vestibulitis syndrome. Gynecol Obstet Invest 1998; 46:256–260.
34. Cervero F. Sensory innervation of the viscera: peripheral basis of visceral pain. Physiol Rev 1994; 74:95–138.
35. Chadha S, Gianotten WL, Drogendijk AC, Weijmar Schultz WC, Blindeman LA, van der Meijden WI. Histopathologic features of vulvar vestibulitis. Int J Gynecol Pathol 1998; 17:7–11.
36. Bohm-Starke N, Falconer C, Rylander E, Hilliges M. The expression of cyclooxygenase 2 and inducible nitric oxide synthase indicates no active inflammation in vulvar vestibulitis. Acta Obstet Gynecol Scand 2001; 80:638–644.
37. Weström LV, Willén R. Vestibular nerve fiber proliferation in vulvar vestibulitis syndrome. Obstet Gynecol 1998; 91:572–576.
38. Bohm-Starke N, Hilliges M, Blomgren BO, Falconer C, Rylander E. Increased blood flow and erythema in the posterior vestibular mucosa in vulvar vestibulitis. Obstet Gynecol 2001; 98:1067–1074.
39. Bohm-Starke N, Hilliges M, Brodda-Jansen G, Rylander E, Torebjörk E. Psychophysical evidence of nociceptor sensitisation in vulvar vestibulitis syndrome. Pain 2001; 94:177–183.
40. Bohm-Starke N, Hilliges M, Falconer C, Rylander E. Neurochemical characterization of the vestibular nerves in women with vulvar vestibulitis syndrome. Gynecol Obstet Invest 1999; 48:270–275.
41. Pukall CF, Binik YM, Khalifé S, Amsel R, Abbott FV. Vestibular tactile and pain thresholds in women with vulvar vestibulitis syndrome. Pain 2002; 96:163–175.
42. Bergeron S, Binik Y, Khalifé S, Pagidas K. Vulvar vestibulitis syndrome: a critical review. Clin J Pain 1997; 13:27–42.
43. Baggish MS, Miklos JR. Vulvar pain syndrome: a review. Obstet Gynecol Surv 1995; 50:618–627.
44. Mann MS, Kaufman RH, Brown D, Adam E. Vulvar vestibulitis: significant clinical variables and treatment outcome. Obstet Gynecol 1992; 79:122–125.
45. Marinoff SC, Turner ML. Vulvar vestibulitis syndrome: an overview. Am J Obstet Gynecol 1991; 165:1228–1233.
46. Schover LR, Youngs DD, Cannata R. Psychosexual aspects of the evaluation and management of vulvar vestibulitis. Am J Obstet Gynecol 1992; 167:630–636.
47. Stewart EG, Spencer P. V Book: A Doctor's Guide to Complete Vulvovaginal Health. New York: Bantam Books, 2002.
48. Bouchard C, Brisson J, Fortier M, Morin C, Blanchette C. Use of oral contraceptives and vulvar vestibulitis: a case–control study. Am J Epidemiol 2002; 156:254–261.
49. Jeremias J, Ledger WJ, Witkin SS. Interleukin 1 receptor antagonist gene polymorphism in women with vulvar vestibulitis. Am J Obstet Gynecol 2000; 182:283–285.
50. Mansfield JC, Holden H, Tarlow JK, DiGiovine FS, McDowell TL, Wilson AG, Holdsworth CD, Duff GW. Novel genetic associations between ulcerative colitis

and the anti-inflammatory cytokine interleukin-1 receptor antagonist. Gastroenterology 1994; 106:637–642.

51. Heresbach D, Alizadeh M, Dabadie A, LeBerre N, Colombel JF, Yaovanq J, Bretagne JF, Semana G. Significance of interleukin-1 beta and interleukin-1 receptor antagonist genetic polymorphism in inflammatory bowel disease. Am J Gastroenterol 1997; 92:1164–1169.

52. Foster DC, Hasday JD. Elevated tissue levels of interleukin-1 beta and tumor necrosis factor-alpha in vulvar vestibulitis. Obstet Gynecol 1997; 89:291–296.

53. Gerber S, Bongiovanni AM, Ledger WJ, Witkin SS. A deficiency in interferon-alpha production in women with vulvar vestibulitis. Am J Obstet Gynecol 2002; 186:361–364.

54. Gerber S, Bongiovanni AM, Ledger WJ, Witkin SS. Defective regulation of the proinflammatory immune response in women with vulvar vestibulitis syndrome. Am J Obstet Gynecol 2002; 186:696–700.

55. Granot M, Friedman M, Yarnitsky D, Zimmer EZ. Enhancement of the perception of systemic pain in women with vulvar vestibulitis. Br J Obstet Gynecol 2002; 109:863–866.

56. Danielsson I, Eisemann M, Sjöberg I, Wikman M. Vulvar vestibulitis: a multi-factorial condition. Br J Obstet Gynecol 2001; 108:456–461.

57. Reid R, Greenberg MD, Daoud Y, Husain M, Selvaggi S, Wilkinson E. Colposcopic findings in women with vulvar pain syndromes: a preliminary report. J Reprod Med 1988; 33:523–532.

58. Ashman RB, Ott AK. Autoimmunity as a factor in recurrent vaginal candidosis and the minor vestibular gland syndrome. J Reprod Med 1989; 34:264–266.

59. McCormack WM. Two urogenital sinus syndromes: interstitial cystitis and focal vulvitis. Br J Obstet Gynecol 1990; 98:703–706.

60. Jantos M, White G. The vestibulitis syndrome: medical and psychosexual assessment of a cohort of patients. J Reprod Med 1997; 42:145–152.

61. Glazer HI, Rodke G, Swencionis C, Hertz R, Young AW. Treatment of vulvar vestibulitis syndrome with electromyographic biofeedback of pelvic floor musculature. J Reprod Med 1995; 40:283–290.

62. Reissing ED, Binik YM, Khalifé S, Cohen D, Amsel R. Vaginal spasm, behaviour and pain: an empirical investigation of the reliability of the diagnosis of vaginismus. Arch Sex Behav 2004; 33:5–17.

63. Pukall CF, Strigo IA, Binik YM, Amsel R, Khalifé S, Bushnell MC. Neural correlates of painful genital touch in women with vulvar vestibulitis syndrome. Submitted.

64. Talbot J, Marrett S, Evans AC, Meyer E, Bushnell MC, Duncan GH. Multiple representations of pain in human cerebral cortex. Science 1991; 251:1355–1358.

65. Casey KL, Minoshima S, Morrow TJ, Koeppe RA. Comparison of human cerebral activation patterns during cutaneous warmth, heat pain, and deep cold pain. J Neurophysiol 1996; 76:571–581.

66. Rainville P, Duncan GH, Price DD, Carrier B, Bushnell MC. Pain affect encoded in human anterior cingulate but not somatosensory cortex. Science 1997; 277:968–971.

67. Bingel U, Quante M, Knab R, Bromm B, Weiller C, Buchel C. Subcortical structures involved in pain processing: evidence from single-trial fMRI. Pain 2002; 99:313–321.

68. van Lankveld JJ, Weijenborg PT, Ter Kuile MM. Psychologic profiles of and sexual function in women with vulvar vestibulitis and their partners. Obstet Gynecol 1996; 88:65–70.
69. Gates EA, Galask RP. Psychological and sexual functioning in women with vulvar vestibulitis. J Psychosom Obstet Gynaecol 2001; 22:221–228.
70. Janssen SA. Negative affect and sensitization to pain. Scand J Psychol 2002; 43:131–137.
71. Asmundson GJG, Taylor S. Role of anxiety sensitivity in pain-related fear and avoidance. J Behav Med 1996; 19:577–586.
72. McCaul KD, Malott JM. Distraction and coping with pain. Psychol Bull 1984; 95:516–533.
73. Payne KA, Binik YM, Amsel R, Khalifé S. When sex hurts, anxiety and fear orient attention towards pain. Eur J Pain. In press.
74. Barlow DH. The causes of sexual dysfunction: the role of anxiety and cognitive interference. J Consult Clin Psychol 1986; 54:140–148.
75. Dove NL, Wiederman MW. Cognitive distraction and women's sexual functioning. J Sex Marital Ther 2000; 26:67–78.
76. van den Hout M, Barlow D. Attention, arousal and expectancies in anxiety and sexual disorders. J Affect Disord 2000; 61:241–256.
77. Bergeron S, Bouchard C, Fortier M, Binik Y, Khalifé S. The surgical treatment of vulvar vestibulitis syndrome: a follow-up study. J Sex Marital Ther 1997; 23:317–325.
78. Meana M, Binik I, Khalifé S, Cohen D. Affect and marital adjustment in women's rating of dyspareunic pain. Can J Psychiatry 1998; 43:381–385.
79. Meana M, Binik I, Khalifé S, Cohen D. Psychosocial correlates of pain attributions in women with dyspareunia. Psychosomatics 1999; 40:497–502.
80. Wesselmann U, Burnett AL, Abramovici H, Heinberg LJ. The urogenital and rectal pain syndromes. Pain 1997; 73:269–294.
81. McKay M. Vulvodynia: a multifactorial clinical problem. Arch Dermatol 1989; 125:256–262.
82. McKay M. Subsets of vulvodynia. J Reprod Med 1988; 33:695–698.
83. Oldenhave A. Some aspects of sexuality during the normal climacteric. In: Berg G, Hammer M, eds. The Modern Management of the Menopause. Carnforth: Parthenon Publishing, 1994:605–615.
84. Hurd WW, Amesse LS, Randolph JF Jr. Menopause. In: Berek JS, ed. Novack's Gynecology. 13th ed. Philadelphia: Lippincott Williams & Wilkins, 2002:1109–1142.
85. Willhite LA, O'Connel MB. Urogenital atrophy: prevention and treatment. Pharmacother 2001; 21:464–480.
86. Weber AM, Walters MD, Schover LR, Mitchinson A. Vaginal anatomy and sexual function. Obstet Gynecol 1995; 86:946–949.
87. Laan E, van Lunsen RHW. Hormones and sexuality in postmenopausal women: a psychophysiological study. J Psychosom Obstet Gynecol 1997; 18:126–133.
88. Kao A, Binik YM. Cause and symptom or separate syndromes? Reviewing the association between urogenital atrophy and dyspareunia in postmenopausal women. Submitted.
89. American College of Obstetricians and Gynecologists. Vulvar nonneoplastic epithelial disorders. Int J Gynecol Obstet 1998; 60:181–188.
90. Njirjesy P, Sobel JD, Weitz MV, Leaman DJ, Small MJ, Gelone SP. Cromolyn cream for recalcitrant vulvar vestibulitis: results of a placebo controlled study. Sex Transm Inf 2001; 77:53–57.

91. Bornstein BJ, Livnat G, Stolar Z, Abramovici H. Pure versus complicated vulvar vestibulitis: a randomized trial of fluconazole treatment. Gynecol Obstet Invest 2000; 50:194–197.

92. Zolnoun DA, Hartmann KE, Steege JF. Overnight 5% lidocaine ointment for treatment of vulvar vestibulitis. Obstet Gynecol 2003; 102:84–87.

93. Abramov L, Wolman I, David MP. Vaginismus: an important factor in the evaluation and management of vulvar vestibulitis syndrome. Gynecol Obstet Invest 1994; 38:194–197.

94. ter Kuile MM, Weijenborg ThM. A cognitive-behavioral group programme for women with vulvar vestibulitis syndrome: factors associated with treatment success. Sexual Pain Disorder Symposium, Amsterdam, Holland, Oct 20–24, 2003.

95. Weijmar Schultz WCM, Gianotten WL, van der Meijden WI, van de Wiel HBM, Blindeman L, Chadha S, Drogendijk AC. Behavioral approach with or without surgical intervention to the vulvar vestibulitis syndrome: a prospective randomized and non-randomized study. J Psychosom Obstet Gynecol 1996; 17:143–148.

96. Bergeron S, Brown C, Lord M-J, Oala M, Binik YM, Khalifé S. Physical therapy for vulvar vestibulitis syndrome. J Sex Marital Ther 2002; 28:183–192.

97. Bergeron S, Binik Y, Khalifé S, Pagidas K, Glazer HI, Meana M, Amsel R. A randomized comparison of group cognitive behavioral therapy, surface electromyographic biofeedback, and vestibulectomy in the treatment of dyspareunia resulting from vulvar vestibulitis. Pain 2001; 91:297–306.

98. Bergeron S, Meana M, Binik Y, Khalifé S. Painful genital sexual activity. In: Levine SB, Risen CB, Althof SE, eds. Handbook of Clinical Sexuality for Mental Health Professionals. New York: Brunner-Routledge, 2003:131–152.

99. Danielsson I, Sjöberg I, Östman C. Acupuncture for the treatment of vulvar vestibulitis: a pilot study. Acta Obstet Gynecol Scand 2001; 80:437–441.

100. Kandyba K, Binik YM. Hypnotherapy as a treatment for vulvar vestibulitis syndrome: a case report. J Sex Marital Ther 2003; 29:237–242.

101. Max M. Antidepressants as analgesics. In: Fields H, Liebeskind J, eds. Progress in Pain Research and Management. Seattle: IASP Press, 1992:229–246.

102. Glazer HI. Dysesthetic vulvodynia: long term follow-up with surface electromyography-assisted pelvic floor muscle rehabilitation. J Reprod Med 2000; 45:798–802.

103. Sarrel PM. Sexuality and menopause. Obstet Gynecol 1990; 75:26S–30S.

104. Walling M, Anderson BL, Johnson SR. Hormonal replacement therapy for postmenopausal women: a review of sexual outcomes and gynecological effects. Arch Sex Behav 1990; 19:119–137.

105. Cardozo L, Bachmann G, McClish D, Fonda D, Birgerson L. Meta-analysis of estrogen therapy in the management of urogenital atrophy in postmenopausal women: second report of the hormones and urogenital therapy committee. Obstet Gynecol 1998; 92:722–727.

106. Iddenden DA. Sexuality during the menopause. Med Clin North Am 1987; 71:87–94.

11

Vaginismus

W. C. M. Weijmar Schultz and H. B. M. Van de Wiel
Groningen University Medical Centre, Groningen, The Netherlands

INTRODUCTION

Vaginismus is defined as recurrent or persistent involuntary spasm of the musculature of the outer third of the vagina that interferes with vaginal penetration, which causes personal distress (1). Vaginistic women vary widely in their sexual behavior repertoire: from very limited to very extensive. In some cases, the desire to have children is first and foremost, without there being any real motivation to work on the sexual relationship. The complaint can be situational or generalized. Vaginismus is not part of the sexual response cycle.

Prevalence rates for vaginismus are scant, without the benefit of multiple studies on specific populations. Prevalence estimates for vaginismus range from 1% to 6% (2). Vaginismus is a supreme example of the mandatory blending of mind and body. The precise etiology is often unclear. There are various theories on the causes of vaginismus, each with its own therapeutic approach. In this chapter, first, the literature on the concept of vaginismus is reviewed; secondly, the different views on the origination of vaginismus are discussed, followed by the various treatments. The chapter is concluded with a diagnostic and treatment protocol.

THE DEFINITION

The assumption that dyspareunia and vaginismus are distinct types of sexual pain disorders has recently been challenged (3–8). Research has demonstrated persistent problems with the sensitivity and specificity of the differential diagnosis of these two phenomena. Both complaints may comprise, to a smaller or larger extent: (1) problems with muscle tension (voluntary, involuntary, limited to vaginal sphincter, or extending to pelvic floor, adductor muscles, back, jaws, or entire body), (2) fear of sexual pain (either specifically associated with genital touching/intercourse or more generalized fear of pain, or fear of sex), and (3) propensity for behavioral approach or avoidance. All these three phenomena are typical of vaginismus, but may also be present in dyspareunia.

Also, differentiation between vaginismus and dyspareunia using clinical tools is difficult, or nearly impossible (3,7,8), and vaginal spasms cannot be diagnosed reliably (3). Only physical therapists can differentiate vaginismic women from matched controls on the basis of muscle tone or strength differences (3,9,10). In addition, for the treatment of vaginismus, despite strong clinical support, vaginal "dilatation" plus psycho-education, desensitization, and so on is not to date supported by scientific study (5,10–13). Finally, there is accumulating basic research to support the idea that the pelvic floor musculature, like other muscle groups, is indirectly innervated by the limbic system and therefore highly reactive to emotional stimuli and states (14–16). On the basis of this emerging knowledge of the underlying pathophysiologic mechanisms, it is obvious that current diagnostic categories of vaginismus and dyspareunia may overlap, and need to be reconceptualized. The same goes for the spasm-based definition of vaginismus despite the absence of research confirming this spasm criterion.

At the 2nd International Consultation on Erectile and Sexual Dysfunctions in July 2003 in Paris, a multidisciplinary group of experts in the field has proposed new definitions of vaginismus and dyspareunia (2,17). Vaginismus is defined as: *The persistent or recurrent difficulties of the woman to allow vaginal entry of a penis, a finger, and/or any object, despite the woman's expressed wish to do so. There is often (phobic) avoidance and anticipation/ fear of pain. Structural or physical abnormalities must be ruled out/addressed.* It is emphasized that reflexive involuntary contraction of the pelvic muscles as well as thigh adduction, contraction of the abdominal muscles, muscles in the back and limbs, associated with varying degrees of fear of pain and of the unknown, typically precludes full entry of a penis, tampon, speculum, or finger. However, discomforting or painful vaginal entry may occur.

Dyspareunia is defined as: *Persistent or recurrent pain with attempted or complete vaginal entry and/or penile vaginal intercourse.* The authors clarify that the experience of women who cannot tolerate full penile entry and the movements of intercourse because of pain needs to be included in the definition of dyspareunia. Clearly, they state, it depends on the woman's pain tolerance and her partner's hesitance or insistence. A decision to desist the attempt at full entry of the penis or its movement, within the vagina, should not change the diagnosis. Finally, they recommend that the diagnoses be accompanied by descriptors relating to associated contextual factors and to the degree of distress.

VIEWS ON THE CAUSES OF VAGINISMUS

Vaginismus is treated in various ways. Interventions vary from surgery to relational therapy. There are various theories on the causes of vaginismus and each has its own therapeutic approach. We elaborate on the psychoanalytical view, the psychological view, the behavioristic view, the interactional view, the sociocultural view, the pain view, the overactive pelvic floor muscle view, the somatic view, and the multidimensional view.

The Psychoanalytical View

Musaph defined vaginismus as a hysterical symptom, or a conversion symptom (18). In other words, a psychological complaint (anxiety) is changed into a physical symptom (a vaginistic reaction). According to Musaph, why some women are vaginistic whereas other are not depends on whether they have a primary disposition towards suppression as a defense mechanism; this might be towards a disrupted mother–child relationship, or other stressful situations that occurred in the oral and oedipal phase of emotional development.

Although psychoanalysis has paid a great deal of attention to the development of sexuality, very few analysts have written about treatment for vaginismus. Musaph distinguished between two forms of psychoanalytical therapy: dynamic-oriented therapy and classical psychoanalysis. The dynamic-oriented therapy form is a method to heal the symptoms, that is, the aim of therapy is to cure the neurotic reaction, in this case the vaginistic reaction. Some analysts use other resources besides the usual psychoanalytical methods, such as psychopharmaceuticals and hypnosis. Important elements in classical psychoanalysis are regression and reliving the traumatic experiences that are related to the sexual problem.

More recent research revealed that women with vaginismus have significantly increased comorbid anxiety disorders, whereas depression rates are not found to be increased (4,19,20). The role of childhood sexual trauma is unclear, since different frequency rates are found (3,4), and the presence of increased rates of posttraumatic stress disorder has not been investigated as yet. Psychological characteristics, measured with self-report instruments, do not unequivocally corroborate the presence of anxiety disorders. Personality traits found to be more often present in this group suggest the presence of self-focused attention and negative self-evaluation in the etiology or maintenance of vaginismus (3,20). Sexual functioning may be impaired with regard to sexual desire and arousal response during sexual activity. Psychopathology and impaired psychological functioning may be caused as well as effect of vaginismus. Experimental evidence thus far documented the role of experienced threat in increased pelvic floor muscle tension, but did not discriminate between women with and without vaginismus (10,21,22). The causation and maintenance of vaginismus by psychological factors thus remain unresolved although fear of penetration and associated attentional bias may play a role. So far, no randomized controlled trials of psychological treatment for vaginismus have been published.

The Behavioristic View

Another view on the origination of vaginistic reaction comes from the behavioristic angle. Although the majority of authors with this point of view agree that vaginismus is a conditioned anxiety reaction that results in spasm of the entrance to the vagina (23–26), only a small minority give an explanation for the origination of this behavior. Brinkman, for instance, gave an explanation model (27). He assumed that vaginismus is the end result of a classic conditioning process in which painful sexual intercourse took place. As a consequence of this process, the penis is conditioned into an aversion stimulus that when an approach is made, gives rise to tension and avoidance behavior, which once again leads to painful spasm of, in particular, the vaginal and anal sphincter muscles. Brinkman assumed that conditioning of the vaginistic reaction can occur in various ways. Sometimes one negative experience is enough, particularly in the case of incest or rape. Often, conditioning takes place over several experiences and such influences are far more difficult to establish.

Treatment according to the behavioristic view, which has been gaining popularity over the past 20 years, is based on the learning principle. In other words, a reaction that has been learned can also be unlearned. To resolve vaginistic complaints, various therapy forms have been developed within behavioral therapy: systematic desensitization, muscle exercises, and counter-conditioning. These therapy forms are not mutually exclusive and are often used in combination.

Systematic desensitization was originally developed by Wolpe and it appears to be effective in reducing various forms of tension (28). Wolpe made two basic assumptions:

1. A certain stimulus (e.g., an approaching penis) causes anxiety (response).
2. When a response can be generated that is antagonistic to anxiety (e.g., relaxation in the presence of an anxiety-invoking stimulus), then the relationship between the stimulus (the approaching penis) and the anxiety response will diminish.

There are two forms of systematic desensitization: *in vitro* and *in vivo*. *In vitro* means that the desensitization takes place in a fantasy situation, whereas *in vivo* means that it takes place in the real situation. Systematic desensitization *in vivo* is the more commonly used method for the treatment of women with vaginistic complaints. First, the woman learns to relax. Then she learns to gradually accept objects of increasing diameter in her vagina, such as fingers or vaginal rods. She starts with the smallest size and finishes with the largest size that matches the size of the partner's penis in erection. Many therapists employ systematic desensitization (23,25,27,29–33). It is often combined with other techniques, such as muscle exercises (23,34–36), stroking exercises (29,34–37), discussing difficult relational aspects (34), and cognitive therapy (33). Some therapists exchange the relaxation exercises for tranquillizers or hypnosis. The aim of muscle exercises is to teach women to become conscious of their vaginal muscles and to practice contracting and relaxing them. Consciousness is important, because vaginistic women contract their pelvic floor muscles convulsively, without being aware of doing so.

An often used method to gain control of the vaginal muscles was described by Luyens (34). According to this author, a woman can become conscious of her vaginal muscles by looking at her genitals using a hand-mirror and then making squeezing and bearing-down motions with the vagina. Often, first attempts are unsuccessful, because many women are unable to localize these muscle groups and pull in their stomach instead. However, this can be learned by means of pelvic floor muscle exercises. An additional advantage of pelvic floor muscle exercises is that these exercises have a positive effect on the intensity with which genital sensations are experienced during sexual arousal.

The Interactional View

The interactional view assumes that vaginistic complaints have a function in maintaining the balance between partners, or in the emotional functioning of the woman herself. In this sense, the complaint can form a solution! There are very few authors who explain the phenomenon of vaginismus fully on the basis of this view. However, much of the literature mentions the behavior and the personality structure of the male partner. He comes forward as a low self-confidence, anxious, passive, dependent person who is afraid of failure and for whom sex is a loaded subject (27,38,39). The partners of vaginistic women are believed to often suffer from sexual problems themselves, such as impotence and premature ejaculation (29,35,39,40). Despite these problems, the couple usually look very harmonic on the outside. They give the impression of being very well suited (18,37). In a recent study, rates of parital discord were equal to the general population (3). It speaks for itself that within the interactional view, partner-relational therapy and sexual therapy are not considered to be two clearly distinguishable specialties. Both concern the same system of two persons. Although the majority of therapists agree that the partner can play a major role in maintaining the complaints, very few actually involve the male partner in the therapeutic process. This is where we pay the price for the fact that *in vivo* observation is missing from the sexual anamnesis.

The Sociocultural View

Sjenitzer believes that vaginismus is caused by the social position of women in our society and their dissatisfaction with their role (41). According to this author, vaginismus is a protest against the patriarchal norms that reduce women to either a lust object or a mother. In addition, she makes a stand against sexist ideas in the treatment of vaginismus, particularly against placing coitus in the central position in the sexual relationship. The feminist view states clearly that women often seek something in sexuality that is completely different from what men seek. In women, the experience of emotional intimacy is generally a prerequisite for them to enjoy sex. Bezemer developed group therapy for women with vaginistic complaints (42). At the same time, group therapy was organized for the male partners of these patients, led by male therapists. The aim of this therapy was to restore the woman's power over her body and her physical reactions. Thus, a therapy aim such as "coitus" was totally taboo! When a woman has power over her body, she can decide equally well *not* to have sex. A clear example of this view is given in the study by Van Ree who sometimes regards vaginismus as an adequate reaction to an inadequate way of life (43).

The Pain View

In a recent review article, Reissing et al. have raised the question as to the extent to which the existing concept of vaginismus is correct (5). Is the increased pelvic floor muscle tension actually characteristic of vaginismus? In their view, the role of the pelvic floor muscles in vaginismus is identical to the role of the muscles in chronic tension headaches: an important symptom, but not of decisive importance to the diagnosis. Does this apply to the experience of pain? They believe that in vaginistic patients, until now the pain or the changed sensations (dysesthesia) have been unjustly bypassed. Is vaginismus therefore a phobic reaction to penetration? This is indeed the case in some vaginistic women, but it is not clear whether this fear is cause or consequence. In their view, women with vaginismus are suffering from an aversion/phobia for vaginal penetration, or from a genital pain problem, or both. If the aversion/phobia lies in the forefront, then cognitive behavioral therapy and pharmacological intervention are the obvious choice. In contrast, a genital pain problem requires a multidisciplinary approach, such as is also the case with other chronic pain syndromes.

The Overactive Pelvic Floor Muscle View

More than half of the women with vaginismus also report complaints related to urination and/or defecation (44). According to Van de Velde, vaginismus should be regarded as a pelvic floor muscle problem (hyperactivity) and not primarily as a sexual problem. She considers that conditioning is the most likely mechanism behind the involuntary contractions of the pelvic floor muscles, which makes pelvic floor muscle physiotherapy an important part of the treatment.

The Somatic View

From a purely somatic point of view, constriction or an obstruction can be solved by using a scalpel. Although Walthard rejected surgical intervention for the treatment of vaginismus as early as in 1909 (45), and Sikkel-Bufinga (46), who performed a follow-up study found that only one vaginistic patient had benefitted from the surgical knife, until recently a few doctors could still be found who opted for such a surgical approach (47). The least vigorous method is dilatation plasty, in contrast with the far more drastic perineal plasty or levator plasty, in which part of the pelvic floor muscles are also cleaved through the midline. The emotional consequences of such an operation can be enormous. The most important consequence is that the woman loses control of her pelvic floor muscles, together with the control over her body and her right to self-determination. This is even more painful when the phenomenon vaginismus is used as a solution for relationship problems. It is remarkable that although this form of therapy was commonplace until recently, very little has been published on it. Treatment with pharmacotherapy including benzodiazepines and Botulinum toxin injections has been mentioned in the literature but no controlled trials are available (48,49).

The Multidimensional View

According to this vision the two categories of sexual pain disorders, dyspareunia and vaginismus, are heterogenous, multisystemic, and multifactorial disorders that should not be characterized as simply a "disorder of the pelvic floor" or as a "pain problems" or as a "vestibulum problem" or as a "psychological problem." From this point of view for treatment, an integrated approach is recommended (2).

Specific attention is needed for six areas: the mucous membrane, the pelvic floor, the experienced pain, sex and partner therapy, the emotional profile, and the genital mutilation/sexual abuse.

In this vision, there is no "one size fits all" approach and no or–or approach but an and–and approach. The treatment should be individualized to each women, after carefully listening to her story and after she has been well informed about the disease and its natural course and about possible treatments or ways of handling it: care made to measure. It is up to the woman and her partner to decide which treatment they wish to embark on.

TREATMENT FOR VAGINISMUS

The above-described views and treatment models show that there is wide variation in the causal attributes of vaginismus and that this "diagnostic" variety leads to an even wider variety of therapeutic interventions. In itself this is not particularly surprising when we consider that in order to have sexual intercourse in a satisfactory manner, obviously apart from the physical conditions that have to be met, there must also be special knowledge, expertise, attitudes and, last but not least, emotional moods. All this is overruled by motivation: Do I really want to?

A thorough diagnostic procedure in which an inventory is made of somatic, psychological, and social aspects, therefore seems vital in order to choose the best approach. During such a procedure, it is often difficult to say when the diagnostics end and the therapy begins.

The literature shows that it is impossible to make a direct comparison of the effectiveness of the different treatment methods (5,11–13). It is also striking that no studies have appeared that used a pre–post design or a between-groups design, in which for example, a treatment was compared to a waiting list condition (50).

Prediction of treatment by means of psychological variables has thus far been investigated in noncontrolled studies only (51–53). Irrespective of the type of treatment and the specific therapeutic aims, an average success rate of 60–80% is reported. However, if we only look at the examinations that more or less pass the methodological criticism test then the success rate would be about 60% or less (54,55).

These rates suggest that all treatment forms achieve results and as far as this aspect is concerned, they vary very little. This indicates a nonspecific treatment effect. In terms of attention, validation of her complaint, and the patient's feeling of control and competence, the active constituents seem to be effective on a meta level than on a content level. Cost/effectiveness ratios of the diverse treatment forms then become interesting. Behavioral therapy, in comparison with other psychotherapeutic approaches, can be regarded as relatively efficient (56). This finding in combination with the fact that behavioral therapeutic techniques can also be transferred to non-psychotherapists, make the behavioral therapeutic treatment of vaginismus interesting in more than one respect. Each care provider will choose a therapeutic strategy for vaginistic couples on the basis of his or her training. For example, for gynecologists and urologists, in most cases without any specific sexological training, the behavioral therapeutic approach will be the most obvious choice. It works and it is efficient too! However, its application requires more intense effort than just the acquisition of a set of vaginal rods. It is a treatment that is very time-consuming, requires great patience, great empathy, sensitivity to nonverbal signals, and insight into relational interactions. A care provider who intends to treat vaginismus has to be able to take a good sexual history. He or she must be able to signal or interweave ambivalent feelings regarding coitus, sex, the partner, their own body, the desire to have children. He or she must be able to bring to light serious relational problems or severe traumatic experiences (sexual violence!) and he or she has to realize that being able to have sex does not automatically mean that the coitus is enjoyed. Thus in brief, the same applies to every care provider who intends to treat vaginismus as it applies to the patient: Do I really want to?

If the answer is no, then it is better to refer the patient elsewhere. If the answer is yes, then it is highly recommended to follow a suitable training course first.

Treatment Protocol

Introduction

Treatment according to protocol comprises an, at the start, unknown number of sessions. The first session takes ~45–60 min. Subsequent sessions take 20 min. Sessions are held once every 2–4 weeks. Major components of the treatment include information about vaginismus, a physical examination, explanation of the treatment, behavioral therapy, sensation focus exercises, pelvic floor muscle exercises, systematic desensitization, and cognitive therapy. These components do not have a fixed order; they are applied electively. During the exercises and during the consultations, underlying factors (causes and/or problems) can become clear.

It is worthwhile to administer a measurement instrument before and after treatment. With the aid of a measurement instrument, possible comorbidity can be detected and the effect of the intervention can be evaluated. Questionnaires in the English language have the advantage that they are well known in the international literature, which facilitates comparisons of international publications, and that they have been used often in research, which facilitates comparisons between results and populations. However, for local use these questionnaires have to be translated and validated again but this is recommended because of cultural differences. A simple but effective instrument to obtain measurement data is the Visual Analogue Scale. From time to time during the treatment, the woman marks a score on a sliding scale to represent the amount of progress that has been made.

Information About Vaginismus

Categorically, information is given about what vaginismus is, the types of vaginismus (complete, situational, primary, secondary), the difference from dyspareunia, the vicious circle, how often it occurs, the reaction of the partner, the consequences on sexual satisfaction, the wish to have children, pregnancy, delivery, possible causes (psychological, relational, social, physical), the role of the pelvic floor muscles, the relationship between vaginismus and complaints related to micturition and/or defecation, and treatment methods (education, psychological approach, relational therapy, group therapy, treatment with artificial aids, physical treatment). In addition, the aim of treatment is discussed; this could be the realization of pregnancy without coitus, or making coitus possible.

Explanation of the Treatment

Explain that the treatment protocol depends on the aim of treatment. If the aim solely concerns the wish to have children, then treatment can comprise learning to insert a 1 cc syringe into the vagina, filled with semen obtained by masturbation (artificial insemination). This technique can be applied at home at a time during the menstrual cycle that gives the best chance of conception. For every woman with vaginismus, but particularly for a woman who chooses solely for artificial insemination, it is important to realize that vaginismus does not have any predictive value regarding the course of possible childbirth. They have just as much chance as any other woman of an easy or difficult delivery with or without the aid of technical gadgetry. However, it is of great importance that the person who is supervising the delivery is well informed about the problems and takes them into consideration, that is, as little internal examination as possible and, if necessary, as carefully as possible whereby the patient is given control of the situation.

If the aim is coitus, or to be able to insert a tampon or speculum, then treatment will comprise various elements: information about vaginismus, a physical examination, behavioral therapy, self-exploration, pelvic floor muscle exercises, systematic desensitization, and cognitive therapy. Explain precisely what these elements entail. Make it clear to the patient that she must now do things that she will find very unpleasant and would rather avoid. There is going to be hard work, especially at home with the homework assignments. Explain the importance of the homework assignments. Make it clear to the patient that you are trying to teach her to come to terms with her fear of penetration, but that overcoming the fear will not necessarily mean a more satisfactory sex life. Coitus can be very nice, but it is not of overriding importance for the quality of the sexual interaction. As part of the first consultation, a written report may be very helpful.

Physical Examination

In order to detect or exclude physical causes, the nonphysician and physician will have to work together. Especially in the case of vaginismus, it is not always desirable or practical to perform a medical examination straight away. The patient and care provider must make the decision together and also agree when it will take place and who will be there. The medical examination can best be described as an "educative gynecological sexological examination." In a nutshell, it can be described as an examination with "accessories." Although the doctor is gathering information (where do the patient's boundaries lie), he or she also tells the patient about the anatomy of the external genitals and points out what is normal, or shows the patient possible abnormalities. In this way, the examination can sometimes correct a negative self-image, or the doctor can explain to the patient and ideally also to her partner how physical changes and reactions are correlated with sexual problems.

It is extremely important that the patient knows in advance that she has total control over the situation, knows exactly what is going to happen and that she is the one who decides who is going to be there and who is not, and that she knows that during the examination, her boundaries will be respected and safe-guarded. Through this examination, the foundations are laid for a meaningful discussion afterwards, in which all the findings are repeated and it often happens that sexual complaints come to light that the patient has been concealing.

The Context

In concrete terms: Seat yourself comfortably and have the examination couch adjusted for the woman to be sitting. Give the patient a hand-mirror. Also give her the freedom not to look if she does not want to. Allow her partner to look over your shoulder. Take a moistened cotton bud and tell the patient (and her partner if he is present) what you see, what details you are paying close attention to, what is normal, what is abnormal and whether you consider this is playing a role in the patient's complaints. By conducting the examination in this way, you force yourself to make a thorough inspection. In the case of vaginismus, examining the patient using a speculum or the fingers do not form part of the physical examination. Tell the patient before you start that you are not going to do these things. This will save her from anticipatory anxiety and the examination will go more smoothly, which will promote better results. It is also important to ask the patient about her actual experience of the examination while you are busy and not to just assume that she is picking up your reassuring words and signals. An important aspect of the examination is the nonverbal communication: the patient's behavior and that of her partner during the examination often say much more than words can express. Obviously, the nonverbal communication works in both directions—the doctor also constantly sends out signals.

Adequate Spreading

In order to achieve a good view, you should ask the patient's permission to spread the vulva and then ask her to bear-down. The physician might also ask her to spread her vulva herself with her fingers. Adequate spreading is of great importance, otherwise, for example, you might not be able to see hyperaemic foci at the base of the hymen, which form a symptom of the most common cause of dyspareunia in young women, the vulvar vestibulitis syndrome. Adequate spreading also enables the patient to experience the consequences of pelvic floor muscle activity: by bearing-down or coughing, she will be able to see that the entrance to her vagina becomes larger.

Subsequently, you can ask the patient's permission to insert the cotton bud through the hymen while she is bearing-down and assure her that you will stop the procedure immediately if she wishes. If the cotton bud can be inserted easily without any problem (which is very often an eye-opener!), the procedure can be repeated with a finger or with a smooth metal rod that is the slightly thicker than the cotton bud. Hegar rods are extremely useful for this purpose because they are available in many small diameters. If it is possible to proceed to larger diameters during the procedure, you can switch over to vaginal rods. These are plastic rods with different diameters to match the natural situation, that is, the size of the partner's penis.

Measuring of Pain

To measure vulvar pain, the cotton-swab test is widely used (57,58). Pain is diagnosed by palpating different sites around the vulvar vestibule in a clockwise fashion and noting the patient's verbal and physical reactions. However, the cotton-swab test is prone to measurement error when used for experimental purposes or to measure treatment outcome (59). Ideally, the degree of pain should be documented with a diagnostic tool, for example, the vulvalgesiometer (60). It can be used as a diagnostic tool capable of differentiating among women with different types of genital pain, and because of its large range of exertable pressures, it may aid in quantifying the severity of pain (mild, moderate, and severe) experienced by these women. This device also has applications in quantifying changes in vestibular sensitivity as a result of treatment.

The Pelvic Floor

The sheet of pelvic floor muscles can be easily translated for the patient by describing it as a sort of trampoline: an elastic sheet that closes off the lower pelvis and has two openings, the anus and the vagina. The pelvic floor muscles contain both these openings in loops and they determine the discharge diameter of the anus and access diameter of the vagina. Women with dyspareunia or vaginismus contract these muscles in order to voluntarily or involuntarily control the accessibility of the vagina. This results in an inability to relax at times when this would be desirable, for example, during love-making or when being examined on the gynecology couch. Involuntary contraction on the gynecology couch does not infer that this also happens at home.

Inversely, some women can undergo a gynecological examination without any problem, but have vaginistic reactions in other circumstances, depending on what they find threatening. In many cases, the pelvic floor muscles are chronically contracted and feel like "steel cables." Muscles that are constantly contracted will start to cause pain, especially if pressure is also exerted from the other side, such as during an attempt at coitus.

In order to find out pelvic floor muscle problems, the physician places his or her finger between the woman's labia just in front of the vaginal opening and see how that feels. At the same time, she can be advised to reduce the tension in her pelvic floor muscles by repeatedly contracting or relaxing them and giving reversed pressure. This reversed pressure creates room to continue pushing or contracting the muscles, which is followed by relaxation. At the moment of relaxation, the physician moves the finger slowly inside. As the finger moves, keep it dorsally curved to feel the pelvic floor muscle without touching any painful areas at the vestibulum. In the end of the examination, the finger is slowly withdrawn. The use of a lubricant will facilitate the examination and also prevent tissue damage (Sensilube, Sonogel).

If physical abnormalities are found that can cause pain, for example, a stiff hymen or epithelial defects, then the patient may have dyspareunia with secondary pelvic floor muscle hypertonia that contributes to maintaining the complaints. All forms of physical illness or abnormality that cause vaginismus or pain during coitus require medical treatment by a doctor. If the patient has general pelvic floor muscle problems with impaired micturition or defecation, then attention must also be paid to these aspects by means of learning to adopt a correct toilet position and micturition frequency, and breaking the habit of bearing-down during micturition. In the case of the irritable bowel syndrome, dietary measures can be discussed.

Behavioral Therapy

The aim of group or individual behavioral therapy is to break the stimulus–response pattern and regain optimal control over the situation. For the group therapy protocol, the reader is referred to centers where group therapy is given. The protocol described below is for individual behavioral therapy.

Treatment comprises self-exploration, relaxation of the pelvic floor muscles, and systematic desensitization. This can be achieved in a step-by-step exercise program that consists of self-exploration, muscle relaxation exercises, and gradually learning to accept penetration in situations where it is the woman's own expressed wish to do so. Each step requires a great deal of practice; the next step cannot be taken until the previous one has been successfully completed. Every new step can trigger resistance, which manifests itself as anxiety, tension, or pain. Intrapsychological and interpsychological aspects can come to light that require referral to a psychotherapist or relational therapist. It is important to warn the patient right from the start that further referral may be necessary, in order to alert her "not to feel dumped" in a later phase of treatment.

Step 1: Self-exploration

The patient is given the following assignment to do at home in her own peaceful and quiet environment: examine her genitals with a hand-mirror (exposure *in vivo*). A second step is for her to touch her genitals. It is expressly not the aim to experience sexual arousal, but to become accustomed to her genitals. Next she is given the assignment to manipulate her pelvic floor muscles at various intervals, by systematically contracting and relaxing them. In order for her to recognize the feeling, she can be told that the muscles are the same ones that prevent her from inadvertently breaking wind. In this way, assignments are combined with relaxation exercises.

Step 2: Systematic Desensitization

After the successful completion of step 1, the next assignment is for the patient to place her finger between her labia just in front of the vaginal opening and to see how that feels. At the same time, she can be advised to reduce the tension in her pelvic floor muscles by repeatedly contracting or relaxing them and giving reversed pressure. This reversed pressure creates room to continue pushing or contracting the muscles, which is followed by relaxation. At the moment of relaxation, she can push her finger inside, or a cotton bud, hegar rod, vaginal rod, or a vibrator. Disadvantages of cotton buds, hegar rods, vaginal rods, and vibrators are that they are alien to the body and they give an awfully mechanical and coitus-oriented impression. Thus, if the patient has a history of indecent assault, rape, or incest, old fears can be rekindled. Advantages are the variety of diameters that enable gradual habituation. All the advantages and disadvantages of whether or not to use artificial aids in the exercises should be discussed fully prior to any decision-making about this issue. Ultimately, it is the patient's decision. In addition, there is nothing against exercising in a variety of ways, or first with the fingers and if that is unsuccessful, with artificial aids or vice versa.

The patient can do the exercises on her own, in the presence of her partner or together with her partner. She is asked to make time to do the exercises at least two or three times per week. However, a prerequisite is that when she decides to try the exercises, she is feeling relaxed, at peace with herself and is certainly not thinking "I will just do them quickly to get them over with".

Once she has managed to accept penetration of her finger or an artificial aid, she can keep it in place for a period of time and experience what feelings arise on a conscious level and how the tissues feel. Careful movement of the pelvic floor muscles, fingers, or artificial aid will increase the sensations. Then it is the end of the exercise for the moment and the fingers or artificial aid are slowly withdrawn. Short exercise sessions prevent the patient from becoming obsessively preoccupied and also prevent tissue irritation. The use of a lubricant will facilitate the exercises and also prevent tissue damage. Quite apart from this, there is no change in the advice to continue love-making with the partner, albeit with a strict ban on coitus or attempts at coitus.

Step 3

Once the patient is successfully able to insert one finger or an artificial aid (i.e., without anxiety, tension, or pain), the next step is to insert two fingers (at the moment of insertion, one above the other, then moved next to each other) or an artificial aid with a slightly larger diameter. This procedure is repeated until the fingers or artificial aid can be inserted in a relaxed manner and, once inserted, can be moved without anxiety, tension, or pain. If artificial aids are being used and the patient has a male partner, then if she so desires, the procedure can be continued until she can successfully (i.e., in a relaxed manner) insert and move an artificial aid with a diameter that matches the partner's penis. If the patient has a female partner, then being able to insert a finger or dildo in a relaxed manner will suffice. Sometimes when a patient is using vaginal rods, she experiences the progression from one rod to another as being too big. In such cases it is useful to wrap the rod in more and more condoms during each exercise session, in order to make the transition more gradual. In addition, this makes the rod more user-friendly.

Step 4

During treatment, the partner can gradually become more involved in the exercises. All the steps are repeated, starting with the discussion about genital anatomy. In some cases, it is necessary to start with genital "look and feel exercises." Each new step is always discussed thoroughly and tailored to incorporate attention to the thoughts and feelings that arise. Between steps, this usually requires a number of individual and/or relationship-oriented interventions. Sometimes the exercises prove to be a bridge too far and it is necessary to refer the patient to a psychotherapist, relational therapist, or physiotherapist (electrofeedback).

Step 5

It is the patient herself who indicates when she feels the time is right to experiment with her partner. She can choose a moment within or outside the context of love-making, or choose a moment in extension of an exercise session with fingers or artificial aids. In order to prevent the male partner from insisting on penetration while the patient is not yet ready, it can be worthwhile only to tell *her* that the coitus ban has been lifted. When the patient is ready, she takes the leading role (i.e., determines the timing and position) and he makes himself totally subservient. The penis is inserted in exactly the same manner as that employed in the penetration exercises. Both partners should be warned that in the initial stages, love-making will seem rather technical or mechanical, but that gradually the technicalities will sink into the background.

Cognitive Therapy

The cognitive therapeutic approach is based on the notion that between stimulus and response, there are factors within the individual that determine the nature and intensity of the response. Interventions in this field aim to change the behavior and feelings of the woman by teaching her to think and behave differently. To achieve this, the doctor as primary treating physician of vaginistic patients, will probably require the assistance of a psychologist/sexologist, psychotherapist, or relational therapist.

Owing to the fact that vaginismus is often a conditioned response, the role of cognitive therapy is small. The active ingredient in cognitive therapy is therefore to break the conditioned response, that is, "just get on with things" (exposure *in vivo*). Women with vaginismus will undoubtedly have irrational thoughts of "too thick," "does not fit," and so on, especially when the complaints have been present for some time. Although such thoughts can be removed cognitively by means of good patient education, in principle, this will have little or no effect on the occurrence of the complaints. Many patients have followed this path of little success. The most important aspect of cognitive therapy therefore is not so much removing the complaint, but instead motivating the patient, offering insight into the origination of the complaint, and further tackling the problem if it appears to contain a strong rational component. Particularly if the woman's body is expressing what she cannot put into words, cognitive therapy is suitable in the form of:

> cognitive restructuring; whether or not with the aid of RET techniques, detecting, and changing dysfunctional thought patterns;
> increasing the patient's ability to solve problems, for example, in the form of social expertise training in which she learns to better express her

sexual feelings and motives towards her partner, particularly the dictation of her boundaries.

In summary we can say that in the treatment of vaginismus, diverse interventions can play a role at any time in the treatment process.
Generally, areas for special focus are:

increasing sexual knowledge;
reformulating (aspects of) the complaint;
decreasing inhibiting thoughts;
increasing positive thoughts;
learning to tune into positive physical feelings;
learning to use one's imagination for sexual fantasies.

In relationship-oriented sexual counseling, attention can also be paid to:

increasing mutual assertiveness;
improving communicative expertise.

REFERENCES

1. Basson R, Berman J, Burnett A, Derogatis L, Ferguson D, Fourcroy J et al. Report of the international consensus development conference on female sexual dysfunction: definitions and classifications. J Urol 2000; 1163(3):888–893.
2. Lu TF, Basson R, Rosen R, Guiliano F, Khoury S, Montorsi F (eds). Sexual Medicine. Sexual Dysfunctions in Men and Women. 2nd International Consultation on Sexual Dysfunctions. Health Publications, Paris, 2004:932. ISBN 0-9546956-0-7.
3. Reissing ED, Binik YM, Khalifé S, Cohen D, Amsel MA. Etiological correlates of vaginismus: sexual and physical abuse, sexual knowledge, sexual self-schema, and relationship adjustment. J Sex Marital Ther 2003; 29:47–59.
4. Van Lankveld JJDM, Grotjohann Y. Psychiatric comorbidity in heterosexual couples with sexual dysfunction assessed with the Composite International Diagnostic Interview. Arch Sex Behav 2000; 29(5):479–498.
5. Reissing ED, Binik YM, Khalifé S. Does vaginimus exist? A critical review of the literature. J Nerv Ment Dis 1999; 187(5):261–274.
6. Meana M, Binik YM, Khalife S, Cohen D. Dyspareunia: sexual dysfunction or pain syndrome? J Nerv Ment Dis 1997; 185(9):561–569.
7. Kruiff de MD, Ter Kuile MM, Weijenborg PThM, Van Lankveld JJDM. Vaginismus and dyspareunia: is there a difference in clinical presentation? J Psychosom Obstet Gynaecol 2000; 21:149–155.
8. Van Lankveld JJDM, Brewaeys AM, Ter Kuile MM, Weijenborg PThM. Difficulties in the differential diagnosis of vaginismus, dyspareunia and mixed sexual pain disorder. J Psychosom Obstet Gynaecol 1995; 16(4):201–209.
9. Van der Velde J, Everaerd W. Voluntary control over pelvic floor muscles in women with and without vaginistic reactions. Int Urogynecol J 1999; 10:230–236.
10. Van de Velde J, Laan E, Everaerd W. Vaginismus, a component of a general defense mechanism: an investigation of pelvic floor muscle activity during exposure to

emotion-inducing fil excerpt in women with and without vaginismus. Int Urogynecol J Pelv Floor Dysfunct 2001; 12:328–331.

11. Van de Wiel HBM, Jaspers JPM, Weijmar Schultz WCM. Treatment of vaginismus; a review of concepts and treatment modalities. J Psychosom Obstet Gynecol 1990; 1:1–18.

12. Heiman JR, Meston CM. Empirically validated treatment for sexual dysfunction. Ann Rev Sex Res 1997; 8:148–194.

13. O'Donohue W, Dopke CA, Swingen DN. Psychotherapy for female sexual dysfunction. A review. Clin Psych Rev 1997; 17:537–566.

14. Holstege G. The emotional motor system in relation to the supraspinal control of micturition and mating behavior. Brain Res 1998; 92:103–109.

15. Blok BFM, Sturms LM, Holstege G. A PET study on cortical and subcortical control of pelvic floor muscles. J Comp Neurol 1997; 389:535–544.

16. Blok BFM, Sturms LM, Holstege G. Brain activation during micturition in women. Brain 1998; 121(Pt 11):2033–2042.

17. Basson R, Leiblum S, Brotto L, Derogatis L, Fourcroy J, Fugl-Meyer K, Graztiottin, Heiman J, Laan E, Meston C, Van Lankveld J, Weijmar Schultz W. Definitions of women's sexual dysfunction reconsidered: advocating expansion and revision. J Psychosom Obstet Gynecol 2003; 24(3).

18. Musaph H. Vaginisme. Een seksuologische beschouwing [Vaginismus, a Sexological View]. Haarlem: De Erven F. Bohn N.V. 1965.

19. Derogatis LR, Meyer JK, King KM. Psychopathology in individuals with sexual dysfunction. Am J Psych 1981; 138:757–763.

20. Kennedy P, Doherty N, Barnes J. Primary vaginismus: a psychometric study of both partners. Sex Marital Ther 1995; 10:9–22.

21. Van de Velde J, Everaerd W. The relationship between involuntary pelvic floor muscle activity, muscle awareness and experienced threat in women with and without vaginismus. Behav Res Ther 2001; 39:395–408.

22. Van der Velde J, Everaerd W. Vaginismus, a component of a general defensive reaction. An investigation of pelvic floor muscle activity during exposure to emotion-inducing film excerpts in women with and without vaginismus. Int Urogynecol J 2001; 12:183–192.

23. Haslam MT. The treatment of psychogenic dyspareunia by reciprocal inhibition. Br J Psych 1965; 3:280–282.

24. DeMoor W. Vaginismus: etiology and treatment. Am J Psychother 1972; 26:207–215.

25. Kaplan HS. The classification of female sexual dusfunctions. J Sex Marital Ther 1974; 2:124–239.

26. Jackman LS. Differentating between dyspareunia and vaginismus. Med Aspect Hum Sex 1976; 2:113–114.

27. Brinkman W. Langdurige gedragstherapie in een geval van vaginisme [Longlasting behavioral therapy for vaginismus]. Tijdschrift voor Gedragstherapie 1975; 1:54–69.

28. Wolpe J. Psychotherapy by Reciprocal Inhibition. Stanford: University Press, 1958.

29. Masters WH, Johnson VE. Human Sexual Inadequacy. Boston: Little, Brown, 1970.

30. Malleson J. Sex problems in marriage, with particular reference to coital discomfort and the unconsummated marriage. Practitioner 1954; 172:389–396.

31. Gaafar A. Vaginismus: a simple effective office procedure for its treatment. Alex Med J 1962; 6:566–571.

32. Cooper AJ. An innovation in the behavioral treatment of a case of non-consummation due to vaginismus. Br J Psych 1969; 1:721–722.
33. Shahar A, JaffeY. Behavior and cognitive therapy in the treatment of vaginismus: a case study. Cognit Ther Res 1978; 1:57–60.
34. Luyens M. Behandeling van vaginisme [Treatment of vaginismus]. Tijdschrift voor Seksuologie 1980; 3:77–91.
35. Lamont JA. Vaginismus. Am J Obstet Gynecol 1978; 131:632–636.
36. Reamy K. The treatment of vaginismus by the gynecologist: an eclectic approach. J Obstet Gynecol 1982; 59:58–63.
37. Thoben A, Moors J. Vaginisme. Een behandelingsvorm en een discussie over een aantal aspecten [Vaginismus. A treatment modality and a discussion about several aspects]. Deventer: Van Loghum Slaterus, 1977.
38. Friedman U. Virgin Wives: A Study of Unconsummated Marriages. London: Tavistock, 1984.
39. Drenth J, Bezemer W. Angst en pijn [Fear and pain]. In: Drenth J, ed. Seks als probleem (Sex as a Problem). Haarlem: Holland, 1979.
40. Steege JF. Dyspareunia and vaginismus. Clin Obstet Gynecol 1984; 3:750–759.
41. Sjenitzer T. Dichtzitten: een protest tegen verplicht neuken [Being closed: a protest against compulsory fucking]. Psychologie en Maatschappij 1980; 29–39.
42. Bezemer W. Een groepsbehandeling van vaginisme [Group therapy for vaginismus]. Tijdschrift voor Seksuologie 1985; 1:16–24.
43. Van Ree F. 'Gezond' (secundair) vaginisme; een casuïstische mededeling [A case of 'Healthy' (secundary) vaginismus]. Tijdschrift voor Psychotherapie 1985; 4:285–292.
44. Van der Velde J. The Pelvic Floor, the Mechanism of Vaginismus. Thesis Amsterdam, 1999.
45. Walthard M. Die psychogene Atiologie und die Psychotherapie des Vaginismus. Münchener Medizinische Wochenschrift 1909; 39:1998–2000.
46. Sikkel Buffinga AJ. Nogmaals: vaginisme [Once again: vaginismus]. Tijdschrift voor Seksuologie 1986; 10:152–156.
47. Frenken J, Van Tol P. Seksuele problemen in de gynaecologenpraktijk [Sexual problems in gynecological practice]. Med Contact 1987; 5:150–154.
48. Mikhail AR. Treatment of vaginismus by i.v. diazepam (Valium®) abreaction interviews. Acta Psychiatr Scand 1976; 53:328–332.
49. Brin MF. Treatment of vaginismus with botulinum toxin injections. Lancet 1997; 349:252–253.
50. McGuire H, Hawton K. Interventions for vaginismus (Cochrane Review). In: The Cochrane Library. Issue 1, 2002. Oxford: Update Software.
51. Scholl GM. Prognostic variables in treating vaginismus. Obstet Gynecol 1988; 72:231–235.
52. Hawton K, Catalan J. Sex therapy for vaginismus: characteristics of couples and treatment outcome. Sex Marital Ther 1990; 4:39–48.
53. Schnyder U, Schnyder-Lüthi C, Ballinari P, Blaser A. Therapy for vaginismus: *in vivo* versus *in vitro* desensitization. Can J Psychtr 1998; 43:941–944.
54. Clement U, Pfafflin F. Changes in personality scores among couples subsequent to sex therapy. Arch Sex Behav 1983; 90:908–913.
55. Hawton K, Catalan J. Sex therapy for vaginismus: characteristics of couples and treatment outcome. Sex Marital Ther 1990; 5:39–48.

56. DiLoreto AO. Comparitive Psychotherapy: An Experimental Analysis. Chicago: Aldine-Atherton, 1971.
57. Friedrich EG Jr. The vulvar vestibule. J Reprod Med 1983; 28:773–777
58. Friedrich EG Jr. Vulvar vestibulits syndrome. J Reprod Med 1987; 32:110–115
59. Pukall CF, Payne KA, Binik YM, Khalifé S. Pain measurement in vulvodynia. J Sex Marital Ther 2003; 29(s):110–120.
60. Pukall CF, Binik YM, Khalifé S. A new instrument for pain assessment in vulvar vestibulitis syndrome. Submitted.

12

Paraphilias

Cynthia S. Osborne and Thomas N. Wise

Johns Hopkins University School of Medicine, Baltimore, Maryland, USA

INTRODUCTION

One literal translation of paraphilia—love beyond the usual—casts a benign, if not romantic, hue over a subject that has been marked by considerable professional dissidence (1). Although this chapter will not provide a critique of the paraphilia construct, any responsible discussion of the paraphilias must acknowledge the cultural underpinnings of efforts to define normality vs. abnormality in human behavior. This theoretical debate plays out in the literature, where a range of positions are evident, from loyal adherence to traditional definitions of pathological sex to advocacy for the elimination or radical revision of the paraphilia diagnostic category (2–4). Only a greater empirical base will resolve this controversy and provide a reasonably objective basis on which clinicians can define the boundary between "normal" and "abnormal" sexuality.

The focus of this chapter is not to engage the debate regarding normalcy, but to provide a clear conceptualization of the paraphilias, a review of etiological theories, and an articulation of current treatments. A core assumption throughout the chapter is that the most reasoned understanding of the paraphilias is one that integrates both biological and psychological perspective.

DEFINING AND CONCEPTUALIZING THE PARAPHILIAS

Paraphilias are defined as psychosexual disorders in which significant distress or impairment in an important domain of functioning results from recurrent, intense sexual urges, fantasies, or behaviors generally involving an unusual object, activity, or situation (5). Although the DSM-IV-TR lists eight specific paraphilias, paraphilia as a broad category represents a heterogeneous group of disorders and diverse behavioral expressions. The DSM-IV-TR defines three subtypes of paraphilias:

> those involving nonhuman objects,
> those involving the suffering or humiliation of oneself or one's partner,
> those involving children or other nonconsenting persons.

The minimum time duration for a fantasy, urge, or behavior to qualify as a disorder is 6 months. Recurrent by definition, the paraphilias are generally chronic and lifelong, although the associated fantasies, urges, and behaviors diminish over the life span in some adults. Paraphilic fantasies and urges may vary in frequency and intensity over time, often beginning in childhood or adolescence and intensifying in adulthood. Acute episodes may occur and, in some individuals, resolve quickly with treatment. The paraphilic fantasy or behavior may be obligatory, or required for arousal, or nonobligatory, where an individual experiences arousal in response to other erotic stimuli as well. It may be nonobligatory in early life but become increasingly obligatory over time or with increased engagement with the pattern. Individuals with one paraphilia may be prone to develop others, and multiple paraphilias in one individual appear to occur with high frequency (6,7).

The present diagnostic categorizing system, in which paraphilias are defined according to the specific deviant focus, implies that each paraphilia represents a distinct disease process. Difficulties stemming from this conceptualization are apparent in the common scenario of multiple paraphilias co-occurring in one individual, where the multiple paraphilia conceptualization suggests that each paraphilic interest in the individual represents a distinct pathological phenomenon. No clear evidence exists for such an assertion and, further, it is more clinically useful to conceptualize the scenario as multiple paraphilic variations reflecting a shared underlying phenomenon. Lehne and Money proposed the term "multiplex paraphilia," noting variations of paraphilic content expressed over an individual's life span, but all influenced by a common underlying deficit or etiological process (7,8).

Prevalence

There is little reliable data regarding the prevalence of the paraphilias. As individuals with paraphilias rarely present in mental health or medical facilities, it is assumed that the prevalence in the general population is higher than estimates based on clinical samples. A 1983 review of psychiatric hospital records revealed a 0.08% incidence of fetishism (9). In contrast, a 10-year review of the records from the authors' specialty clinic showed a 5.4% incidence of fetishism, highlighting the variation in patient samples depending on contextual variables.

The same review revealed an overall prevalence rate of 24% for the paraphilias and paraphilia not otherwise specified relative to sexual dysfunction, sexual pain, and gender identity disorder diagnoses. For the specific paraphilias, the following rates were revealed: transvestic fetishism 35%, paraphilia NOS 31%, sexual masochism 8%, exhibitionism 7.4%, pedophilia 6.7%, fetishism 5.4%, voyeurism and sexual sadism 2.7% each, and frotteurism <1%. Again, it is important to note that patient samples are not representative of the general population and patient samples in specialty clinics are not representative of general medical or psychiatric samples.

Much of the prevalence data for the offending paraphilias have been drawn from sexual offender arrest or treatment records. Such records often do not distinguish between paraphilic and nonparaphilic offenders. As a result, the prevalence of specific paraphilias among sex offenders or in the general population is unknown and data gathered from arrest records likely under-reflect the incidence of paraphilias (10).

Gender and the Paraphilias

As far as is known, the paraphilias occur predominantly in males, with the exception of sexual masochism, which is also commonly observed in females, although still with less frequency than in males. Exceptions have been reported, including single case reports of female genital exhibitionism and female fetishism (11–13). Two recent reports described, collectively, five cases of accidental autoerotic death in females, with evidence strongly suggesting the presence of the paraphilia asphyxiophilia, in which cerebral hypoxia is induced for the purpose of generating or intensifying sexual arousal (14,15). Gosink reported that autoerotic deaths occur differentially in males and females at a ratio of more than 50:1. It is not known to what extent this figure reflects gender differences in the prevalence of other paraphilias. Another recent report described multiple paraphilias in a female, including fetishistic arousal to men in diapers as well as sexual sadism characterized by extreme preoccupation with sexual torture and a collection of detailed plans to murder young males to whom she was sexually attracted (16). Another report described a female sex offender who displayed elements of hypersexuality, sexual sadism, sexual masochism, and pedophilia, including violent sexual fantasies involving children (17).

Pedophilia in females is rare but has been reported. A recent review of records in the authors' clinic revealed, among 149 individuals diagnosed with one or more paraphilias, one female was diagnosed with pedophilia, one with sexual sadism, and five with paraphilia NOS. All other subjects were male. Chow and Choy recently reported on the positive response to treatment with the SSRI sertraline in a female diagnosed with pedophilia (18). True prevalence of pedophilia is difficult to determine from sex offender records, as offenders are not commonly assessed for deviant sexual interests and many studies fail to differentiate between sexually deviant and nondeviant offenders. Therefore, the relative occurrence of pedophilia in male and female sex offenders is not known.

A 1991 review by Wakefield and Underwager revealed that, among female sex offenders who were assessed for sexual deviancy, most were determined to not have pedophilia, suggesting that factors other than sexual gratification often motivate the behavior (19). Some gender differences in clinical character-istics between males and females with pedophilia have been suggested. Most sig-nificantly, while history of sexual victimization is reported with some frequency by both males and females with pedophilia, the higher frequency in females suggests that history of sexual abuse may have greater etiological significance in the development of pedophilia in females than in males (F. Berlin, personal communication, 2003) (19).

In summary, while the literature strongly supports the assumption that the paraphilias occur predominantly in males, there are increasing reports of paraphilias in females. The occurrence of paraphilias in females may be a less rare clinical phenomenon than previously assumed.

Comorbidity

There is considerable co-occurrence of other paraphilias in patients diagnosed with one (7,20–24). A recent study of men with pedophilia showed the following comorbidity patterns with additional paraphilias: voyeurism 13.3%, frotteurism 11%, exhibitionism, transvestic fetishism, and paraphilia NOS 6.7% each, and fetishism and sexual sadism 4.4% each (25).

Kafka and Prentky conducted a study of lifetime comorbid nonsexual diag-noses in males with paraphilias and paraphilia-related disorders (26). Almost 72% had a lifetime prevalence of a mood disorder, with dysthymic disorder occurring most frequently. Interestingly, there were no significant differences in comorbidity patterns between men with paraphilias and men with paraphi-lia-related disorders, with the exception of retrospectively diagnosed childhood ADHD, which was identified in 50% of the paraphilia group but in only 17% of the paraphilia-related group. Similar comorbidity patterns were found in a later study (27).

It is known that many individuals with fetishistic cross-dressing have comorbid psychiatric disorders. A sample of transvestites who sought psychiatric evaluation in a sexual behaviors clinic were found to have high rates of mood or substance abuse disorders (28). This was consistent with a previous study wherein 80% of gender dysphoric transvestites qualified for a concurrent Axis I diagnosis, generally an affective disorder (29). A recent study of comorbidity between alcoholism and specific paraphilias found that >50% of sexual sadists were alcohol dependent, with the lowest association between transvestism and alcoholism (30).

A recent study of the co-occurrence of personality disorders in sex offen-ders revealed that 72% of the sample had at least one personality disorder (31).

The most prevalent was antisocial personality disorder. All subjects had impulse control disorder and a paraphilia, but it is not clear how many of the offenders in the study had a diagnosis of pedophilia or other specific paraphilias.

In another recent study, Raymond et al. (25) found that 93% of individuals with pedophilia had at least one lifetime comorbid axis I diagnosis. Highest were comorbid mood and anxiety disorders. There was high co-occurrence of alcohol and cannabis use disorders, and 60% had comorbid personality disorders, in particular obsessive-compulsive, antisocial, avoidant, and narcissistic. Contrary to commonly held assumptions, there was a relatively low incidence—23%—of antisocial personality disorder.

THE DSM-IV-TR LISTED PARAPHILIAS

The eight specifically listed paraphilias and paraphilia NOS are summarized in Fig. 12.1. They are discussed here in logically grouped form.

Voyeurism, Exhibitionism, and Frotteurism

Voyeurism, exhibitionism, and frotteurism have also been found to frequently co-occur. It has been proposed that they may be fundamentally related through shared underlying mechanisms (32). Voyeurism and exhibitionism involve visual processing of sexual stimuli from a distance, without direct physical contact with a partner, whereas in frotteurism physical contact is made. The voyeur "looks" in order to "receive" an alluring sexual image, the exhibitionist "shows" in order to "transmit" a sexual invitation, and the frotteur touches in order to "feel" intimate (33).

Voyeurism

The paraphilic focus in voyeurism is sexual fantasies, urges, or behaviors involving observing unsuspecting persons, usually unclothed and/or engaged in sexual activity. Federoff has described the "requirement" aspect of voyeurism and the other paraphilias as the central feature distinguishing them from nonparaphilic equivalents (34). It is not simply the act of watching a women naked, undressing, or engaging in sex that arouses the paraphilic voyeur; the victim's lack of suspicion that she is being observed and the risk of being discovered are central to the voyeur's arousal. Like the exhibitionist, the voyeur rarely makes contact with his victim. His ritual often is accompanied by masturbation during or after the voyeuristic episode.

Money has described variants of voyeurism (33). They include pictophilia, or dependence on viewing pornography for arousal, and troilism, or dependence for arousal on observing one's partner "on hire or loan" to a third party while engaged in sexual activity. The internet provides increasing opportunities for such paraphilia variants to thrive.

A paraphilia involves, over at least a 6-month period, recurrent, intense sexually arousing fantasies, sexual urges or behaviors. The targets of the fantasies, urges or behavior reflect three subtypes of paraphilia:
1) non-living objects
2) suffering or humiliation of self or partner
3) children or other nonconsenting persons

Paraphilia	Subtype	Criterion A *Focal content of fantasies, urges, behaviors*	Criterion B *Action on urges or distress or impairment*	Criterion C *Other criterion*
Fetishism	1) Nonliving objects	Arousal involving use of nonliving objects	Resultant distress or impairment	*Type of Object Criterion:* Objects not limited to female attire or devices used for tactile genital stimulation, e.g. vibrator
Transvestic Fetishism	1) Nonliving objects	Arousal involving cross-dressing	Resulting distress or impairment	No age criteria
Sexual sadism	2) Suffering or humiliation of partner or 3) Children or other nonconsenting persons	Arousal involving psychological or physical suffering of others	Action on urges with unconsenting person or resulting distress	None
Sexual masochism	2) Suffering or humilation of self	Arousal involving being made to psychologically or physically suffer	Resulting distress or impairment	None
Exhibitionism	3) Other unconsenting persons	Arousal involving exposing one's genitals	Action on urges or resulting distress	None
Voyeurism	3) Other unconsenting persons	Arousal involving observing others naked, disrobing or engaging in sexual activity	Action on urges or resulting distress	None
Frotteurism	3) Other unconsenting persons	Arousal involving touching or rubbing against others	Action on urges or resulting distress	None
Pedophilia	3) Children	Arousal involving prebuscent child	Action on urges or resulting distress	*Age criterion:* Individual is at least 16 years old and at least 5 years older than the child
Paraphilia NOS	1), 2) or 3) Any category of focus	Any focal content not already described in a listed paraphilia	Resulting distress of impairment*	No age criteria

*While the DSM-IV-TR does not list any Criterion B requirements, the authors assume the intent of consistency with the 8 listed paraphilias

Figure 12.1 Summary of DSM-IV-TR criteria for paraphilia.

Exhibitionism

In exhibitionism, the individual displays his genitals to an unsuspecting person. The exhibitionist ordinarily becomes aroused in response to the shocked response of a stranger or to the fantasy that the stranger becomes aroused in response to his display. A response of indifference may fuel a conpulsion to repeat the behavior until the craving is satisfied.

Exhibitionism must be distinguished from "nudist" interests, such as enjoyment of vacationing at nude beaches and resorts, and from prank behaviors, such as flashing and mooning. While sometimes offensive or illegal, these do not involve sexual arousal. Fedoroff has stated that exhibitionists have no interest in experiences such as nude beaches, where social norms are intolerant of overt expressions of sexual arousal (34). However, in the authors' research, a small number of diagnosed exhibitionists have reported such overlapping interests and behaviors. A exhibitionistic variant that reflects this overlap is the seeking of approval or validation, such as in the form of applause, as the exhibitionist perceives his victims more as an audience, as does the flasher, than as individuals upon whom he perpetrates harm.

Most exhibitionists and voyeurs are heterosexual men who seek out female victims. Some seek audiences of particular age ranges, such as children or adolescents. In these cases, it is critical to assess for a primary or co-occurring diagnosis of pedophilia. Some seek only adult victims and others are indiscriminate regarding age of their audience.

Frotteurism

Frotteurism is a paraphilic preference for rubbing one's genitals against an unsuspecting person. This paraphilia most often occurs in crowded public places where the frotteur disguises his behavior as an accidental result of crowd or vehicle motion. The frotteur tries to escape after accomplishing contact, to avoid confrontation or arrest. He may fantasize about an intimate, exclusive relationship with his victim (35). He may also fondle his victim's genitals or breasts, a variant of frotteurism known as toucherism (33). Sexual arousal in response to watching other men engage in frotteurism is described as another variant (36).

Like other sexual offenders, exhibitionists, voyeurs, and frotteurs may use cogtive distortions to rationalize, justify, and minimize the negative impact of their behaviors. The voyeur may blame the victim for leaving a window open to outside view, claiming that she wants to be seen; the exhibitionist may believe that others find his display funny rather than offensive; voyeurs and exhibitionists may perceive a harmlessness to their acts because no one is physically touched; the frotteur, who denies intentionality, believes that no harm is done because no one is "meant" to be touched.

Sexual Sadism and Sexual Masochism

Sexual sadism denotes sexual arousal and excitement in response to the psychological or physical suffering of another, whereas sexual masochism denotes a preferred fantasy of selfsuffering. The term sexual sadism derives from the name of the 18th century French aristocrat and pornographic author, Marquis de Sade, who reportedly lived a disreputable adult life abusing young prostitutes. The term sexual masochism was coined by the 19th century psychiatrist Richard von Krafft-Ebing, who derived the term from the name of the well-known German novelist Leopold von Sacher-Masoch, who was reported to have high interest in images of brutality, and in fantasies of being enslaved by a beautiful and torturing woman. Freud was the first to combine both terms—sadism and masochism—into the expression sadomasochism.

The term sadomasochism suggests a fundamental link between sexual sadism and sexual masochism. Although not all masochists also practice sadism and vice versa, factors distinguishing sadism from masochism in any one individual may be subtle and paradoxes may be inherent to both the masochist's and the sadist's positions. The supposedly submissive masochist holds control and defines the limits of activity, whereas the sadist suffers a dependence on control (34). For example, the man who erotically enjoys being beaten appears at first glance to be a masochist. Thorough assessment, however, may reveal that he is most aroused by the sadistic experience of controlling his partner by pushing her as far as he can, against her will, to inflict pain on him. The more she resists, the more aroused he is. Only a keen understanding of these subtleties and a detailed investigation of the partners' overt behaviors and internal experiences elucidate an accurate diagnostic formulation.

The incidence of either sexual sadism or sexual masochism is unknown but both appear to be more common in individuals of middle and upper socioeconomic groups. Some utilize prostitutes to act out their fantasies (37). Baumeister estimates that between 5% and 10% of the population engage in some form of recreational sadomasochistic activity, where light discomfort, but not severe pain or injury, is commonly inflicted (38). Far fewer have engaged in sex play where sadomasochistic fantasies are acted out on a regular and preferred basis. Nevertheless, the prevalence of sadomasochistic social clubs suggests that these preferences are not rare. Surveys of sadomasochistic magazine readers and club members suggest that masochistic interests are more common than sadistic interests.

The actual behaviors, as well as their intensity, associated with sadomasochistic preferences vary greatly (39). Spanking or being spanked is common, often using implements such as whips, canes, or hairbrushes. Also common are tying, blindfolding, or handcuffing, or the masochistic reciprocal of being tied, blindfolded, or handcuffed. More rarely, acute pain is inflicted, such as by applying burning candles to bare skin or piercing the skin with sharp objects. Although it is commonly asserted that sadomasochistic partners maintain tightly controlled parameters to avoid serious injury, activities can get out of control and occasionally do lead to injury. In S&M clubs, individuals may be suspended from ceilings or confined in cages. Such behaviors underscore, in the eyes of some theorists, both control and hostility as core elements in sadomasochism. Among the most dangerous of activities are those that involve choking and strangling. Even the most liberal advocates of recreational S&M warn against "breath control play" or asphyxiophilia, asserting that no amount of care can reliably prevent death (40).

Fetishism and Transvestic Fetishism

Fetishism

Fetishism was first described in 1886 by Richard von Krafft-Ebing and in 1887 by French psychologist Alfred Binet (41–43). The essential feature is the necessity for an inanimate object to achieve or maintain sexual arousal, either in fantasy or in actual behavior. The fetish is often preferred or required for arousal, egosyntonic, and rarely the cause of personal distress. Individuals may experience sexual dysfunction when engaging sexually without use of the fetishistic object or fantasy.

Fetishism is demarcated from paraphilia not otherwise specified by the exclusion of body parts from the definition of fetishism. Fetishism is definitionally limited to the use of nonliving objects and often features masturbation while holding, rubbing, or smelling the object, whereas fetish-like preferences related to the human body or other living creatures are generally coded as paraphilia not otherwise specified (5). These categorical distinctions and their rationale are unclear and are also the source of professional debate (44). According to DSM-IV-TR nosology, for example, what is commonly referred to as "foot fetishism" is a form of partialism and is coded, therefore, as paraphilia NOS (302.9). Many clinicians and researchers, however, conceptualize fetishism as not limited to nonliving objects but, rather, including arousal to part objects (body parts) as well. In this conceptualization, foot fetishism and other part object paraphilias are coded as fetishes (302.81) (20,45).

There is very limited data about fetishistic individuals, since they rarely seek treatment. Many studies are in the form of single case reports. A review by Chalkley and Powell examined the clinical characteristics of 48 fetishists (9). The sample was predominantly male; 22% were homosexual; the majority described preferences for multiple fetishistic objects; and soft textured fabrics were more arousing than hard textures such as rubber.

In his study of Internet chat groups, Junginger found feminine underwear, rubber objects, and body parts such as feet, toes, legs, hair, and ears to be among the most common, although it also appears quite common to fetishize the form or texture of an object, such as silk or rubber. Discussion groups related to diapers and enemas were also found to be common (46). An interesting phenomenon is the shifting of fetish trends over time. Mason has pointed out that a century ago objects made of velvet and silk were preferred, whereas today rubber and leather appear to be more common (44).

A brief Internet search dispels any doubt regarding the high prevalence and diversity of fetishistic curiosity in modern culture. A search, during the summer of 2003, of the word "fetish" drew a list of 359 possible sites and 1192 possible pages, offering both the curious and the desperate virtual buffet of fetishistic opportunities.

Transvestic Fetishism

In transvestic fetishism, cross-dressing in feminine apparel is fetishistically used, or the fantasy of such via autogynephilic—meaning love of self—imagery. The term transvestism was coined by the German sexologist Magnus Hirschfeld (47). DSM-IV-TR criteria require that a heterosexual male experience "recurrent, intense sexually arousing fantasies, sexual urges, or behaviors involving cross-dressing" (5,48). The fantasies and behaviors must cause distress or impairment in psychosocial or occupational functioning. The diagnosis is subcategorized to specify whether gender dysphoria, or discomfort with one's biologic sexual designation, is or is not present. This dimension varies greatly among the cross-dressing population. Some transvestites develop marked distress about their biologic designation and seek sexual reassignment, whereas others express no such wish. Blanchard used the term transvestic autogynephilia, literally meaning "love of oneself as a woman," to refer to the core feature of sexual excitement in response to cross-gender behaviors or fantasies, which include but are not limited to cross-dressing, in the transvestic fetishist (49).

Cross-dressing itself is not diagnostic of transvestic fetishism. Early investigators found cross-dressers to report a wide range of behaviors. The nuclear transvestite clearly and exclusively fulfills DSM diagnostic criteria. Other cross-dressers engage in some bisexual or homosexual experiences, although their basic orientation is heterosexual (50). Still others are effeminate homosexuals whose cross-dressing is in no way fetishistic.

Many transvestic individuals do not seek psychiatric evaluation or do so only if discovered by a spouse or family member or if they become gender dysphoric. Thus, knowledge is extremely limited regarding the phenomenological features of fetishistic cross-dressers who do not seek psychiatric assistance. When fetishistic cross-dressers seek evaluation for gender dysphoria or for sexual reassignment surgery, they often minimize their arousal patterns when cross-dressed. Resources such as local transsexual support groups and Internet sites may counsel individuals to minimize disclosures that might jeopardize their hopes for surgical or hormonal reassignment. Thus, patients are increasingly savvy about what is expected during psychiatric assessment. The clinician must be aware of these phenomena and that fetishistic arousal is often denied.

A survey of subscribers to a magazine for transvestites offers a broader picture of men reporting themselves to be cross-dressers (51). The vast majority were heterosexual, although almost one-third had some homosexual experiences. Cross-dressing was reported to begin before the age of 10 in two-thirds and the majority noted that cross-dressing allowed them to express a different and preferred side of their personality. The respondents, 57% of whom were above the age of 40, reported that they experienced sexual excitement and orgasm while cross-dressed only occasionally. In total, 75% had experienced the need to purge cross-dressing by throwing out all of their feminine clothes and attempting to renounce the need to cross-dress; 83% reported that their wives were aware of the cross-dressing but only 28% experienced their wives as accepting of it. A distinct minority felt themselves to be a woman trapped inside a man's body, while three-quarters felt that they were men with a feminine side. The majority felt that they were equally masculine and feminine and almost one-half were interested in utilizing female hormones. Only 17% would have sexual reassignment, if possible, and 45% had at some time consulted a psychologist or psychiatrist. Two-thirds of those who had sought therapy reported it as helpful. When compared with a similar survey 25 years earlier, this figure reflected a dramatic difference in those endorsing help by psychotherapy, perhaps suggesting greater understanding of the disorder by the mental health profession (52). The majority of cross-dressers in both surveys were primarily heterosexual. Some males, colloquially designated as "drag queens," cross-dress to mimic feminine behavior satirically rather than fetishistically. Such individuals do not meet criteria for the diagnosis of transvestic fetishism (53).

Transvestic fetishists report a spectrum of behaviors and cognitions. It is important to note that for some, the need for erotic arousal abates over time. As the erotic cross-dresser ages, his cross-dressing may be used more to reduce anxiety than to produce sexual arousal (54).

The content of transvestic fantasy varies. It may be of the self with female genitals and breasts, partially or entirely nude; dressed in female attire; as a pregnant woman; engaged in nonsexual feminine activities such as house cleaning; or engaged in sexual activity, in the role of a woman, with a partner (55).

The personality profiles of fetishistic cross-dressers who present as patients reveal elevated rates of neuroticism as well as lower rates of agreeableness. This may suggest a vulnerability for affective distress and the propensity for disagreeableness, which may foster marital discord (56). In a nonclinical cohort of cross-dressers attending a weekend seminar, personality characteristics were found to be no different than normal controls, with the exception of higher reported levels of openness to fantasy (57). These data suggest that the cross-dresser who seeks treatment may be significantly different from the nonpatient transvestite. If so, data from clinical cohorts may not be generalized to all cross-dressers.

Studies indicate that ~50% of applicants for surgical sex reassignment have histories of transvestic fetishism (58). The gender dysphoric transvestite may make a dramatic presentation with acute gender dysphoria and the wish for sexual reassignment. Therefore, thorough understanding of these disorders is critical for clinicians (58,59). It must be considered that gender dysphoria is a transient "state phenomenon" related to loss, trauma, or comorbid state (29). Such cases demand consideration of aggressive antidepressant treatment and restraint from supporting sex reassignment as a first line solution. For some transvestites, an initial optimism about reassignment is replaced by depression when issues of loss emerge or if illusions about the financial feasibility of reassignment are shattered. Clinicians are advised to avoid simplistic short-term solutions and to remain cognizant of the possibility of emergent deeper levels of dysphoria and self-destructive thoughts. Not uncommonly, complex underlying themes and comorbid conditions become more apparent as treatment progresses, suggesting the pursuit of a long-term treatment approach combining psychotherapy and medication.

Pedophilia

Pedophilia, which literally means "love of children," is a complicated and distressing disorder encompassing both psychiatric and forensic spheres. It is a paraphilic syndrome characterizing individuals who experience recurrent and intense erotic fantasies, urges, or behaviors involving a prepubescent (13 years of age or younger) child. To meet DSM-IV-TR criteria, the individual has either acted upon such urges, or the urges cause significant distress or interpersonal difficulty. Also, to be diagnosed with pedophilia, an individual must be at least 16 years of age and at least 5 years older than the victim. Excluded from this category are older adolescents who are involved sexually with 12- or 13-year-olds. Specifiers denote whether the individual is sexually attracted to males, females, or both; whether the behavior is limited to incestual relationships; and whether the attraction to children is exclusive or non-exclusive. These specifiers are best viewed as descriptive as opposed to reflecting discreet categories (10).

Sexual behaviors with children, unfortunately, are not uncommon. In a general population survey, 12% of men and 17% of women reported that as a child they were sexually touched by an adult (60). The perpetrators of this behavior were often parents or other caretakers. Not all child abuse is motivated by a preferred attraction to younger individuals. Some individuals sexually abuse children in an opportunistic manner, when intoxicated, or secondary to dementia or mental retardation. Still others are indiscriminate in their partner choice due to excessive drive and loss of impulse control. These individuals may have sex with any available or exploitable person, regardless of age, but are not motivated by a nonnormative age attraction.

Therefore, it is critical for clinicians to note that not all child sexual offenses are pedophilic. The essential feature of pedophilia is a primary erotic attachment to children, not criminal-mindedness. Many individuals with pedophilia suffer from fantasies and urges but never engage sexually with a child. Many pedophilic individuals describe romantic love and affection for the children to whom they are also sexually attracted and may fantasize about being in a committed, loving relationship with the child. As abhorrent as this may be to others, an individual with pedophilia is also a sex offender *only* if he engages in the illegal act of sexual behavior with a child. In and of itself, pedophilia is an unfortunate psychosexual affliction, but not criminal. Most individuals with pedophilia would be grateful to experience more normative sexual attractions.

Approximately 90% of sexual abuse offenses with children are perpetrated by males (61). Consistent with that figure, it appears that individuals with pedophilia are predominantly but not exclusively male (62).

Behavioral manifestations of pedophilia vary widely. Some individuals endorse primary erotic fantasies of children but never act upon such urges, including by the use of pornography. Others limit their behavior to viewing child pornography. For some, use of child pornography appears to fuel the underlying pedophilic urges and increases the risk of escalation from urge to action. However, while clinical observation suggests such as association, only objective research will clarify the correlation, if there is one at all, between exposure to pornography and behavioral manifestation of any paraphilia.

The growth of the Internet and electronic access to child pornography has led to recent legal quagmires regarding exploitation of real vs. virtual children. Possession of child pornography, including in a downloaded format on one's personal computer, is a criminal felony. However, a recent supreme court decision reversed some aspects of the Child Pornography Prevention Act by ruling that there is no evidence that computer-generated images of children are linked to harm to real children and that regulation of such images is an infringement of protected free speech (63). Similarly, in a recent case involving a patient of one of the authors, in the course of soliciting sex with a supposed minor via the Internet, the individual was entrapped by a federal agent posing as the minor. The charges were later dismissed on grounds of their being no real victim and that prosecution could not be justified on the basis of a "virtual" victim.

Paraphilia Not Otherwise Specified

When the defining characteristics of a nonnormative pattern of erotic interest meet the DSM-IV-TR general criteria for paraphilia but fall outside the diagnostic criteria for the eight listed paraphilias, the interest is categorized as a paraphilia not otherwise specified. Presumably because the number of possible paraphilias and fetishes is virtually limitless, the DSM-IV-TR lists as specific paraphilias those most commonly observed and reported in clinical and forensic practice. The paraphilia NOS category includes the many other nonstandard sexual interests, and lists seven as examples: telephone scatologia (obscene phone calls), necrophilia (corpses), partialism (exclusive focus on part of the body), zoophilia (animals), coprophilia (feces), klismaphilia (enemas), and urophilia (urine).

Definitional problems regarding the paraphilias become particularly apparent in the NOS category. There are dozens of paraphilias described in the literature, including some listed in the DSM-IV-TR as examples of paraphilia NOS, that fail to meet any of the three subtype criteria for paraphilia: erotic focus on nonhuman objects, suffering or humiliation of self or partner, or children or other nonconsenting persons (64). Partialism, coprophilia, urophilia, and numerous other atypical interests described in the literature involve a human focus and do not inherently involve suffering, humiliation, or nonconsenting persons.

Kafka proposed that some problematic sexual behaviors, while they meet DSM-IV-TR criteria for paraphilia NOS, are more accurately conceptualized as a distinct disorder, for which he proposed the category "paraphilia-related disorders" (65,66). Paraphilia-related disorders involve fantasies, urges, or behaviors that do not meet DSM-IV-TR criterion A for paraphilia because they are normative in content by societal standards but occur with pathological frequency or intensity.

Like the paraphilias, they are repetitive, intrusive, and persist for at least 6 months. Kafka's suggested paraphilia-related disorders include egodystonic compulsive masturbation, protracted promiscuity, and dependence on pornography. This conceptualization has not met with consensus and it remains unclear how such categorical distinctions improve the current classification system. Hopefully, future iterations of the DSM will resolve some of the nosological confusion.

ETIOLOGY OF THE PARAPHILIAS

The etiology of the paraphilias remains largely unknown at this time. Studies have identified broad areas of influence as well as some specific risk factors, but precise underlying mechanisms and comprehensive theories of causality await elucidation. What follows are the dominant explanatory theories and identified risk factors. The most current thinking assumes that etiology is based in a complex multifactorial equation reflecting both biology and environment.

Psychoanalytic Models of Etiology

Psychoanalytic writers posit that early life experiences are fundamentally related to the development of the paraphilias. Stoller asserted that vengeful hostility, in response to the young child's ambivalent struggle to separate from his mother, is the core of all perversion (67). Many variations of this theme have been proposed.

Psychoanalytic View of Fetishism

Psychoanalytic theory suggests that fetishism is due to unconscious fears and a sense of inadequacy related to early childhood experience (68,69). Freud proposed that fetishism originates in the phallic phase of psychosexual development as a male child experiences anxiety about his mother's missing penis, for which he finds a symbolic object, thus resolving his fear and restoring an erotic attachment to his mother (70). The memory of sexual pleasure as a mechanism to cope with stress becomes fixated and eventually transmutes into repetitive behavior.

Psychoanalytic View of Transvestic Fetishism

In the orthodox psychoanalytic view, cross-dressing is a defense against castration anxiety. Some proposed that transvestism represents an unconscious wish for the father's attention by identification with the mother (71,72).

Greenacre described transvestism as an effort at reparation of a flawed body image in early life (73). Stoller described transvestism as a "hostile mastery" of early trauma and humiliation by the mother (74). In contrast, Oversey and Person suggested anxiety as the central theme in transvestism, caused by flawed maternal bonding and consequent incomplete sense of self (75).

Psychoanalytic View of Exhibitionism

To the psychoanalyst, exhibitionism is associated with childhood experiences with a dominant, seductive mother and a distant father (69,76). The assault on the male child's developing sense of masculinity and adequacy is resolved in the feelings of gratification and power when a female reacts to his genital displays.

Psychoanalytic View of Sadomasochism

Stoller described sexual masochism as the neurotic eroticization of maternal hatred, a narcissistic solution to early life trauma (74), although in later writings, after observing many higher functioning individuals and couples who engaged in recreational S&M practices, he questioned his earlier assumptions (77,78). Kernberg suggested that masochists experience narcissistic gratification in the grandiose view of the self associated with high tolerance for pain (79). Waska described the masochist as alternating between compulsion toward servitude and rage at the internalized possessive, rejecting, or neglectful maternal object (80). The masochist suffers a core incapacity to self-soothe and, therefore, deep cravings to be soothed by others. The cravings, and accompanying rage, explain the masochist's inherently ambivalent position, in which self-suffering disguises feelings of anger and yearning for maternal soothing. Ultimately, his compensatory style is one of the expecting to be hurt by those from whom he needs love, and one of the confusing pain and humiliation with longed-for love. He tolerates pain and suffering in order to remain attached to the needed but pain-causing mother, a stance that is preferable to no attachment at all. In Lebe's formulation, the masochist is sensitive to others but cannot be to himself because as a child he was unable to differentiate between self and the punishing or rejecting mother (81). A more recent formulation proposed that sexual desire itself is a driving force in masochism, and that sadomasochistic aggression is, paradoxically, an attempt to find safety under the primitive lure of sexual feelings and preoedipal yearnings (82).

Psychoanalytic interpretations assist the clinician in formulating a sense of the early life experiences of individuals seeking treatment and in understanding their developmental vicissitudes. Most clinicians who treat individuals with paraphilias can provide testimony to the life stories that offer convincing anecdotal evidence for the relevance of psychoanalytic constructs to our efforts to explain unusual erotic interests.

Family Dysfunction Models of Etiology

Other etiological theories, while not based specifically in psychoanalytic thought, view paraphilias as developing out of adverse early life experience and dysfunctional family processes. Studies have found varying degrees of association between the childhood experiences such as emotional and sexual abuse, family dysfunction, behavior problems, and the paraphilias. In a recent study, childhood sexual abuse was determined to be a specific developmental risk factor for pedophilia, whereas emotional abuse and other adverse experiences were found to be general risk factors for the paraphilias (83). Other studies have contradicted this finding (84–86). However, most have concluded that, at the least, adverse childhood experiences increase the risk of developing pedophilia (83,87–91). In particular, based on the higher rates of sexual abuse in the life histories of many, although not all, individuals with pedophilia, sexual abuse is now widely recognized as a risk factor in the development of pedophilia (89,92,93). Berlin has observed that of the females diagnosed with pedophilia in his clinic over the past 15 years, all reported histories of childhood sexual abuse, leading him to conclude that childhood sexual abuse may play a particularly significant role in the development of pedophilia in females (F. Berlin, personal communication, 2003).

A recent study of the perceptions of sexual offenders found a significant positive association between child sex offending and offender self-reports of childhood neglect and abuse, including sexual abuse and early exposure to sexually deviant behavior (94). As in many studies, the sample population was described in nonspecific categorical language such as "child molesters," leaving ambiguity regarding how many of the offenders were pedophilic. Nevertheless, the results are consistent with the hypothesis that negative early interpersonal experiences may play a contributing role in the development of problematic adult sexuality, including pedophilia.

A study of five adolescent males who practiced autoerotic asphyxia revealed early histories of physical abuse, sexual abuse, and, more specifically, choking in each of the five boys. The investigators hypothesized that choking had become paired with sexual arousal and that the pairing, along with the abusive early experiences, were etiologically relevant to the development of a paraphilia in four of the five boys (95).

Behavioral Models of Etiology

Conditioning Theories of Paraphilia

Theorists of classical conditioning have proposed that some forms of fetishism can be explained by early learned associations between sexual stimulation and common objects of infancy such as diapers, bottles, and pacifiers (22). One early study using aversion techniques with sexual offenders provided modest support for conditioning theories, in that frequency of masturbation to exhibitionist fantasies, implying stronger conditioning, was associated with treatment failure (96). However, etiological explanations based on responses to treatment have limited validity.

Clinical work in the Internet era provides observational support for the role of conditioning in the paraphilias. Exposure to Internet-based sexually explicit material and accompanying high levels of sexual arousal appear to, in some individuals, profoundly influence the development of conditioned sexual fantasy and arousal responses. However, there is a wide range of responses to comparable levels of exposure. Therefore, caution must be exercised in drawing conclusions about any direct causative effects of exposure—Internet or otherwise—on the development or latensification of psychosexual pathology. Fisher and Barak have presented eloquent reviews on the effects of exposure to pornography, concluding that it is difficult to distinguish between the effects of exposure and the effects of pre-existing underlying personality factors in individuals who seek such exposure (97).

In contrast to classic conditioning is the theory of imprinting, which proposes that early childhood is a critical period in which animals instinctually grow attached to a primary object. Species such as precocial birds are thought to become "imprinted," or physiologically programed to follow whatever creature or object they see shortly after hatching (98). Binet hypothesized pathological imprinting in humans as a possible explanation for the development of fetishes (41). Owing to events in sensitive developmental periods, an association between arousal and a particular object or experience becomes imprinted. Study of nonhuman species suggests that behavior learned through imprinting is extremely difficult, if not impossible, to unlearn, whereas in classic conditioning models deconditioning and reconditioning are, theoretically, possible. Overall, empirical attempts to validate conditioning theories in the etiology of paraphilias have produced mixed results.

Junginger pointed out the possible relevance of the two-process learning theory, which has earned acceptance as an explanation of avoidance behavior in obsessive-compulsive disorder, to the development of fetishism (46). In this conceptualization, a formerly neutral object, when paired with sexual stimulation, acquires the power to elicit sexual arousal, leading to an operant response of stimulation and approach, rather than fear and avoidance as in OCD. The rewards inherent in sexual arousal and orgasm then serve as positive reinforcement.

Deviant Arousal Theory of Paraphilia

Some behaviorists have examined the role of deviant arousal—arousal in response to deviant or nonnormative stimuli—in the etiology of sexual offending behaviors. Some have found evidence of deviant arousal in pedophilia and others have found deviant arousal in exhibitionism, although with concurrent higher arousal to normative stimuli (99–101). Still other studies have failed to find deviant arousal in exhibitionism. The inconsistent findings suggest that deviant arousal is present in some men with paraphilia and less so or not at all in others (102). Why that is the case is unknown and there is no current explanation for the presence or development of the deviant arousal.

Courtship Disorder Theory of the Paraphilias

Courtship Disorder theory has been proposed as an etiological explanation for three frequently co-occurring paraphilias—voyeurism, exhibitionism, and frotteurism—and preferential rape, defined as preferred arousal to coercive sex, based on the assumption that they are fundamentally related (103). In this theory, normal sexual interaction has four sequential phases: (1) finding a partner; (2) non-physical interaction; (3) physical nongenital contact; and (4) sexual intercourse. Voyeurism is viewed as a disturbance in the first phase, exhibitionism as a disturbance of the second, frotteurism of the third, and preferential rape as a disturbance of the fourth phase. Although this theory has logical appeal, it is not clear from the research whether specific paraphilias tend to co-occur with statistical consistency, or whether, as has been asserted, individuals with one paraphilia suffer from an underlying deficit that predisposes them to the development of others (104).

Personality Theories of the Paraphilias

Efforts to identify associations between personality and variant sexual behavior have been inconsistently fruitful. Some studies, but not all, have found exhibitionists to be unassertive (88). One of the authors' own studies compared personality profiles of men diagnosed with a paraphilia with those of men with sexual dysfunction and with a normative sample (105). Profiles of men diagnosed with a paraphilia showed a distinctive group profile marked by higher neuroticism, lower agreeableness, and lower conscientiousness than those of sexually dysfunctional men, whose profiles were comparable with the normative group. Detailed analysis of the facet scores demonstrated that the paraphilic men were significantly higher than sexually dysfunctional or normals in depression, hostility, impulsiveness, excitement-seeking, and openness to fantasy, while significantly lower in warmth. These findings are consistent with earlier suggestions that men with paraphilias have difficulty with attachment and intimacy, and are commonly self-centered, antagonistic, and autonomically prone to distress (106–109). Consistent with the finding by Fagan and colleagues that the paraphilia group was higher in openness to fantasy, others have observed that men with paraphilias often experience fantasy as a central aspect of their sexuality (110,111).

A recent study of pedophilic sex offenders found that 60% of the sample met criteria for a personality disorder (25). However, contrary to the commonly asserted hypothesis that antisocial personality disorder is etiologically fundamental to pedophilia, <23% of the sample met criteria in this study. Others have also found limited evidence to support such hypotheses (112).

Biological Theories of the Paraphilias

Understanding of the neurobiology of sexual functioning, both normal and deviant, is incomplete. Nevertheless, it is clear that sexual interest and function derive from both the central nervous system and endocrine factors. In normal sexual arousal, central nervous system involvement includes a cascade of connections from the neocortex to the limbic system and the hypothalamus, particularly the preoptic area and the brainstem (113). Sexual arousal begins via either sensory input, such as tactile, visual or olfactory stimulation, or via fantasy in the neocortex. This cortical arousal propagates through the limbic system and hypothalamus to enable a progression of physiologic events that promote sexual behaviors and orgasm. Subcortical brain areas are important for sexual functioning and include the limbic system and the preoptic nuclei in the hypothalamus. Both peptides, such as beta endorphin and oxytocin, and LHRH modulate sexual behavior in animals.

The role of monoamines is also important in normal sexuality. Dopamine appears to enhance sexual arousal with particular activity in the mesolimbic system, whereas serotonin diminishes sexual drive and arousal (114,115). Prolactin inhibits dopamine, resulting in diminished libidinal drive. Lowering prolactin levels via bromocriptine in women with pituitary adenomas has been shown to increase libidinal drive.

Endocrine factors are also relevant to libidinal drive. The role of estrogen in normal sexuality is not fully elucidated but it is evident that estrogen affects serotonin receptors as well as regulates beta endorphin, a peptide that has reduced sexual drive in animal studies (116). Progesterone may also lower sexual drive.

Regarding understanding paraphilic dysregulation from a biological perspective, the most compelling data is found in studies with androgens. It is known that testosterone levels strongly correlate with sexual drive in women, and aggressive sexual offenders often are found to have higher androgen levels than controls (117,118). Among the most robust data supporting biological factors underlying sexually deviant behavior is the elevation of androgen levels found in convicted rapists (119). However, the implications of these findings for the paraphilias are unclear at this time.

Early biological hypotheses regarding the paraphilias included Epstein's theory of phylogenetic preparedness of fetishism (120). He observed that a rubber boot, but not leather, evoked penile erection and ejaculation in a chimpanzee, suggesting that the fetishistic attraction to an unusal object is not limited to humans. Epstein speculated that the wet surface of the boot bore a relationship to the female chimpanzee's genitalia during rear mount sexual behavior.

There have been reports of elevated plasma epinephrine and norepinephrine levels in individuals with pedophilia (121,122). Whether such abnormalities are related to underlying anxiety disorders rather than specific to pedophilia has not been discerned.

A recent well-designed large-scale study comparing the brain functioning of men with pedophilia to men with other atypical sexual interests or behaviors found significant correlation between pedophilia and poorer than average brain functioning, as measured by Full-Scale IQ and verbal and visuospatial memory (123). The study also found a significant association between pedophilia and lower rates of right-handedness, consistent with earlier reports of decreased right-handedness in child sex offenders (124). The study's findings suggest that early (prebirth) neurodevelopmental perturbations of the developing brain may account for some cases of pedophilia. Future studies may clarify what parts of the brain are affected, whether such perturbations reflect an independent pathological process or a general risk factor, and whether such findings have relevance to the development of other paraphilias.

In another recent study, an association was identified between pedophilia and retrospectively recalled childhood accidents resulting in unconsciousness (125,126). Twice as many pedophiles as nonpedophiles reported head injuries with unconsciousness before the age of 6, suggesting that neurodevelopmental perturbations occurring in a window of time after birth may also increase the risk of pedophilia. The authors of these studies cautiously point out that more data are needed before the findings can be interpreted with confidence. Whether head injury causes a neurodevelopmental abnormality that increases the risk of pedophilia or whether a pre-existing neurodevelopmental problem increases the risk of both head injury and pedophilia is unknown.

Although most studies regarding possible etiological associations between childhood head injury and the paraphilias have focused on pedophilia, some single case studies have been cited suggesting that some fetishistic behavior may also be related to childhood head injury (127).

A study of 477 adult males with traumatic brain injury identified 27 men, or almost 6% of the sample, who, with no prior histories of sexual offending, committed sexual offenses following their head injuries (128). Some but not all of the offending behaviors were paraphilic in nature. The authors concluded that traumatic brain injury was a significant etiological factor underlying the offending behaviors. Such studies support the hypothesis that head injury is related to the development of some adult onset cases of paraphilia.

Left temporal lobe lesions have been known to result in sexual disinhibition and compulsivity in some individuals. Similarly, is evidence that temporal lobe epilepsy may cause some cases of fetishism and other paraphilias, most commonly exhibitionism (104,129). However, the majority of individuals with temporal lobe epilepsy do not have a paraphilia and, in fact, many are hyposexual. Future studies may explain the occurrence of paraphilia in a small subgroup of these individuals.

Although there is little evidence currently of a genetic link in the development of paraphilias, studies have found an association between pedophilia and Klinefelter's syndrome, a rare chromosomal variant in men (130–132).

Kafka has suggested that serotonergic factors may provide a biologic explanation for all paraphilias, but there is limited data to confirm this (133). There are also reports of fetishistic cross-dressing across generations in families (134,135). Whether such behaviors indicate biologic or social modeling underpinnings remains to be demonstrated.

TREATMENT OF THE PARAPHILIAS

Treatment of the paraphilias may be biological or psychological. Although there are case reports of success based solely on one, state-of-the-art treatment today is most often a thoughtful integration of both. This section of the chapter reviews the research on pharmacological interventions followed by a discussion of critical variables in the assessment of the paraphilias. The chapter concludes with an overview of the principles of psychotherapeutic treatment. A core assumption of the authors is that paraphilias are most often chronic and incurable but highly manageable. Treatment is a process of determining and implementing those interventions that offer the patient maximal opportunity to control behavior, manage affect and impulses, and reduce distress.

Pharmacological Treatment of the Paraphilias

There is no data to suggest that pharmacological intervention cans specifically target or ameliorate underlying paraphilic mechanisms. Rather, pharmacological interventions are either symptom focused or directed toward ameliorating or managing comorbid conditions. For example, where hypersexuality is a factor, pharmacological treatments are commonly implemented to lower libidinal drive; where concurrent mania fosters hypersexuality, mood stabilizing agents are indicated; where comorbid depression or anxiety exacerbates paraphilic urges and behaviors, pharmacological intervention to lower affective distress may be a crucial early treatment; where paraphilic behavior is driven by underlying psychotic or delusional processes, the obvious first line treatment is pharmacological management of the psychotic state. As exemplified in these scenarios, pharmacological interventions for the paraphilias fall into three primary categories: antidepressants, antiandrogens, and neuroleptics and other agents.

Antidepressants

Some individuals with a paraphilia experience distressingly high drive and hyperarousability. Pharmacological interventions to lower libidinal urges are not only sometimes useful, but frequently essential, particularly the offending disorders such as pedophilia (136). The side-effect of diminished sexual desire, arousability, and behavior has been well documented in the specific serotonin reuptake inhibitors (SSRIs). Although the precise mechanism of action is unknown, it is thought that the SSRIs lower drive by increasing levels of serotonin (10,137,138). The SSRIs are often utilized in cases where high biological drive is a significant contributing factor (139). They are, of course, also helpful in reducing comorbid depressive and anxiety symptoms as well as intrusive sexual preoccupation. The clinical evidence for serotonin agonists include numerous reports of treatment success using fluoxetine, sertraline, and paroxetine for fetishism, voyeurism, exhibitionism, and pedophilia (18,137,140–146).

It has been hypothesized that for a subset of individuals, paraphilias may be secondary to obsessive-compulsive related disorders, for which the SSRIs have been found to be effective. A study comparing the effectiveness of the SSRI fluvoxamine to the heterocyclic desipramine in the treatment of exhibitionism found that fluvoxamine effectively reduced the paraphilic urges and behavior, whereas desipramine was associated with relapse (147). A study comparing the effectiveness of fluvoxamine, fluoxetine, and sertraline in paraphilics found all three effective in reducing the severity of fantasies and no significant differences in overall efficacy (138). Kafka and Hennen reported on the successful use of psychostimulants in combination with SSRIs in the treatment of individuals with paraphilias and comorbid adult symptoms of ADHD (148).

Although most studies regarding the use of antidepressants in the treatment of the paraphilias have focused on the SSRIs, there have been case reports of the effective use of other antidepressants. The tricyclic clomipramine, which has significant serotonin reuptake inhibition, has been reported to be effective in treating exhibitionism (149–151). Another case report described the remission of exhibitionism with trazodone, although the precise mechanism of action in this agent is not fully understood (152).

The number of studies regarding antidepressants in the treatment of the paraphilias remains small and more studies are needed in order to clarify the effects of SSRIs compared with other psychopharmacological interventions. Further, it is unclear whether the SSRIs are selectively useful in individuals with a clear obsessive-compulsive disorder component, comorbid anxiety, or depressive disorder underlying the paraphilia or, rather, they have a more generalized usefulness for the paraphilias.

Antiandrogens

In paraphilias where elevated sexual drive does not remit to other treatments, the use of antiandrogens is indicated. In contrast to the SSRIs and other antidepressants, where the effects on libido are indirect, the antiandrogens have a direct suppressing effect on testosterone levels. Most of the current knowledge regarding the use of antiandrogens stems from research with sex offending populations, although the use of testosterone reducing agents has also been reported in transvestic individuals who cannot control cross-dressing behaviors (153). Use of antiandrogenic medications in the treatment of paraphilias usually must be long-term. Relapse is common upon cessation of the medication. Treatment with antiandrogens may result in erectile dysfunction, although many individuals maintain adequate sexual functioning. As with the SSRIs, the goal of antiandrogen medications is to augment the individual's ability to achieve behavioral control (10).

Methoxyprogesterone acetate (MPA) is the most commonly used hormonal agent for the reduction of sex drive in the United States (140,146,154,155). It does not compete with androgens at the receptor level but blocks levels of testosterone by inducing hepatic testosterone reductase. The goal of this strategy is to reduce baseline testosterone to 50% of initial values. Common dosages are 50–300 mg orally or 300–400 weekly via intramuscular injections with reduction to 100 mg weekly for a maintenance program. Depot preparations of methoxyprogesterone are also available. Side-effects include weight gain, hyperglycemia due to an exaggerated insulin response to a glucose load, headaches and increased risk of deep vain thromboses.

Cyproterone acetate (CPA) is also frequently used to suppress sex drive in individuals with paraphilias. CPA blocks androgen receptors, directly decreasing the biological effects of testosterone. It is not available in the United States and most of the research regarding this agent derives from Germany (156). CPA can be given orally 100 mg daily or 200 mg every other week via intramuscular injection. Reports clearly demonstrate that CPA reduces sexual drive and erectile ability. Possible side effects include weight gain, depression and feminization (157,158).

Some researchers argue that long-acting gonadotropin-releasing hormone (GnRH) agonist analoges are the most potent antiandrogens, have the fewest side-effects, and therefore are the most promising pharmacological treatment for the future (159). Either leuprolide or triptorelin is given intramuscularly in doses of 3.75 or 7.5 monthly. These agents suppress testosterone via decreasing the number of pituitary GnRH receptors and testicular LH receptors, thereby desensitizing the testes to LH. It more completely suppresses androgen than MPA or CPA. In an open trial of 30 sex offenders, triptorelin administered on a monthly basis (3.75 mg per dose) diminished paraphilic fantasies and drives according to self-report at 8-months follow-up. In another report, triptorelin treatment resulted in complete cessation of paraphilic behavior and significant decreases in paraphilic fantasies in five of six subjects (160). Termination of the treatment resulted in relapse to paraphilic fantasies in some subjects and in behavioral relapse in others. When a GnRH agonist is initially given, a "flare" phenomenon may result in that there is a transient rise in testosterone levels before receptor down regulation (161). To manage this, nonsteroidal antiandrogens such as flutamide may be helpful.

Neuroleptics and Other Agents

Neuroleptic agents have been reported to diminish paraphilic behaviors and fantasies. One early report described the successful treatment of a case of familial exhibitionism in Tourette's syndrome with haloperidol (162). Additionally, there have been case reports of other pharmacological interventions for the paraphilias. A report described success in eliminating pedophilic cognitions and behaviors with a combination of the anticonvulsant carbamazepine and the benzodiazepine clonazepam (163). These were selected to specifically target the patient's mixed depression and anxiety as well as his sexual impulsivity. Lithium has also been reported to be effective in reducing inappropriate sexual behaviors. However, the diagnostic classification of subjects in many studies has been vague and the use of mood stabilizers may reflect a comorbid mania or other psychotic state as the actual target of intervention (164,165).

Although more research is needed, the current knowledge base regarding reduction of sexual drive and sexual preoccupation through pharmacological means is compelling. Further, due to the high comorbidity between the paraphilias and other psychiatric disorders, the need for pharmacological support in the treatment of the paraphilias is significant. In sum, pharmacological interventions are today a critical component of state-of-the-art treatment of paraphilias, especially the offending paraphilias. Most often, these medications are coupled with, and signifiantly enhance the effects of, concomitant psychological treatment, to be discussed in the following section.

Psychological Treatment of the Paraphilias

As earlier research has demonstrated, medication may modify target symptoms such as anxiety, depression, obsessionality, or hypersexual drive, but cannot "cure" the paraphilia or interpersonal problems (166). Psychotherapy is essential to foster compliance with medication, ameliorate attitudinal problems, and to develop cognitive skills in resisting and managing paraphilic fantasies and urges. Because concurrent treatment modalities may demand the involvement of multiple clincians, issues of communication, transference and countertransference, legal risks, and ethical challenges should be familiar to clinicians before embarking on the multimodal treatment of paraphilias (167).

The empirical evidence regarding outcomes of psychological treatment of the paraphilias is limited. To date, most studies have been conducted with heterogeneous sex offender populations that include but are not limited to paraphilic offenders. The extent to which paraphilic offenders, nonparaphilic offenders, and non-offending paraphilics are the same or different in terms of etiological factors or treatment needs is unknown. Further, while there are no studies convincingly demonstrating the superiority of one psychotherapeutic methodology to another, there is growing evidence that cognitive-behavioral and relapse prevention models are effective in reducing recidivism of sexual offending behaviors (168). These models, with their focus on behavior, related cognitions, and development of self-regulatory skills, demonstrate the greatest promise for the psychological treatment of the paraphilias.

From a cognitive-behavioral perspective, the paraphilias are primary and chronic. Although fundamentally altering a sexual interest is not viewed as possible, managing the interest is. Therefore, treatment does not focus on cure, but on management of associated thoughts, fantasies, and urges, reduction of associated distress, and conscious choices about behavior. In this framework, exploration of underlying life history themes takes place *after* behavioral goals have been achieved and relapse prevention strategies learned, and is conceptualized as of secondary importance relative to the need for behavioral control.

The current classification system, the multitude of etiological theories and their inferred treatment approaches, and the tendency for outcome studies to focus on specific paraphilias imply that specific paraphilias require specific treatments. To the contrary, a general rule of thumb is that the paraphilias are more alike than different and, regardless of the specific manifestation, reflect common underlying mechanisms, such as disordered capacity to regulate affect and impulses, that become the target of treatment.

Psychiatric Assessment of Paraphilias

Assessment informs the clinician regarding necessary intensity of treatment and which psychotherapeutic modalities—individual, group, or conjoint couple—are called for. It is beyond the scope of this chapter to detail the components of the full psychiatric-psychosexual evaluation. Rather, those assessment components uniquely related to the paraphilias are highlighted.

Defining the impairment: Because psychological treatment focuses on those aspects of the disorder most related to functional impairment, identification of the specific nature of impairment is essential. The following impairment-related variables, summarized in Figure 12.2, are crucial aspects of assessment.

Cognitive impairment. Sexual thoughts may be as or more distressing than urges or cravings. An individual can have low or average biological drive and still experience frequent distressing and intrusive sexual cognitions. He may be distressed by the content of the fantasies and/or by their intrusive effects, including, for example, guilt, despair, or distraction during efforts at partnered sexual activity. Distorted cognitions that promote denial or minimization or blame others for the problematic behavior contribute to impaired judgment and increase the risk of behavior, particularly in the offending paraphilias. As along as distortions are present, internal motivation to control behavior is minimal and the risk of paraphilic behavior remains significant.

Drive impairment. High biological drive may fuel sexual urges or cravings that are preoccupying, distressing, and difficult to control, increasing the risk of behavioral escalation. Drive assessment inquires about an individual's ability to control his urges, his subjective experience of his drive, frequency of masturbation, and amount of time spent feeling sexually preoccupied. The presence of high drive and/or preoccupying urges and cravings demands consideration of a pharmacological intervention early in treatment. In the

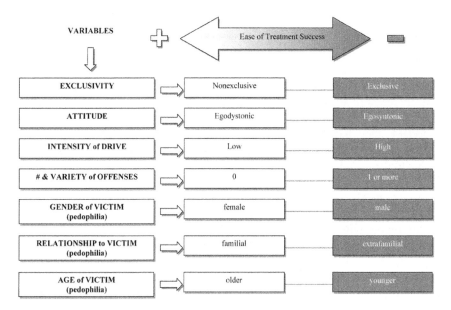

Figure 12.2 Variables effecting treatment success in paraphilias.

authors' clinic, excessively high drive has been identified as a significant component of the disorder in 10% of patients diagnosed with a paraphilia or nonparaphilic problematic sexuality. Although most patients describe themselves as sexually obsessed and preoccupied, and most endorse impairment in controlling their urges, only a fraction experiences difficulty in the form of high drive or genital hyperarousability. This highlights the importance of assessing the nature and intensity of sexual cravings from a psychological as well as biological perspective.

Behavioral impairment. In some individuals, the problem is limited to urges and fantasies. In others, the urges and fantasies have escalated to paraphilic behavior. Problematic behaviors may include frequent masturbation, masturbation in inappropriate contexts, excessive use of or preoccupation with paraphilic pornography, placing undue sexual demands on a partner, seeking inappropriate partners with whom to act out a paraphilic interest, unsafe sexual practices, and deceitfulness. As a paraphilia escalates behaviorally, partnered sex may become impaired. Some individuals suffer extreme financial consequences due to purchasing online sexual services, phone sex activities, or hiring sex workers. Most significantly, some paraphilias lead to severe legal consequences and harm to others.

Exclusivity vs. nonexclusivity. Exclusivity is associated with poorer treatment outcomes. The more exclusive the paraphilia, the more likely it precludes sexual intimacy with an appropriate partner. Treatment then focuses on management of urges and fantasies, behavioral control, minimizing the risk of harm to others, acceptance of one's sexual differences and grieving related losses rather than return to a previous level of nonparaphilic functioning. Although the DSM-IV-TR includes a specifier for exclusive/nonexclusive types only for pedophilia, identifying how this variable contributes to impairment is important in any paraphilia.

Egodystonic vs. egosyntonic attitude. Some individuals seek help because they have been discovered engaging in paraphilic behavior by a spouse, partner, or employer. This individual may have an egosyntonic relationship to the paraphilia, in that he experienced no apparent distress other than that associated with being discovered. Although this may reflect an underlying antisocial or narcissistic personality component that will contribute to poor treatment outcome, this conclusion should be resisted until objective evidence is presented. Distorted cognitions that enable an egosyntonic attitude are common in paraphilias that have been enacted secretly over time and may resolve with successful treatment. However, the real presence of underlying sociopathy results in a rigidly egosyntonic attitude and carries significant negative implications for treatment outcome. Without rigorous assessment, the degree to which personality factors are contributing to disordered attitude will remain unclear.

Level of risk. Paraphilic expression may be limited to fantasies, with little immediate risk of behavioral escalation. On the other hand, there may be an immediate danger, as in the offending paraphilias, autoerotic asphyxiation, and some cases of sexual sadism or masochism. Danger may be symbolic and benign or real and potentially lethal, as in cases reflecting loss of control or confusion regarding the boundary between consent and coercion. Assessment of self-mutilating behaviors is particularly critical in transvestic fetishism, where gender dysphoric transvestites may report attempts at auto-castration.

In pedophilia, the number and variety of prior offenses, relationship to victim, age, and gender of victim have been shown to be strong predictors of reoffense (169). Therefore, these variables comprise a critical aspect of risk assessment in pedophilia. Hanson and colleagues, in their excellent reviews, have pointed out that structured assessment of these specific risk factors is more effective than unstructured clinical assessment.

Comorbidity. Comorbid multiple paraphilias, depressive, anxiety, and substance abuse disorders are common. Although there is no empirical evidence that paraphilias are commonly associated with particular personality disorders, personality disorders may co-occur. Comorbidity assessment clarifies the nature and extent of functional impairment, identifies potential obstacles to treatment success, and informs pharmacological decisions and decisions about initial treatment focus.

Cognitive-Behavioral Treatment

Cognitive-behavioral treatment integrates cognitive and behavioral interventions to assist individuals in gaining control of the paraphilic cognitions, urges, and behaviors. Group psychotherapy is often the modality of choice, particularly in severe or offending paraphilias. Although individual treatment can target paraphilia related impairments, the potency of group therapy to do so, through both therapeutic support and therapeutic confrontation, is greater. Recent outcome studies, using rates of recidivism, suggest that treatment outcomes in pedophilia are relatively positive (169–171). This is contrary to common myth that sexual offenders are untreatable and has positive implications for the application of similar treatments to other paraphilias (172).

The development of insight is not central to the cognitive-behavioral model, but insight oriented strategies may be integrated in order to achieve particular goals. Because the paraphilias represent a heterogeneous group, treatment must be individualized and the basic framework adjusted in order to accommodate individual presentations. It is beyond the scope of this chapter to detail cognitive-behavioral treatment protocols. Rather, a skeleton of treatment guidelines is presented. Overall treatment objectives include the following.

Control and management of problematic thoughts, affects, urges, impulses, and behaviors
Modification of paraphilic arousal
Amelioration or management of comorbid conditions
Resolution of other life issues
Relapse prevention

Strategies commonly used to promote the development of self-control in thoughts, feelings, urges, and behavior include *thought substitution, redirection, distraction, affect and urge tolerance, behavioral rehearsal, behavioral abstinence*, and *positive conditioning*. Treatment addresses the cognitions, feelings, urges, and behaviors that are related to the cycle of paraphilic regression. Any factor that increases the odds of paraphilic behavior occurring is conceptualized as a "trigger" or high risk association. The identification of triggers, an understanding of the relative risk associated with each, and the development of concrete strategies to manage them are central components of early treatment. Making decisions about complete or partial avoidance of triggers is a critical aspect of treatment and, later, relapse prevention.

Cognitive distortions provide justification for inappropriate behavior and allow the individual to minimize or deny the negative effects on self and others. Facilitated by cognitive interventions such as *thought substitution, redirection*, and *distraction*, the individual learns to replace problematic cognitions with rational thought and to redirect his thinking in alternative directions. Similarly, after identifying those feeling states and sexual urges that serve as triggers, the individual learns to use *redirection, distraction*, and *affect and urge tolerance*. This includes the skill of tolerating feelings without acting on them, and learning to trust that feelings, including sexual feelings, pass if not enacted. Whether particularly high or not, sexual drive must be managed in the treatment of paraphilias. Treatment promotes concrete strategies for mediating sexual feelings and for learning behavioral alternatives to indulgence in paraphilic behaviors.

Modifying paraphilic sexual arousal: As noted in the discussion on etiology, treatment regarding paraphilic arousal generally emphasizes behavioral control as opposed to unlearning or relearning. There is considerable disagreement about the effectiveness and ethical basis of such techniques, and little empirical evidence that deconditioning strategies are effective in modifying a core paraphilic pattern. However, many individuals enter treatment in the hope that such a possibility exists. Behavior modification strategies are used to challenge the paraphilic fixedness or rigidity. *Behavioral rehearsal* uses mental imagery of paraphilic scenes reported by the patient, but with alternative, nonparaphilic outcomes. *Positive conditioning* is the use of nonparaphilic sexual fantasy during masturbation. The more exclusive the paraphilic arousal, the more difficult is modification. However, if used as one among many strategies, and if neither the patient nor the clinician holds unrealistic expectations, it may have benefits in controlling, not eradicating, sexual arousal.

Relapse prevention: The risk of relapse in chronic behavioral disorders is high. The core of relapse prevention is the use of cognitive-behavioral strategies learned in treatment to manage triggers and high risk situations with competence. An individual is ready for this stage of treatment when he has achieved behavioral control, demonstrated capacity to function without cognitive distortions, demonstrated capacity to manage his own affect and impulses, and shown consistent motivation to maintain abstinence from paraphilic behaviors. He has become exquisitely familiar with the repeating sequences of thoughts, urges, and behaviors associated with his own paraphilic regressive cycle. In relapse prevention, he develops a clear personal plan for self-management and for management of high risk situations.

CONCLUSION

The human capacity to eroticize is vast and the boundary between normal and abnormal diffuses. When sexual interests are conceptualized on a continuum rather than as rigid categories, many sexually healthy adults recognize nonproblematic but "beyond the usual" aspects of their own erotic preferences. Diagnostis is uncomplicated toward the far end of the continuum, where sexual interests are exclusive, or nearly so, and where either others are harmed or suffering is apparent as a result of the interest. Complexity and ambiguity characterize clinical scenarios where the interest is nonexclusive, no one has been harmed, and where, while suffering may be present, it has profound contextual or relational dimensions that make distinctions between the pathological and the incompatible less clear. The accessibility, via the world wide web, of sexual stimuli ranging from the traditional and acceptable to the bizarre and abhorrent, has, in one short decade, brought human sexuality into a spotlight that illuminates, embarrassingly, the lack of empirically based knowledge regarding the nature and causes of human sexual interest and behavior. The implications of this cultural phenomenon for the paraphilias are profound. Never before has the mandate been greater to conduct rigorous scientific inquiry to define the line between sexual recreation and sexual pathology, to develop an empirically based and clinically useful taxonomy, to identify specific etiological mechanisms, and to identify those treatments, both biological and psychological, that offer the most efficacious results.

REFERENCES

1. Rogers JE. Sex: A Natural History. 1st ed. New York: Henry Holt and Company, LLC, 2002.
2. Moser M. Paraphilia: a critique of a confused concept. In: Kleinplatz PJ, ed. New Directions in Sex Therapy: Innovations and Alternatives. Philadelphia: Brunner-Routledge, 2001:91–108.
3. Suppe F. Classifying sexual disorder: the diagnostic and statistical manual of the American Psychiatric Association. J Homosex 1984; 9(4):9–28.
4. Gert B. A sex caused inconsistency in DSM-III-R: the definition of mental disorder and the definition of paraphilias. J Med Philos 1992; 17(2):155–171.
5. American Psychiatric Association. Diagnostic and Statistical Manual of Mental Disorders. 4th text revision ed. Washington, DC: American Psychiatric Association, 2000.
6. Bradford JM, Boulet J, Pawlak A. The paraphilias: a multiplicity of deviant behaviors. Can J Psychiatry 1992; 37(2):104–108.
7. Abel GG, Osborn C. The paraphilias: the extent and nature of sexually deviant and criminal behavior. Psychiatric Clin North Am 1992; 15(3):675–687.
8. Lehne GK, Money J. Multiplex versus multiple taxonomy of paraphilia: case example. Sex Abuse 2003; 15(1):61–72.
9. Chalkley A, Powell G. The clinical description of forty-eight cases of sexual fetishism. Br J Psychiatry 1983; 142:292–295.
10. Fagan PJ, Wise TN, Schmidt CW, Berlin FS. Pedophilia. J Am Med Assoc 2002; 288(19):2458–2465.
11. Hollender MH, Brown CW, Roback HB. Genital exhibitionism in women. Am J Psychiatry 1977; 134:436–438.
12. Zavitzianos G. The perversion of fetishism in women. Psychoanal Q 1982; 51(3):405–425.
13. Grob CS. Female exhibitionism. J Nerv Ment Dis 1985; 173(4):253–256.
14. Behrendt N, Buhl N, Seidl S. The lethal paraphiliac syndrome: accidental autoerotic deaths in four women and a review of the literature. Int J Legal Med 2002; 116:148–152.
15. Gosink PD, Jumbelic MI. Autoerotic asphyxiation in a female. Am J Forensic Med Pathol 2000; 20:114–118.
16. Litman LC. Sexual sadism with lust-murder proclivities in a female? Can J Psychiatry 2003; 48(2):127.
17. Cooper AJ, Swaminath S, Baxter D, Poulin C. A female sex offender with multiple paraphilias: a psychologic, physiologic (laboratory sexual arousal) and endocrine case study. Can J Psychiatry 1990; 35:334–337.

18. Chow EWC, Choy AL. Clinical characteristics and treatment response to S SRI in a female pedophile. Arch Sex Behav 2002; 31(2):211–215.
19. Wakefield H, Rogers M, Underwager R. Female sexual abusers: a theory of loss. Issues in Child Abuse Accusations 1990; 2:181–195.
20. Bancroft J. Human Sexuality and Its Problems. 2nd ed. London: Churchill Livingstone, 1989.
21. Crepault C, Couture M. Men's erotic fantasies. Arch Sex Behav 1980; 9(5):565–581.
22. Gosselin C, Wilson G. Sexual Variations. New York: Simon & Schuster, 1980.
23. Langevin R. Sexual Strands. Hillsdale, NJ: Erlbaum, 1983.
24. Langevin R. Erotic Preference, Gender Identity, and Aggression in Men: New Research Studies. Hillsdale, NJ: Erlbaum, 1985.
25. Raymond NC, Coleman E, Ohlerking F, Christenson GA, Miner M. Psychiatric comorbidity in pedophilic sex offenders (comment). Am J Psychiatry 1999; 156(5):786–788.
26. Kafka MP, Prentky RA. Attention-deficit/hyperactivity disorder in males with paraphilias and paraphilia-related disorders: a comorbidity study. J Clin Psychiatry 1998; 59(7):388–396.
27. Kafka MP, Hennen J. A DSM-IV Axis I comorbidity study of males ($n = 120$) with paraphilias and paraphilia-related disorders. Sex Abuse 2002; 14:349–366.
28. Fagan PJ, Wise TN, Derogatis LR, Schmidt CW. Distressed transvestites. J Nerv Ment Dis 1988; 176(10):626–632.
29. Wise TN, Meyer JK. The border area between transvestism and gender dysphoria: transvestic applicant for sex reassignment. Arch Sex Behav 1980; 9:327–340.
30. Allnutt SH, Bradford JM, Greenberg DM, Curry S. Co-morbidity of alcoholism and the paraphilias. J Forensic Sci 1996; 41(2):234–239.
31. Borchard B, Gnoth A, Schulz W. Personality disorders and "psychopathy" in sex offenders imprisoned in forensic-psychiatric hospitals—SKID-11 and PCL-R-Results in patients with impulse control disorder and paraphilia. Psychiatr Prax 2003; 30(3):133–138.
32. Freund K, Blanchard R. The concept of courtship theory. J Sex Marital Ther 1986; 12(2):79–92.
33. Money J. Lovemaps: Clinical Concepts of Sexual/Erotic Health and Pathology, Paraphilia, and Gender Transposition in Childhood, Adolescence and Maturity. New York: Irvington Publishers, Inc., 1986.
34. Fedoroff JP. The paraphilic world. In: Levine SB, Risen CB, Althof SE, eds. Handbook of Clinical Sexuality for Mental Health Professionals. New York: Brunner-Routledge, 2003:333–356.
35. American Psychiatric Association. Diagnostic and Statistical Manual of Mental Disorders. 4th ed. Washington, DC: American Psychiatric Association, 1994.
36. Freund K, Seto MC, Kuban K. Frotteurism and the theory of courtship disorder. In: Laws DR, O'Donohue W, eds. Sexual Deviance: Theory, Assessment and Treatment. New York: The Guilford Press, 1997:111–130.
37. Weinberg T, Kamel WL. S and M: Studies in Sadomasochism. Buffalo: Prometheus, 1983.
38. Baumeister RF. Gender differences in masochistic scripts. J Sex Res 1988; 25:478–499.
39. Ernulf KE, Innala SM. Sexual bondage: a review and unobtrusive investigation. Arch Sex Behav 1995; 24:631–654.

40. Wiseman J. SM101. 2nd ed. Greenery Press, 1992.
41. Binet A. Le fetichisme dans l'amour. Rev Philoso Bd 1887; XXIV:252–274.
42. Krafft-Ebing Rv. Psychopathia Sexualis. 12th ed. New York: Stein & Day, 1965.
43. Krafft-Ebing Rv. Psychopathia sexualis with especial reference to the antipathic Sexual instinct: a medico-forensic study. Revised ed. Philadelphia: Physicians and Surgeons, 1928.
44. Mason FL. Fetishism: psychopathology and theory. In: Laws DR, O'Donohue W, eds. Sexual Deviance: Theory, Assessment, and Treatment. New York: Guilford, 1997:75–91.
45. Wise TN. Fetishism: etiology and treatment. Compr Psychiatry 1985; 26(3): 249–257.
46. Junginger J. Fetishism: assessment and treatment. In: Laws DR, O'Donohue W, eds. Sexual Deviance: Theory, Assessment and Treatment. New York: Guilford, 1997:92–110.
47. Hoenig J. Magnus Hirschfield, 1868–1935. In: Money J, Musaph H, eds. Handbook of sexology. Amsterdam: Excerpta Medica, 1977:38–42.
48. American Psychiatric Association. Diagnostic and Statistical Manual of Mental Disorders. 4th text revision ed. Washington, DC: American Psychiatric Association, 2000.
49. Blanchard R. Clinical observations and systematic studies of autogynephilia. J Sex Marital Ther 1991; 17(4):235–251.
50. Buhrich N, McConaghy N. The discrete syndromes of transvestism and transsexualism. Arch Sex Behav 1977; 6:483–495.
51. Docter RF, Prince V. Transvestism: a survey of 1032 cross-dressers. Arch Sex Behav 1997; 26(6):589–605.
52. Prince V, Bentler PM. Survey of 504 cases of transvestism. Psychol Rep 1972; 31:903–917.
53. Zucker KJ. Are transvestites necessarily heterosexual? [comment]. Arch Sex Behav 1997; 26(6):671–673.
54. Buhrich N. Motivation for cross-dressing in heteroSex transvestism. Acta Psychiatr Scand 1978; 57(2):145–152.
55. Blanchard R. Varieties of autogynephilia and their relationship to gender dysphoria. Arch Sex Behav 1993; 22(3):241–251.
56. Wise TN, Fagan PJ, Schmidt CW, Ponticas Y, Costa PT. Personality and Sexual functioning of transvestic fetishists and other paraphilics. J Nerv Ment Dis 1991; 179(11):694–698.
57. Brown GR, Wise TN, Costa PT. Personality characteristic and sexual functioning of 188 cross-dressing men. J Nerv Mental Dis 1996; 184:265–273.
58. Kockott MP, Fahrner E. Transsexual who have not undergone surgery: a followup study. Arch Sex Behav 1987; 16:511–522.
59. Levine SB, Shumaker RE. Increasingly Ruth: toward understanding sex reassignment. Arch Sex Behav 1983; 12:247–261.
60. Laumann EO, Gagnon JH, Michael RT. The Social Organization of Sexuality: Sexuality Practices in the United States. Chicago: University of Chicago, 1994.
61. Sediak AJ, Broadhurst DD. Executive Summary of the Third National Incidence Study of Child Abuse and Neglect. Washington, DC: U.S. Department of Health and Human Services, 1996.
62. Berlin FS. Pedophilia. Med Aspects Hum Sex 1985; 19(8):79, 82, 85, 88.
63. Ashcroft V. The Free Speech Coalition. 00–795. 2002. 198, US. F3d 1083 affirmed.

64. Milner JS, Dopke CA. Paraphilia not otherwise specialized. In: Laws DR, O'Donohue W, eds. Sexual Deviance: Theory, Assessment, and Treatment. New York: The Guilford Press, 1997:394–423.

65. Kafka MP. Paraphilia-related disorders—common, neglected, and misunderstood. Harv Rev Psychiatry 1994; 2(1):39–40.

66. Kafka MP. Compulsive sexual behavior characteristics. Am J Psychiatry 1997; 154:1632.

67. Stoller R. The term perversion. In: Fogel G, Myers W, eds. Perversions and Near Perversions. New Haven, CT: Yale University Press, 1991.

68. Nagler S. Fetishism: a review and case study. Psychiatry Q 1957; 10:713–741.

69. Allen DW. A psychoanalytic view. In: Cox DJ, Daitzman RJ, eds. Exhibitionism: Description, Assessment and Treatment. New York: Garland, 1980:59–82.

70. Freud S. Fetishism. In: Strachey J, ed. The Standard Edition of the Complete Psychological Works of Sigmund Freud. Vol. 3. London: Hogarth Press, 1962.

71. Fenichel O. The psychology of transvestism. In: Anonymous, ed. Collected Papers. New York: W.W. Norton, 1953:167–180.

72. Bak R. Fetishism. J Am Psychoanal Assoc 1953; 1:285–298.

73. Greenacre P. Certain relationships between fetishism and the faulty development of the body image. Emotional Growth. New York: International Universities Press, 1971:9–30.

74. Stoller R. Perverion: The Erotic Form of Hatred. New York: Pantheon, 1975.

75. Oversey L, Person E. Transvestism: a disorder of sense of self. J Psychoanal Psychother 1976; 28(174):193.

76. Mester H. Exhibitionism—acriticism of only biologically oriented interpretations of this sexual disorder. Z Psychosom Med Psychoanal 1985; 31(2):156–171.

77. Baumaster RF. Gender differences in masochistic scripts. J Sex Res 1988; 25:478–499.

78. Stoller R. Oserving Erotic Imagination. New Haven, CT: Yale University Press, 1985.

79. Kernberg OF. Sadomasochism, sexual excitement and perversion. J Am Psychoanal Assoc 1991; 39:333–362.

80. Waska RT. Precursors to masochistic and dependent character development. Am J Psychoanal 1997; 57(3):253–267.

81. Lebe D. Masochism and the inner mother. Psychoanal Rev 1997; 84(4):523–540.

82. Celenza A. Sadomasochistic relating: what's sex got to do with it? Psychoanal Q 2000; 69(3):527–543.

83. Lee JK, Jackson HJ, Pattison P, Ward T. Developmental risk factors for sexual offending. Child Abuse Negl 2002; 26(1):73–92.

84. Finkelhor D, Hotaling G, Lewis IA, Smith C. Sexual abuse in a national study of adult men and women: prevalence, characteristics, and risk factors. Child Abuse Negl 1990; 14:19–28.

85. Murphy WD, Haynes MR, Page IJ. Adolescent sex offenders. In: O'Donohue W, Geer JH, eds. The Sexual Abuse of Children: Clinical Issues. Vol. 2. Hillsdale, NJ: Erlbaum, 1992.

86. Saunders EB, Awad GA. Male adolescent sexual offenders: exhibitionism and obscene phone calls. Child Psychiatr Hum Dev 1991; 21:169–178.

87. Saunders EG, Awad GA, White G. Male adolescent sexual offenders: the offender and the offense. Can J Psychiatry 1986; 31:542–549.

88. Blair CD, Lanyon RI. Exhibitionism: etiology and treatment. Psychol Bull 1981; 89:439–463.
89. Dhawan S, Marshall WL. Sexual abuse histories of sexual offenders. Sexual Abuse 1996; 8:7–15.
90. Dietz PE, Hazelwood RR, Warren J. The sexually sadistic criminal and his offenses. Bull Am Acad Psychiatry Law 1990; 18:163–178.
91. Gratzer T, Bradford J. Offender and offense characteristics of sexual sadists: a comparative study. J Forensic Sci 1995; 40(3):450–455.
92. Cohen LJ, McGeoch PG, Gans SW, Nikiforov K, Cullen K, Galynker II. Childhood sexual history of 20 male pedophilies vs. 24 male healthy control subjects. J Nerv Ment Dis 2002; 190(11):757–766.
93. Freund K, Kuban M. The basis of the abused abuser theory of pedophilia: a further elaboration on an earlier study. Arch Sex Behav 1994; 23(5):553–563.
94. McCormack J, Hudson SM, Ward T. Sexual offenders' perceptions of their early interpersonal relationships: an attachment perspective. J Sex Res 2002; 39(2):85–93.
95. Friedrich WN, Gerber PN. Autoerotic asphyxia: the development of a paraphilia. J Am Acad Child Adolesc Psychiatry 1994; 33(7):970–974.
96. Evans DR. Subjective variables and treatment effects in aversion therapy. Behav Res Ther 1970; 6:17–19.
97. Fisher WA, Barak A. Internet pornography: a social psychological perspective on internet sexuality. J Sex Res 2001; 38(4):312–323.
98. Welty JC, Baptista L. The Life of Birds. 4th ed. New York: Saunders College Publishing, 1988.
99. Langevin R, Paitich D, Ramsey G, Anderson C, Kamrad J, Pope S et al. Experimental studies of the etiology of genital exhibitionism. Arch Sex Behav 1979; 8:307–331.
100. Murphy WD, Barbaree HE. Assessments of Sexual Offenders by Measures of Erectile Response: Psychometric Properties and Decision Making. Brandon, VT: Safer Society Press, 1994.
101. Marshall WL, Payne K, Barbaree HE, Eccles A. Exhibitionists: sexual preferences for exposing. Behav Res Ther 1991; 29(1):37–40.
102. Tichy P. Phalloplethysmography findings in pedophilia and exhibitionism offenders. Cas Lek Cesk 1996; 135(16):521–524.
103. Freund K, Seto MC, Kuban K. Frotteurism and the theory of courtship disorder. In: Laws DR, O'Donohue W, eds. Sexual Deviance: Theory, Assessment and Treatment. New York: The Guilford Press, 1997:111–130.
104. Murphy WD. Exhibitionism: Psychopathology and theory. In: Laws DR, O'Donohue W, eds. Sexual Deviance: Theory, Assessment and Treatment. New York: Guilford, 1997:22–39.
105. Fagan PJ, Wise TN, Schmidt CW, Ponticas Y, Marshall RD, Costa PT. A comparison of five-factor personality dimensions in males with sexual dysfunction and males with paraphilia. J Pers Assess 1991; 57(3):434–448.
106. Eysenck HJ. The Biological Basis of Personality. Springfield, IL: Thomas, 1967.
107. Eysenck HJ. Hysterical personality and sexual adjustment. J Sex Res 1971; 7:274–281.
108. Eysenck HJ. Masculinity–feminity, personality and sexual attitudes. J Sex Res 1971; 7:83–88.
109. Eysenck HJ. Personality and sexual adjustment. Br J Psychiatry 1971; 118:593–608.
110. Abel GG, Blanchard EB. The role of fantasy in the treatment of sexual deviation. Arch Gen Psychiatry 1974; 30:467–475.

111. Money J. Love and Love Sickness. Baltimore: Johns Hopkins University Press, 1980.
112. Berner W, Berger P, Guitierrez K, Berker K. The role of personality disorders in the treatment of sex offenders. J Offender Rehabil 1992; 11:159–169.
113. Herbert J. Sexuality, stress, and the chemical architecture of the brain. Annu Rev Sex Res 1996; 7:1–43.
114. Bitran D, Hull EM. Pharmacological analysis of male rat sexual behavior. Neurosci Biobehav Rev 1987; 11(4):365–389.
115. Segraves RT. Effects of psychotropic drugs on human erection and ejaculation. Arch Gen Psychiatry 1989; 46(3):275–284.
116. Bridges RS, Ronsheim PM. Immunoreactive beta-endorphin concentrations in brain and plasma during pregnancy in rats: possible modulation by progesterone and estradiol. Neuroendocrinology 1987; 45(5):381–388.
117. Riley A, Riley E. Controlled studies of women presenting with sexual drive disorder: I. Endocrine status. J Sex Marital Ther 2000; 26:269–283.
118. Virkkunen M, Rawlings R, Tokola R, Poland RE, Guidotti A, Nemeroff C et al. CSF biochemistries, glucose metabolism, and diurnal activity rhythms in alcoholic, violent offenders, fire setters and healthy volunteers. Arch Gen Psychiatry 1994; 51(1):20–27.
119. Giotakos O, Markianos M, Vaidakis N, Christodoulou G. Aggression, impulsivity, plasma sex hormones and biogenic amine turnover in a forensic population of rapists. J Sex Marital Ther 2003; 29:215–226.
120. Epstein AW. The fetish object: phylogenetic considerations. Arch Sex Behav 1975; 4(3):303–308.
121. Maes M, De Vos N, Van Hunsel F, Van West D, Westenberg H, Cosyns P et al. Pedophilia is accompanied by increase plasma concentrations of catecholamines, in particular epinephrine. Psychiatry Res 2001; 103(1):43–49.
122. Maes M, Van West D, De Vos N, Westenberg H, Van Hunsel F, Hendriks D et al. Lower baselines plasma cortisol and prolactin together with increased body temperature and higher MCPP-induced cortisol responses in men with pedophilia. Neuropsychopharmacology 2001; 24(1):37–46.
123. Cantor JM, Blanchard R, Christensen BK, Dickey R, Klassen PE, Beckstead AL, Blak T, Kuban ME. Intelligence, memory, and handedness in pedophilia. Neuropsychology 2004; 18(1):3–14.
124. Bogaert AF. Handedness, criminality, and sexual offending. Neuropsychologia 2001; 39:465–469.
125. Blanchard R, Kuban ME, Klassen P, Dickey R, Christensen BK, Cantor JM, Blak T. Self-reported head injuries before and after age 13 in pedophilic and nonpedophilic men referred for clinical assessment. Arch Sex Behav 2003; 32(6):573–581.
126. Blanchard R, Christensen BK, Strong SM, Cantor JM, Kuban MK, Klassen P et al. Retrospective self-reports of childhood accidents causing unconsciousness in phallometrically diagnosed pedophiles. Arch Sex Behav 2002; 31(6):511–526.
127. Pandita-Gunawardena R. Paraphilic infantilism: a rare case of fetishistic behavior. Br J Psychiatry 1990; 157:767–770.
128. Simpson G, Blaszcynski A, Hodgkinson A. Sex offending as a psychosocial sequela of traumatic brain injury. J Head Trauma Rehabil 1999; 14(6):567–580.
129. Kolarsky A, Freund K, Machek J, Polak O. Male sexual deviation: association with early temporal lobe damage. Arch Gen Psychiatry 1967; 17:735–743.
130. Knecht T. Pedophilia and diaper fetishism in a man with Klinefelter's syndrome. Psychiatr Prax 1993; 20:191–192.

131. Laverma H. Klinefelter's syndrome and sexual homocide. J Forensic Psychiatry 2001; 12(1):151–157.
132. Serfert D, Windgassen K. Transsexual development in a patient with Klinefelter's syndrome. Psychopathology 1995; 28:312–316.
133. Kaflka MP. A monoamine hypothesis for the pathophysiology of paraphilic disorders. Arch Sex Behav 1997; 26(4):343–358.
134. Green R. Family co-occurrence of "gender dysphoria:" ten sibling or parent-child pairs. Arch Sex Behav 2000; 29(5):499–507.
135. Krueger DW. Symptom passing in a transvestite father and three sons. Am J Psychiatry 1978; 135(739):742.
136. Lehne GK, Thomas K, Berlin FS. Treatment of sexual paraphilias: a review of the 1999–2000 literature. Curr Opin Psychiatry 2000; 13:569–573.
137. Greenberg DM, Bradford JM. Treatment of the paraphilic disorders: a review of the role of the selective serotonin reuptake inhibitors. Sexual Abuse 1997; 9:349–361.
138. Greenberg DM, Bradford JM, Curry S, O'Rourke A. A comparison of treatment of paraphilias with three serotonin reuptake inhibitors: a retrospective study. Bull Am Acad Psychiatry Law 1996; 24(4):525–532.
139. Balon R. Pharmacological treatment of paraphilias with a focus on antidepressants. J Sex Marital Ther 1998; 24(4):241–254.
140. Abouesh A, Clayton A. Compulsive voyeurism and exhibitionism: a clinical response to paroxetine. Arch Sex Behav 1999; 28(1):23–30.
141. Bradford JMW. Pharmacological treatment of the paraphilias. In: Oldham JM, Riba M, eds. Review of Psychiatry. Washington, DC: American Psychiatric Press, 1995:755–778.
142. Emmanuel NP, Lydiard RB, Ballenger JC. Fluoxetine treatment of voyeurism. Am J Psychiatry 1991; 148:950.
143. Kaflka MP, Prentky RA. Fluoxetine treatment of nonparaphilic sexual addiction and paraphilias in men. J Clin Psychiatry 1992; 53(10):351–358.
144. Kaflca MP. Sertraline pharmacotherapy for paraphilias and paraphilia-related disorders: an open trial. Ann Clin Psychiatry 1994; 6(3):189–195.
145. Lorefice LS. Fluoxetine treatment of a fetish (letter). J Clin Psychiatry 1991; 52:436–437.
146. Perilstein RD, Lipper S, Friedman LJ. Three cases of paraphilias responsive to fluoxetine treatment. J Clin Psychiatry 1991; 52(4):169–170.
147. Zohar J, Kaplan Z, Benjamin J. Compulsive exhibitionism successfully treated with fluvoxamine: a controlled case study. J Clin Psychiatry 1994; 55(3):83–88.
148. Kafka MP, Hennen J. Psychostimulant augmentation during treatment with selctive serotonin reuptake inhibitors in men with paraphilias and paraphilia-related disorders: a case series. J Clin Psychiatry 2000; 61(9):664–670.
149. Casals-Ariet C, Cullen K. Exhibitionism treated with clomipramine. Am J Psychiatry 1993; 150(8):1273–1274.
150. Torres AR, Cerqueira AT. Exhibitionism treated with clomipramine. Am J Psychiatry 1993; 150(8):1274.
151. Wawrose FE, Sisto TM. Clomipramine and a case of exhibitionism. Am J Psychiatry 1992; 149(6):843.
152. Terao T, Nakamura J. Exhibitionism and low-dose trazodon treatment. Hum Psychopharmacol 2000; 15(5):347–349.
153. Brantley JT, Wise TN. Antiandrogenic treatment of a gender dysphoric transvestite. J Sex Marital Ther 1985; 11:109–112.

154. Berlin FS, Meinecke CF. Treatment of sex offenders with antiandrogenic medication: conceptualization, review of treatment modalities and preliminary findings. Am J Psychiatry 1981; 138(5):601–607.
155. Gottesman HG, Schubert DS. Low-dose oral medroxyprogesterone acetate in the management of the paraphilias. J Clin Psychiatry 1993; 54:182–188.
156. Hill A, Briken P, Kraus C, Strohm K, Berner W. Differential pharmacological treatment of paraphilias and sex offenders. Int J Offender Ther Comp Criminol 2003; 47(4):407–421.
157. Laschet U, Laschet L. Antiandrogens in the treatment of sexual deviations of men. Steroid Biochem 1975; 6:821–826.
158. Neuman F. Pharmacology and potential use of cyproterone acetate. Horm Metab Res 1997; 9:1–13.
159. Rosler A, Witztum E. Pharmacotherapy of paraphilias in the next millennium. Behav Sci Law 2000; 18(1):43–56.
160. Thibault F, Cordier B, Kuhn JM. Gonadotropin hormone releasing hormone agonist in cases of severe paraphilia: a lifetime treatment? Psychoneuroendrocrinology 1996; 21(4):411–419.
161. Vallis K, Waxman J. Tumour flare in hormonal therapy. In: Stoll BA, ed. Endocrine Management of Cancer 11: Contemporary Therapy. Basel: S. Karger AG, 1988:144–152.
162. Comings DE, Comings BG. A case of familial exhibitionism in Tourett's syndrome successfully treated with haloperidol. Am J Psychiatry 1982; 139:913–915.
163. Varela D, Black DW. Pedophilia treated with carbamazepine and clonazepam. Am J Psychiatry 2002; 159(7):1245–1246.
164. Balon R. Lithium for the paraphilias? Probably not. J Sex Marital Ther 2000; 26(4):361–363.
165. Bartova D, Buresova A, Hajnova R, Svestka J, Tichy P. The effect of oxyprothepine decanoate, lithium and cyproterone acetate on deviant sexual behavior. Cesk psychiatr 1986; 82(6):355–360.
166. Weisman MM, Klerman GL, Prusoff BA. Depressed outpatients: results one year after treatment with drugs and/or interpersonal psychotherapy. Arch Gen Psychiatry 1981; 38:52–55.
167. Riba MB, Balon R. The challenges of split treatment. Annu Rev Psychiatry 2003; 20:143–164.
168. Pithers WD. Relapse prevention with sexual aggressors: a method for maintaining therapeutic gain and enhancing external supervision. In: Marshall WL, Laws DR, Barbaree HE, eds. Handbook of Sexual Assault: Issues, Theories, and Treatment of the Offender. New York: Plenum Press, 1990:343–361.
169. Hanson RK, Bussiere MT. Predicting relapse: a meta-analysis of sexual offender recidivism studies. J Consult Clin Psychol 1998; 66:348–362.
170. Hanson RK, Gordon A, Harris AJ, Marques JK, Murphy W, Quinsey VL et al. First report of the collaborative outcome data project on the effectiveness of psychological treatment for sex offenders. Sex Abuse 2002; 14(2):169–194.
171. Hanson RK, Morton KE, Harris AJ. Sexual offender recidivism rates: what we know and what we need to know. Ann NY Acad Sci 2003; 989:154–166.
172. Berlin FS, Malin HM. Media distortion of the public's perception of recidivism and psychiatric rehabilitation. Am J Psychiatry 1991; 148:1572–1576.

Index

About the Editors

RICHARD BALON is Professor of Psychiatry, Associate Director of Residency Training, and Director of Master of Science in Psychiatry Program at the Department of Psychiatry and Behavioral Neurosciences, Wayne State University School of Medicine, Detroit, Michigan. He has published widely in the areas of psychopharmacology, sexual dysfunction associated with medications, and the biology of anxiety and psychiatric education and has authored or edited four books including Practical Management of Psychotropic Drug Side Effects (Marcel Dekker). He is a member of editorial board of several psychiatric journals including the Journal of Sex and Marital Therapy.

ROBERT TAYLOR SEGRAVES is Professor of Psychiatry at Case Western Reserve University School of Medicine, Cleveland, Ohio and Chairperson of the Department of Psychiatry, MetroHealth Medical Center, Cleveland, Ohio. He has published over 100 articles and has authored or edited four textbooks on human sexuality. He served on the American Psychiatric Association workgroups of psychosexual disorders for DSM III and DSM IV. He is a past President of the Society of Sex Therapy and Research and is editor of the Journal of Sex and Marital Therapy.